Forgiveness and Health

Loren L. Toussaint • Everett L. Worthington, Jr.
David R. Williams
Editors

Forgiveness and Health

Scientific Evidence and Theories Relating Forgiveness to Better Health

Springer

Editors
Loren L. Toussaint
Department of Psychology
Luther College
Decorah, IA, USA

Everett L. Worthington, Jr.
Department of Psychology
Virginia Commonwealth University
Richmond, VA, USA

David R. Williams
Harvard T.H. Chan School of Public Health
Boston, MA, USA

ISBN 978-94-017-7895-4 ISBN 978-94-017-9993-5 (eBook)
DOI 10.1007/978-94-017-9993-5

Springer Dordrecht Heidelberg New York London

Softcover re-print of the Hardcover 1st edition 2015

Printed on acid-free paper

Springer Science+Business Media B.V. Dordrecht is part of Springer Science+Business Media (www.springer.com)

Endorsements

The world being what it is, there is no shortage of circumstances where the worst of human behaviors provides the opportunity for one of the best, namely, forgiveness. Philosophers have long wrestled with the question of whether forgiveness is better for the forgiver or the forgivee. Remarkably, this question has become a subject of careful scientific research in recent years, and this excellent, important book presents the first thorough overview of the subject. Naturally, the answer to the question "Is forgiveness good for you?" is mighty complicated.

Robert M Sapolsky
John A. and Cynthia Fry Gunn, Professor
Departments of Biology, Neurosurgery, and Neurology and Neurological Sciences

How we experience life's challenges can profoundly affect our well-being. In this outstanding book, Toussaint, Worthington, and Williams open our eyes to the power of forgiveness, which may be one of the most important tools we have for reducing disease and improving human health. Their review of the subject is the best to date and a must-read for scientists, practitioners, and laypeople alike.

George M. Slavich
Director, Laboratory for Stress Assessment and Research
Cousins Center for Psychoneuroimmunology
University of California, Los Angeles

This volume contains a treasure-trove of insights into the complex relationships between forgiveness and health. The editors have brought together a superb cast of contributors from multiple disciplines to produce an extremely valuable and important work. This combination of theoretical, conceptual, empirical, and applied chapters promises to shape agendas on forgiveness and health for years to come.

Anyone interested in this burgeoning field of inquiry will want to have this book on their shelves.

Christopher G. Ellison
Professor of Sociology
Dean's Distinguished Professor of Social Science
University of Texas at San Antonio

This volume is cutting-edge. All that is currently known on forgiveness, unforgiveness, and health is covered between these covers. This book is a remarkable compilation of chapters that review research findings on the relationship between forgiveness and medical and mental health and is of great significance in this emerging area.

Leslie Greenberg
Professor
Department of Psychology
York University

Forgiveness and Health is the definitive volume on the role of forgiveness in human health. Scholarly, creative, and user-friendly, the chapters in this book are likely to steer the field for many years to come.

Michael McCullough
Professor
Department of Psychology
University of Miami

This book is a comprehensive and carefully crafted resource for researchers, teachers, students, and anyone looking to better understand the science of how forgiveness can improve one's health. Leading contributors offer deep insight and useful recommendations about forgiveness and well-being. This book is the best answer to date of the important question "How and why is forgiveness good for you?"

Frederic Luskin
Director of the Stanford Forgiveness Projects

Research on forgiveness has seen an explosion of interest and activity over the past several years. In *Forgiveness and Health*, Toussaint, Worthington, and Williams have done the burgeoning field an important service by bringing together top scholars in the field to assess the current state of theory, measurement, and findings on the topic. As important, their volume provides crucial insights for helping to guide future research efforts on forgiveness and its consequences. There is little doubt that *Forgiveness and Health* will be an essential resource for scholars in the field for years to come.

Marc Musick
Professor, Department of Sociology
Mike Hogg Professor in Liberal Arts
Senior Associate Dean, College of Liberal Arts

This volume signals a coming-of-age of forgiveness theory, research, and practice. Written by leaders in the field, the chapters in *Forgiveness and Health* report on the latest advances in the definition, theory, and measurement of forgiveness. In rich detail, they describe how forgiveness is fully interwoven into physical health, mental health, culture, and context. The volume cements the vital role of forgiveness in efforts to understand and enhance health and well-being and is highly recommended for researchers and practitioners alike.

Kenneth I. Pargament, Ph.D.
Professor, Department of Psychology
Bowling Green State University

This volume provides a welcome and comprehensive approach to understanding forgiveness and its role in health. It is well known that social ties are key determinants of good health and well-being and that social isolation is a risk. But there are strains in every relationship and a need for restoration. Forgiveness is a mechanism for the repair of social relationships – and it is available to everyone.

Ellen L Idler, Ph.D.
Samuel Candler Dobbs Professor of Sociology
Director, Religion and Public Health Collaborative
Department of Epidemiology, Rollins School of Public Health
Emory University

Drs. Toussaint, Worthington, and Williams are, of course, three of the leading experts on the topic of forgiveness and how it relates to, and impacts, both mental and physical health. Consequently, it is not surprising that they assembled a true all-star collection of authors in this comprehensive volume on forgiveness. Though the research literature is not as plentiful in this area as in others with longer histories, through examination of this book, I found it rather amazing how much work has been done in a relatively short amount of time. There is currently no better source for a thorough survey of the work on forgiveness and health than this book. All scholars interested in this area will want to have this volume on their shelf.

Kevin S. Masters, Ph.D.
Professor and Program Director, Clinical Health Psychology
Editor-in-Chief, Annals of Behavioral Medicine
Past President, Division 38 (Health Psychology) American Psychological Association
University of Colorado Denver

Contents

1 **Introduction: Context, Overview, and Guiding Questions** 1
Loren L. Toussaint, Everett L. Worthington, Jr., and David R. Williams

Part I Definition, Measurement, and Models

2 **Defining Forgiveness: Historical Roots, Contemporary Research, and Key Considerations for Health Outcomes** 13
Jeritt R. Tucker, Rachel L. Bitman, Nathaniel G. Wade, and Marilyn A. Cornish

3 **A Conceptual Model of Forgiveness and Health** 29
Caroline R. Lavelock, Daniel J. Snipes, Brandon J. Griffin, Everett L. Worthington, Jr., Don E. Davis, Joshua N. Hook, Eric G. Benotsch, and James Ritter

4 **Measuring Forgiveness in Health-Related Contexts** 43
Charlotte van Oyen Witvliet, Daryl R. Van Tongeren, and Lindsey Root Luna

Part II Empirical Evidence of Forgiveness-Health Connections

5 **Forgiveness and Physiological Concomitants and Outcomes** 61
Kevin T. Larkin, Carol Goulet, and Casey Cavanagh

6 **Forgiveness and Mental Health** 77
Brandon J. Griffin, Everett L. Worthington, Jr., Caroline R. Lavelock, Nathaniel G. Wade, and William T. Hoyt

7 **Forgiveness and Physical Health in Healthy Populations** 91
Alyssa C.D. Cheadle and Loren L. Toussaint

8 Forgiveness and Health in Patient Populations 107
Jennifer P. Friedberg, Hillary Lewin Tuvia, and Rose Cha

9 The Role of Forgiveness in Chronic Pain and Fibromyalgia 123
Martin Offenbächer, Jessie Dezutter, Miguel A. Vallejo, and Loren L. Toussaint

10 Forgiveness and Problematic Substance Use 139
Jon R. Webb and Bridget R. Jeter

11 Forgiveness and Subjective Well-Being: Discussing Mechanisms, Contexts, and Rationales 155
Patrick L. Hill, Marie E. Heffernan, and Mathias Allemand

Part III Factors Connecting Forgiveness and Health

12 Sex, Forgiveness, and Health 173
Andrea J. Miller and Everett L. Worthington, Jr.

13 Forgiveness of Others, Race/Ethnicity, and Health: A Nascent Area of Inquiry 189
Cheryl A. Smith and Michael J. McFarland

14 Aging, Forgiveness, and Health 205
Neal Krause and R. David Hayward

15 Culture, Forgiveness, and Health 221
Mark M. Leach and Stephanie Parazak

Part IV Applications Regarding Forgiveness and Health

16 Forgiveness and Health in Nonmarried Dyadic Relationships 239
Jody L. Davis, Jeffrey D. Green, Chelsea A. Reid, Jaclyn M. Moloney, and Jeni Burnette

17 Forgiveness, Family Relationships and Health 255
Frank D. Fincham

18 Forgiveness Interventions to Promote Physical Health 271
Barbara Elliott

Part V Conclusion

19 Concluding Thoughts: Summary and Integration, Models, and Research Agendas 289
Loren L. Toussaint, Everett L. Worthington, Jr., and David R. Williams

Index 303

Chapter 1
Introduction: Context, Overview, and Guiding Questions

Loren L. Toussaint, Everett L. Worthington, Jr., and David R. Williams

In the past couple of decades, we have witnessed rapid growth in scientific investigations of forgiveness from many perspectives within psychology and in other disciplines. Many peer-reviewed journal articles, scholarly chapters and books have been published each year. Interest in forgiveness continues to grow both among scientists and the lay public (Worthington, 2005). Despite continuing interest in forgiveness and its benefits, few attempts have been made to systematically organize research describing the extent of positive psychological and health benefits of forgiveness. The question remains, is forgiveness good for you? Under what conditions are the positive effects of forgiveness observed? These important questions remain unanswered even though some of the earliest theoretical attempts to connect forgiveness to health and well-being posited its beneficial effects for major societal health problems such as cardiovascular disease and cancer (e.g., Kaplan, 1992).

Without a central organizing source for thinking about forgiveness and health connections, scholars pursuing this work have nevertheless made inroads into this area of inquiry. A catalyst for the growth of research in this area was the John Templeton Foundation's Campaign for Forgiveness Research that was established in 1998 under the leadership of Everett Worthington. For example, a large nationally representative study funded by this initiative documented that forgiveness was

L.L. Toussaint (✉)
Department of Psychology, Luther College, Decorah, IA, USA
e-mail: touslo01@luther.edu

E.L. Worthington, Jr.
Department of Psychology, Virginia Commonwealth University, Richmond, VA, USA
e-mail: eworth@vcu.edu

D.R. Williams
Harvard T.H. Chan School of Public Health, Huntington Ave. 677, 02115-6096 Boston, MA, USA
e-mail: DWILLIAM@hsph.harvard.edu

L.L. Toussaint et al. (eds.), *Forgiveness and Health*,
DOI 10.1007/978-94-017-9993-5_1

positively related to mental and physical health (Toussaint, Williams, Musick, & Everson, 2001). Similarly, initiative-funded laboratory investigations documented that forgiveness was related to physiological response parameters (Lawler et al., 2003; Witvliet, Ludwig, & Vander Laan, 2001). These studies, and many others, set the stage for continued investigation of the health and well-being benefits of forgiveness. Recent work has also sought to understand mechanisms of action and to extend connections between forgiveness and health to chronic health conditions such as cardiovascular disease, substance use, and chronic pain (Carson et al., 2005; Toussaint & Cheadle, 2009; Toussaint et al., 2014).

In this volume, we collect the state-of-the-art research reviews on forgiveness and mental health, physical health, and well-being. Forgiveness has been examined from moral, ethical, and philosophical perspectives. Other discussions of forgiveness consider ways to become more forgiving. Still others postulate evolutionary theories of revenge and forgiveness. In most of these descriptions of forgiveness, there is some attention paid to the benefits of forgiveness, but it is not central to the work. In the current volume, we focus specifically on connections between forgiveness and its health and well-being benefits.

We organize the book to offer an understanding of the theories, methods, and research used in understanding the connections between forgiveness and health and well-being. Furthermore, we consider trait and state forgiveness, emotional and decisional forgiveness, and interventions to promote forgiveness all with an eye toward the positive effects of forgiveness for a victim's (and in some cases offender's) health and well-being. We will consider health to involve social and relational aspects, mental symptoms or disorders, and self-reported physical health, as well as, physiological indicators of good health, well-being/happiness, chronic health conditions, and adjustment to disease or disorder. In addition to documenting the breadth and diversity of the connections between forgiveness and health and well-being, we also include chapters in this volume that consider key moderators such as gender, race, and age, as well as, explanatory mechanisms that might mediate links between forgiveness and key outcomes.

Important to any scientific investigation is a basic understanding of the topic under consideration. Hence, Chap. 2 begins with reflections on the definition of forgiveness. Tucker, Bitman, Wade, and Cornish examine the history and scope of forgiveness, and they compare definitions of forgiveness from psychological, theological and lay perspectives. They summarize early definitions focusing mainly on interpersonal forgiveness and highlight recent advances in defining forgiveness as multidimensional. Their chapter also discusses trait and state definitions, emotional-versus decisional-forgiveness, and philosophical arguments for the uniqueness of the forgiveness construct. They outline what forgiveness involves and what it does not involve. Forgiveness is also contrasted with justice and reconciliation.

In Chap. 3, Lavelock et al. provide an overview of how to conceptualize of the forgiveness, health, and well-being relationships. They offer a macro-level consideration of factors contributing to these relationships. They consider multiple lines of evidence linking forgiveness to health and well-being in a qualitative review of 95 studies. Their review identifies several key areas of interest for investigators interested in the forgiveness-health connection. These areas are succinctly described in a model that offers heuristic value for future research. Both precursors and mechanisms of forgiveness and its connection to proximal and distal health outcomes are described. For new researchers in the field or the casually interested lay-reader, this is an efficient and cogent model to structure the forgiveness and health connection.

The main focus of Chap. 4 is how to measure forgiveness efficiently and effectively in settings where health and medical issues are of utmost importance and the opportunities for learning about the contribution of forgiveness to health is likely greatest. Witvliet, Van Tongeren, and Root Luna offer a review of existing measures. They supplement that with suggestions for additional measurement considerations that are relevant in clinical healthcare settings. The challenges of assessing forgiveness reliably and validly in the health context are numerous, especially because measurement in health and epidemiological settings often requires great efficiency and ease of understanding. Few existing measures are brief enough or are easily understood by patients who might be physically, cognitively and emotionally burdened. Measures that meet efficiency and understandability criteria have not always been carefully evaluated. Witvliet and her colleagues' chapter provides a balanced review of the strides that have been made in forgiveness assessment in general, and specific to health-related studies. It also includes a careful discussion of what new measures might be viable options.

Larkin, Goulet, and Cavanagh provide a review in Chap. 5 of evidence linking forgiveness to physiological outcomes including parameters indicative of systemic arousal, such as electrodermal activity and heart rate variability; neuro-endocrine outcomes, such as cortisol and oxytocin; immune functioning, such as cytokines and CD4 cell percentage; and other proximal indices of physiological health including blood pressure and electromyographic activity. Their chapter also provides an update and comprehensive review of what is known regarding forgiveness and brain activity. They include measures of electro-encephalographic activity, positron emission tomography, and functional magnetic resonance imaging.

In Chap. 6, Griffin, Worthington, Lavelock, Wade, and Hoyt review the research on connections between forgiveness and mental health. Their review builds on and extends a previous review when there were only about a dozen published studies (Toussaint & Webb, 2005). At present, Griffin et al., review an additional 55 studies published since 2003. This provides an invaluable update to our understanding of the work in this area, and it reflects the substantial growth in interest in forgiveness and mental health. Griffin et al. develop four theoretically meaningful propositions and evaluate the empirical evidence in favor of or against each one. Reading this chapter provides answers to key questions including: (1) Is unforgiveness a stress-reaction related to poor mental health? (2) Is forgiveness a coping strategy related to improved mental health? (3) Do individual differences moderate the relationship between forgiveness and health? and (4) Do psychological states mediate the relationship between forgiveness and health?

For the average reader, Chap. 7 might be one of the more helpful chapters. It surveys how forgiveness is related to physical health in healthy populations. Cheadle and Toussaint consider theories of forgiveness and health that are most applicable to individuals in the general population. They review empirical research related to those theories. Given that those populations are not health-compromised, much of the research reviewed uses self-reported physical health, somatic symptoms, and health symptoms as the key health outcomes. A good deal of epidemiological research focuses on these indicators of health status and researchers outside the interest area of forgiveness might also make use of this chapter as it offers an opportunity to compare effect sizes of forgiveness with other well-known psychosocial and biological correlates and determinants of health in generally healthy individuals. For instance, some researchers might compare the effect of forgiveness to that of pessimism, social support, religious attendance, and obesity. In brief, several studies have investigated forgiveness in healthy general population samples, and the distillation of key findings from this work could inform researchers, practitioners and the public of the benefits of forgiveness for healthy individuals.

In contrast, in Chap. 8, Friedberg, Tuvia, Alanson, and Cha consider the forgiveness-health connection in patient populations. Patient populations can be difficult to access, for obvious ethical reasons, but a small and growing literature has developed around the potential benefits of forgiveness for patients. While the study of cardiac patients is common, other populations—like patients with cancer, chronic pain, physical and mental injuries, Parkinson's, and HIV—have also been studied. Terminally ill as well as other patients have also been studied. Friedberg et al. offer insightful recommendations for health enhancement, medicine, and integrative treatment suggestions for how forgiveness could be offered to patients as a coping mechanism in dealing with chronic disease.

Chronic pain is a growing problem in the United States and worldwide (Institute of Medicine, 2011). In Chap. 9, Offenbächer, Dezutter, Vallejo, and Toussaint review what has been perhaps one of the most overlooked connections between forgiveness and holistic health—its connection with pain. Offenbächer et al. begin with a brief review of two common forms of chronic pain: (1) chronic widespread pain, and (2) fibromyalgia. After considering the symptom characteristics and basic epidemiology of these conditions, Offenbächer et al. argue that stress is a central biopsychosocial agent involved in pain and outline several highly relevant sources of stress for these individuals. The authors integrate a biopsychosocial stress model of fibromyalgia and forgiveness. They specifically address how forgiveness could be used as a coping mechanism to mitigate the harmful results of stress for people struggling with chronic pain. Given the increasing prevalence of pain, the extent to which forgiveness might offer an effective coping strategy that provides pain relief should receive more attention among researchers and practitioners.

Webb and Jeter provide, in Chap. 10, a comprehensive and integrative review of forgiveness and substance use/abuse intervention models and empirical research on the topic. They discuss Twelve-Step Facilitation Therapy, Motivational Enhancement Therapy, and Cognitive-Behavioral Coping Skills Therapy and delineate how forgiveness is inherent in each of these evidence-based psychosocial treatments. A good empirical literature has also begun to develop showing that forgiveness is generally associated with less substance use/abuse. Empirical data exist for college students, general population, and treatment seeking individuals. Webb and Jeter provide an up-to-the-minute review of the empirical evidence. They include a table that offers a clear delineation of forgiveness intervention models and substance use intervention models, and they supply a figure that integrates theory and research and offers heuristic value for future work. Both practitioners and scholars interested in forgiveness and substance use/abuse issues will find this a useful chapter for guiding their work.

Hill, Heffernan, and Allemand provide an introduction to the Scaffolding Self and Social Systems (4S) Model in Chap. 11. Their model provides a new conceptualization of how forgiveness can not only help alleviate suffering but also help to facilitate well-being. The Scaffolding Self and Social Systems Model begins by establishing that forgiveness is associated with enhanced well-being. It elaborates mechanisms by which the beneficial association might be supported. Hill et al. outline four critical mechanisms. First, forgiveness can enhance relationship harmony. Second, forgiveness can increase relationship mastery and maintenance skills. Third, forgiveness can promote adaptive identity development. Fourth, forgiveness can increase self-acceptance and self-worth. Each of these mediators in turn promotes enhanced well-being. The authors specifically discuss applications in romantic relationships and family life, but readers are likely to find many other applications of this model in the workplace, friendships, churches, volunteering, and other organized groups.

Chapter 12 addresses an important issue in our understanding of forgiveness. Who are more forgiving, men or women? Two recent meta-analyses in this area have returned opposing results (Fehr, Gelfand, & Nag, 2010; Miller, Worthington, & McDaniel, 2008), but Miller and Worthington provide a truly insightful dissection of the critical issues and potential resolutions to this debate. Their chapter provides an extensive review of literature bearing on the relationships between forgiveness and mental and physical health and how these associations can vary for males or females. Reading this chapter offers insights into not only the research findings showing that women are generally a bit more forgiving than men, but also provides some understanding of what to do with this knowledge. That is, Miller and Worthington devote an entire section to practical implications of sex differences in forgiveness and health and how best to use what we know in developing maximally effective interventions for men and women.

The past couple of decades have witnessed a dramatic upsurge in research that shows that racial and ethnic inequalities in health are pervasive (Williams, 2012; Williams & Mohammed, 2013). Research has also established that racial and ethnic influences are present in religiousness, spirituality, and more recently, forgiveness (see Chap. 13). Smith and McFarland focus on how racial and ethnic factors influence forgiveness and health and their relationship. They provide evidence from three separate national studies that shows that Blacks are consistently more forgiving than Whites. They also offer a conceptual model of the influence of race and ethnicity on forgiveness, health, and the forgiveness-health relationship that identifies family structure, social relationships, neighborhood factors, group schemas, economic and social resources, stress and adversity, and group sanctions and norms as key ingredients that may explain the role of race and ethnicity in the forgiveness and health equation. Smith and McFarland provide the necessary empirical groundwork and conceptual framework for a sustained examination of race and ethnicity influences in future research on forgiveness and health.

Older, as compared to younger, individuals are generally more religious and spiritual (Hayward & Krause, 2013; Krause, 2013). Similarly, in Chap. 14, Krause and Hayward discuss how older people might also be more forgiving than their younger counterparts. They first discuss age differences in forgiveness and in the relationship between forgiveness and health. Then they delineate important methodological issues in aging research—the significance of age, cohort, and life course influences on forgiveness and health. Krause and Hayward also discuss theoretical and conceptual models of aging and forgiveness. They consider several explanations for why forgiveness may be associated with health in late life and offer recommendations for developing forgiveness interventions for older adults.

Leach and Parazak devote Chap. 15 to examining what is known about forgiveness and health across cultures and nations. They make a convincing case for studying forgiveness from a multinational perspective. However, they note from the outset that very little of this work has been done. The authors also suggest that much cross-cultural work on forgiveness has focused on only one aspect of cultural differences—individualism-collectivism (as measured using questionnaires). Other differences exist across cultures. Leach and Parazak identify power-distance, masculinity-femininity, indulgence-restraint, and others that could provide interesting insights into forgiveness dynamics and its relationship with health. They suggest that the understanding of forgiveness is not mutual across cultures, and that differences in orientation toward interpersonal versus inter-group forgiveness are not trivial and are worthy of study. They offer some key theoretical insights that may prompt future cross-cultural research.

In Chap. 16, Davis, Green, Reid, Moloney, and Burnette discuss forgiveness and health among non-married dyadic relationships. People have "commitments" to friends and romantic partners, but, let's face it, if things don't work out, the relationships are often ended. Having the termination of a relationship as an option changes the dynamics of forgiving. Davis et al. explore what is known about negotiating these relationships and how forgiveness can help repair friendships and romantic relationships and how this ultimately impacts health outcomes. An important contribution of this chapter is the authors' review of three theories that could inform future research looking at forgiveness and health in relationships. These theories are: (1) the investment model of commitment, (2) evolutionary theory, and (3) attachment theory. Davis et al. illustrate how predictions based on these theories offer additional insights into the forgiveness-health connection across different relationship types.

Fincham (Chap. 17) reviews the research on forgiveness and health in family contexts. He offers useful suggestions for future work in this area. Family relationships are a source of major fulfilment but also a source of major stresses in life. When people are committed, there is motivation to repair relationships that does not exist in the more transient and more easily ended relationships of friends and romantic partners. Relationship status has long been known to be related to physical health disorders and to well-being. Fincham addresses forgiveness in families and how the forgiveness process may influence physical health through mechanisms of stress and depression. He also considers the role of forgiveness in enhancing relationship quality and its consequences on health. The incentives are stronger to reconcile relationships and the bonds are tighter, making ongoing, committed, family relationships a source of health risk when things are not working well. It is also important to understand the health implications of perpetrating offenses in families and the role of self-forgiveness for perpetrators.

In Chap. 18, Elliott situates forgiveness in a bio-psycho-spiritual model of health. She reviews evidence linking unforgiveness, forgiveness, and health with a special eye toward the implications for forgiveness interventions. Her bio-psycho-spiritual model of stress, forgiveness, and health offers insight into the proximal stress-related endocrine-mediated changes in allostasis and links these acute changes to chronic health conditions and outcomes. Most importantly, Elliott's model offers insight into where the effects of forgiveness interventions might arbitrate the process to alleviate negative health outcomes. She then discusses the implications of the model for different patient groups.

In the concluding chapter, we consider the implications of this body of work and point to thematic trends, or lack thereof, that have emerged from the different research teams to inform future directions for the field. We provide a broad overview and synopsis of the cutting edge research and theory presented in the book through the insights of the many authors. We discuss future directions for research, theory and practice.

We hope you find this book to be both interesting and useful. Leading scholars from several disciplines have contributed and offer their unique perspectives on the topic. It is interesting to see the connections and themes across chapters and also to note the unique offerings from each writing team. As you read, there are some key issues to attend to. First, how do the authors *define* forgiveness and health and what aspects of forgiveness seem most central to health. It is no surprise that there is some variability in how scientists define health, but there is some surprising consistency in how they define forgiveness and the different dimensions of this construct that are mentioned. Second, some authors have chosen to explicitly model the relationships between forgiveness and health in tables, figures, diagrams, and such. Some of these models are built from previous work in other areas and extend the proposed relations to the topic of forgiveness and health. Yet other models are novel and will require careful consideration and research to draw conclusions regarding their validity. Undoubtedly, some of these models will provide a stimulus to the empirical research going on in examining the connection between forgiveness and health. Third, the bodies of literature that are summarized and integrated in each chapter vary considerably. Some areas have seen considerable development and the authors were challenged to effectively distil this work into a brief summary. In other areas, less empirical work exists and the greater challenge might be to take what little has been done and use it to fruitfully direct future work. Fourth, a stress-and-coping framework is perhaps the most consistently used theory to conceptualize forgiveness and its relationships to health and to ways of coping (Strelan & Covic,

2006; Worthington, 2006); keep an eye out to how frequently this conceptualization appears. Fifth, each chapter closes with a look toward the future of research in this area. Authors have developed models and research agendas that will guide emerging lines of research. Sixth, perhaps most importantly is to consider the question, what does this all mean for my health or the health of a friend or loved one? This is the challenge that we all face as we consider the implications of this work and attempt to understand how to live better and healthier lives. When you have completed reading this book our hope is that you might better understand the answer to that question. In some cases, the answer might be fairly straightforward. In others, it might require more nuance and depth. In either case, we hope that readers of this volume will come away with a better understanding of how forgiveness can be a very important part of a healthy lifestyle.

References

Carson, J. W., Keefe, F. J., Goli, V., Fras, A., Lynch, T. R., Thorp, S. R., & Buechler, J. L. (2005). Forgiveness and chronic low back pain: A preliminary study examining the relationship of forgiveness to pain, anger, and psychological distress. *The Journal of Pain, 6*(2), 84–91.

Fehr, R., Gelfand, M. J., & Nag, M. (2010). The road to forgiveness: A meta-analytic synthesis of its situational and dispositional correlates. *Psychological Bulletin, 136*, 894–914. doi:10.1037/a0019993.

Hayward, R., & Krause, N. (2013). Patterns of change in religious service attendance across the life course: Evidence from a 34-year longitudinal study. *Social Science Research, 42*(6), 1480–1489. doi:10.1016/j.ssresearch.2013.06.010.

Institute of Medicine. (2011). Committee on Advancing Pain Research, Care, and Education. *Relieving pain in America: A blueprint for transforming prevention, care, education, and research*. Washington, DC: National Academies Press (US). Pain as a public health challenge. Available from: http://www.ncbi.nlm.nih.gov/books/NBK92516/

Kaplan, B. H. (1992). Social health and the forgiving heart: The Type B story. *Journal of Behavioral Medicine, 15*(1), 3–14.

Krause, N. (2013). Religious involvement in the later years of life. In K. I. Pargament, J. J. Exline, & J. W. Jones (Eds.), *APA handbook of psychology, religion, and spirituality (Vol. 1): Context, theory, and research* (pp. 529–545). Washington, DC: American Psychological Association. doi:10.1037/14045-029.

Lawler, K. A., Younger, J. W., Piferi, R. L., Billington, E., Jobe, R., Edmondson, K., & Jones, W. H. (2003). A change of heart: Cardiovascular correlates of forgiveness in response to interpersonal conflict. *Journal of Behavioral Medicine, 26*(5), 373–393.

Miller, A. J., Worthington, E. L., Jr., & McDaniel, M. A. (2008). Gender and forgiveness: A meta-analytic review and research agenda. *Journal of Social and Clinical Psychology, 27*(8), 843–876.

Strelan, P., & Covic, T. (2006). A review of forgiveness process models and a coping framework to guide future research. *Journal of Social and Clinical Psychology, 25*(10), 1059–1085.

Toussaint, L., & Cheadle, A. C. D. (2009). Unforgiveness and the broken heart: Unforgiving tendencies, problems due to unforgiveness, and 12-month prevalence of cardiovascular health conditions. In M. T. Evans & E. D. Walker (Eds.), *Religion and psychology*. New York, NY: Nova Publishers.

Toussaint, L., Vincent, A., Whipple, M., McAllister, S., Finnie, D., Hathaway, J., ... Vickers Douglas, K. S. (2014). A psycho-educational forgiveness program for fibromyalgia patients: Development and preliminary evaluation. *Pain Studies and Treatment*, *2*(1), 11–16. http://dx.doi.org/10.4236/pst.2014.21003

Toussaint, L. L., Williams, D. R., Musick, M. A., & Everson, S. A. (2001). Forgiveness and health: Age differences in a U.S. probability sample. *Journal of Adult Development, 8*(4), 249–257.

Toussaint, L., & Webb, J. R. (2005). Theoretical and empirical connections between forgiveness, mental health, and well-being. In E. L. Worthington (Ed.), *Handbook of forgiveness.* New York, NY: Brunner-Routledge.

Williams, D. R. (2012). Miles to go before we sleep: Racial inequities in health. *Journal of Health and Social Behavior, 53*(3), 279–295.

Williams, D. R., & Mohammed, S. A. (2013). Racism and health I: Pathways and scientific evidence. *American Behavioral Scientist, 57*(8), 1152–1173.

Witvliet, C., Ludwig, T. E., & Vander Laan, K. L. (2001). Granting forgiveness or harboring grudges: Implications for emotion, physiology, and health. *Psychological Science, 12*(2), 117–123.

Worthington, E. L., Jr. (Ed.). (2005). *Handbook of forgiveness*. New York, NY: Brunner-Routledge.

Worthington, E. L., Jr. (2006). *Forgiveness and reconciliation: Theory and practice*. New York, NY: Brunner-Routledge.

Part I
Definition, Measurement, and Models

Chapter 2
Defining Forgiveness: Historical Roots, Contemporary Research, and Key Considerations for Health Outcomes

Jeritt R. Tucker, Rachel L. Bitman, Nathaniel G. Wade, and Marilyn A. Cornish

Forgiveness is a powerful phenomenon in explaining individual wellbeing. It has been related to numerous mental health benefits including reduced stress, anger, depression, and state anxiety; positive relational health including improved social support and marital quality; and an array of physical health benefits including lowered blood pressure and improved cardiovascular health (Berry & Worthington, 2001; Worthington, 2005; Worthington & Drinkard, 2000). The way one *defines* forgiveness, however, has numerous implications for which underlying processes may account for these health outcomes, and which outcomes are likely to occur (Thoresen, Oman, & Harris, 2005).

Definitions of forgiveness depend on long-standing cultural factors impacted by religious, philosophical, and theoretical perspectives. The concept of forgiveness itself dates back thousands of years. Major world religions have long encouraged forgiveness, with religious adherents extolling the numerous benefits of the practice (Rye et al., 2000). Forgiveness also has a history in philosophy as well, with Nietzsche (1887) arguing for the inherent power difference between offender and offended. Yet, forgiveness received little attention in the field of psychology until the 1980s (see McCullough, Pargament, & Thoresen, 2000, for a historical overview). At about this same time, connections between forgiveness and physical health began to be drawn, with numerous potential benefits discussed (e.g. Kaplan, 1992).

Indeed, numerous systems have been proposed for the forgiveness health relationship. These include forgiveness as an emotion-focused coping strategy, as improving immune system functioning, as activating motivational systems (Worthington & Scherer, 2004), as decreasing sympathetic nervous system activity (Berry & Worthington, 2001) as fostering increased social support (Toussaint & Webb, 2005), as increasing feelings of personal control

J.R. Tucker • R.L. Bitman • N.G. Wade (✉) • M.A. Cornish
Department of Psychology, W117 Lagomarcino Hall, Iowa State University, Ames, IA, USA
e-mail: nwade@iastate.edu

L.L. Toussaint et al. (eds.), *Forgiveness and Health*,
DOI 10.1007/978-94-017-9993-5_2

(McCullough & Worthington, 1994), and as decreasing rumination and the subsequent emotions that spring from it (Worthington & Scherer, 2004). In this chapter, we offer not a single definition but a set of five key considerations when reading any given work on forgiveness:

1. Do the researchers implicitly or explicitly hold theological, moral, or lay perspectives?
2. Do the researchers make a distinction between decisional and emotional forgiveness?
3. Do the researchers emphasize reductions in unforgiveness, increases in forgiveness, or both?
4. Do the researchers see the endpoint of forgiveness as involving changes in cognition, affect, and/or interpersonal motivations and behaviors?
5. Do the researchers emphasize situational or dispositional aspects of forgiveness?

These considerations serve as the structure for the present chapter, and, in what follows, we examine how each of the above questions have been answered by various theologians, philosophers, and researchers. Additionally, we discuss proposed links for how a particular definition may be related with health outcomes. In so doing, we hope to provide readers with a more nuanced understanding of the forgiveness-health link and the motivations spurring its study.

Theological Origins

Prior to the formal psychological study of forgiveness, theological explorations of forgiveness were the primary source of scholarship. All of the major world religions as well as numerous other traditions address forgiveness to some degree (Rye et al., 2000). Most of these place forgiveness high amongst their lists of virtues. The specific understanding of forgiveness, however, varies greatly between religions.[1]

Some of the earliest conceptualizations of forgiveness arise from Buddhist, Hindu, and Jewish theologies and philosophies. One of the main philosophical tenets of Buddhism, especially Zen Buddhism, is non-duality; a belief that categories such as right-wrong, black-white, good-bad, and you-me are an illusion. Thus, forgiveness unfolds when individuals see that they are not separate from the offending person but instead that all are connected. One Buddhist teacher described forgiveness in this way,

> When you forgive me for harming you, you decide not to retaliate, to seek no revenge. You don't have to like me. You simply unburden yourself of the weight of resentment and cut the cycle of retribution that would otherwise keep us ensnarled in an ugly samsaric wrestling

[1]Of course, variations in understandings of forgiveness within a given religious tradition are likely to be as great as the variations across religious traditions. However, for the purposes of the present review we provide basic, shared ideas within a given religious tradition.

> match. This is a gift you can give us both, totally on your own, without my having to know or understand what you've done. (Bhikkhu, 2006).

Here, we see one Buddhist conceptualization of forgiveness as attaining the non-reactive mind. Such a mind sees itself as part of the offending person, and recognizes that to be angry with another is to be angry with oneself. Moreover, we see Buddhism's strong *intrapersonal* emphasis, with Bhikku suggesting that forgiveness is a process that can be resolved even in the absence of any other's knowledge.

According to Buddhist traditions, one pathway to attain the wisdom that sees no differentiation of the self from others is through compassion (Walsh-Frank, 1996). Buddhist compassion encourages the type of loving-kindness that wise people would have for themselves (Walsh-Frank, 1996). Just as there are no differences between self and other, Buddhist compassion does not separate subject (the one hurt) from object (the one offending).

Aspects of Hindu philosophy and spiritual teaching similarly emphasize the interconnectivity of all things. One such aspect of Hinduism is the law of karma, or consequences for behaviors in previous or current lives. For devout believers in karma, current suffering (even suffering at the hands of another) is a result of past actions. Thus, to forgive is to understand the offender as providing consequences for one's previous behavior (Hunter, 2007). Like in Buddhism, all people and all living beings are the same, are included in Brahma (god), and thus "there is no 'Other' against whom one could feel angry" (Hunter, 2007, p. 38). When viewed from this perspective, an individual offering forgiveness to a separate other loses conceptual sense. Accordingly, forgiveness under Buddhist and Hindu perspectives hinges largely on the meditative practice of understanding the illusion of self.

Newberg, d'Aquili, Newberg, and deMarici (2000), in their neuropsychological model of forgiveness, suggest that such meditative practices help to reframe interpersonal hurts by reconciling one's understanding of themselves and their relationship to the world. The meditator who focuses on forgiveness engages parasympathetic nervous activity including decreased heart rate, more relaxed breathing, improved immune functioning, and decreased pain perception. Thus, when conceptualized through Buddhist and Hindu traditions, the salutary effects of forgiveness are likely to occur as a result of the same systems implicated in the association between meditation and health.

Judaism also highly values forgiveness, but its tradition and theology lead to a different understanding of what forgiveness is and how it should be used. In the Jewish tradition, people learn about the willingness of God to forgive when people repent (Johansson, 2011). Adherents of Judaism are taught to do the same for others. In fact, when one is hurt there is a religious obligation to forgive if the offending person genuinely apologizes and asks forgiveness (Hunter, 2007). In contrast to Christian and Islamic teaching, however, if an offending person does not ask for forgiveness, the individual is not morally obligated to forgive, though he/she may still choose to forgive. Thus, from a Jewish religious perspective, forgiveness has a significant relational component. As such, forgiveness implies resolving interpersonal relationship stress. Resolution of interpersonal stress is associated with decreased endocrine system activation and healthier levels of stress hormones during interpersonal interactions (Berry & Worthington, 2001). If a person thus holds implicit or explicit Jewish religious perspectives, reductions in social stress and anxiety may largely mediate the forgiveness-health link.

Forgiveness in Christianity and Islam grows out of Judaism, but both theologies encourage a moral obligation to forgive regardless of the offending person's remorse or apology. In most forms of Christianity, adherents are encouraged to forgive the offending person regardless of the offense, the degree of repentance, or the consequences of the offense (Rye et al., 2000). Although similar in its intrapersonal focus to Hindu and Buddhist perspectives, Christianity does not always emphasize non-reactivity. Instead, when asked about forgiveness, Christians often reflect on the life of Jesus Christ, their own sinfulness, and the loving grace of God (McMinn, Meek, Dominguez, Ryan, & Novotny, 1999). This basic encouragement to forgive, what forgiveness means, and how it is achieved appears quite similar in the Muslim tradition. Islam teaches that Allah is "All Forgiving" and that people should follow this example in their interactions with others (Islam Awareness, 2013). Furthermore, if one wishes to experience the forgiveness offered by Allah, one needs to offer forgiveness to others. The Qu'ran states, "... if you pardon and overlook and forgive – then indeed, Allah is Forgiving and Merciful" (64:14).

Both the Christian and Muslim theologies thus encourage a moral imperative to forgive, that is, adherents are strongly encouraged to forgive regardless of their desire to do so. This may have direct implications for health and wellness. On the one hand, by encouraging people to consider and strive for forgiveness, these theologies might counter individual differences in the disposition to forgive (Lawler et al., 2005; Toussaint & Friedman, 2009). Christians and Muslims who are highly committed may take the moral requirement to forgive seriously, hear the message to forgive more often (from peers and during religious services), and therefore be more likely and able to forgive.

Some empirical evidence supports the connection between religious commitment and the disposition to forgive in Christians, showing that the relationship between religious commitment and forgiveness of a specific offense is either partially or fully mediated by trait forgivingness (Wade, Meyer, Goldman, & Post, 2009). Thus, at least for Christians, being more committed to one's religion was related to greater dispositions to forgive, which in turn accounted for forgiveness of a specific transgression. Furthermore, in research on religion and health, increased forgiveness and decreased hostility were suggested as two mediating variables between greater religiosity and greater subjective health (Lutjen, Silton, & Flannelly, 2012).

On the other hand, a moral imperative to forgive might have a detrimental impact on health. Moral imperatives come with moral judgments. When people are offended in very troubling or traumatic ways, forgiveness may not be a simple moral choice. In such situations the development of emotional forgiveness may be a long and difficult process that requires significant time, help, and effort. If during this process one feels inadequate or unacceptable (to others, themselves, or the divine) because they have not yet forgiven, negative consequences for health are possible. Indeed, self-blame after traumatic interpersonal events has been linked with the perpetuation of cycles of retraumatization (Janoff-Bulman, 1979), as well as negative health outcomes such as post-traumatic stress symptoms and psychological distress (see Wade, Tucker, & Cornish, 2014). Moreover, those who report forgiving a transgressor out of a sense of religious obligation, instead of out of a sense of love, report higher levels of systolic and diastolic blood pressure (Huang & Enright, 2000).

Lay Definitions

Along with theological views, the general public has its own perceptions of forgiveness. These definitions are important to understand, for, as Kearns and Fincham (2004) state, lay definitions may not only implicitly inform research but may also impact how forgiveness is perceived by participants in applied settings and how it is used as a therapeutic tool. Moreover, if researchers utilize the term "forgiveness" in their research measures without careful definition, lay definitions will likely serve as the basis of any observed relationship between such measures and health.

There is some support for the notion that persons utilize a "prototype model" of forgiveness, meaning that they rate certain features as most central to the concept and use a single exemplar as a heuristic when answering questions (Kearns & Fincham, 2004). Still, it would appear that there is a great deal of variety with respect to which features individuals see as included in the forgiveness prototype. In a qualitative study of 270 college students' narratives of forgiveness, Lawler-Row, Scott, Raines, Edlis-Matityahou, and Moore (2007) found quite divergent views of the concept. In their study, 46 % defined forgiveness as having an intrapersonal focus only, 31 % included an interpersonal focus only, and 20 % included both intrapersonal and interpersonal features. Additionally, 20 % saw forgiveness as both a passive "letting go" and an active "moving on", while 40 % saw it as passive alone and 40 % saw it as an active process only. Participants were also split between emphasizing emotional (35 %), cognitive (38 %), behavioral (29 %), or attitudinal (7 %) changes. Finally, 16 % included forgetting in their definitions, and reconciliation was included in 12 % of definitions. Given the homogeneity of the sample used, these findings are surprising. Other research has found similar results. For example, in their (2004) qualitative study of undergraduate and community member samples, Younger, Piferi, Jobe, and Lawler found a variety of individual responses. Here, 40 % of undergraduate and 29 % of the community member samples defined forgiveness as accepting and getting over the offense, 33 % and 39 % respectively defined forgiveness as letting go of negative feelings, and 24 % and 16 % respectively emphasized reconciling and restoring the relationship with the offender.

What are the implications for such varying definitions for researchers interested in understanding the health-forgiveness link? First, because lay definitions vary greatly, there may be different "pathways" into the experience of forgiveness for different individuals even within the same population. This is to say that how individuals define forgiveness may actually shape how they experience it (Younger et al., 2004). As such, researchers might either seek to capture the above dimensions of forgiveness or seek to ensure that participants have a shared understanding of the construct prior to conducting their research. Additionally, because researchers have their own religious, moral, or cultural experiences that may shape their understanding and experiences of forgiveness similar to lay individuals, it is important that they understand their own backgrounds when conducting such research.

Conceptual and Empirical Distinctions

Whereas religious scholars, philosophers, and even the general public seek to explain whether and when forgiveness is rational or moral, empirical psychology focuses on operationalizing forgiveness in an effort to understand its psychological properties, conditions of occurrence, and possible health benefits (Exline, Worthington, Hill, & McCullough, 2003). Empirical psychology seeks to understand what distinct set of interpersonal and intrapersonal processes uniquely account for experiences of forgiveness, what predicts these experiences, and what they lead to with respect to important outcomes.

What Forgiveness Is Not

One important way to begin operationalizing forgiveness is to determine what forgiveness is *not*. Indeed, there seems to be more conceptual agreement in the empirical literature on what forgiveness is not than what forgiveness is. First, most researchers agree that forgiveness is distinct from pardoning, condoning, or excusing an offense or offender (McCullough, Fincham, & Tsang, 2003). Enright, Gassin, and Wu (1992) cautioned against seeing forgiveness as condoning or justifying the offense and underscored the importance of seeing committed offenses as serious, relevant, and problematic acts that should not be minimized. Furthermore, McCullough and colleagues note that forgiveness is also not the same as denying or suppressing the emotions induced as a result of the offense. Researchers also generally agree that forgiveness is separate from pardoning; that is forgiveness is not the equivalent of "letting the offender off of the hook."

Forgiveness is also not the same as justice or reconciliation, which often imply a restoration of a damaged relationship (McCullough et al., 2003). However, many researchers argue that forgiveness can be accomplished without restoring the relationship, although reconciliation may occur (Worthington & Wade, 1999). This is particularly applicable in situations where an offender is deceased or no longer a participant in a victim's life (Freedman & Enright, 1996; Hebl & Enright, 1993).

Types of Forgiveness

Through factor analytic and other statistical strategies, more recent research has narrowed these typologies down into two primary "types" of forgiveness: decisional and emotional. This distinction is critical in identifying the relationship between forgiveness and health. Emotional and decisional forgiveness highlight the difference between choosing to not engage in unforgiveness and experiencing emotional forgiveness (cultivating positive other-oriented emotions; Exline et al., 2003). Different researchers appear to conceptualize this distinction in different ways. Whereas some suggest that this is meant to highlight a difference between cognitive and affective processes (Holeman, Dean, DeShea, & Duba, 2011), others suggest that decisional forgiveness includes only the stated intention to forgive with no necessitation of changes in cognition, emotion, or motivation (Worthington & Scherer, 2004).

What seems common to most delineations between decisional and emotional forgiveness, however, is a distinction between motivational processes. Decisional forgiveness appears to be primarily motivated by a principle or religious belief in beneficence or by a desire to start to restore the relationship with the offender (Worthington & Scherer, 2004). Emotional forgiveness, on the other hand, is motivated by empathic attunement with the offender and recognition of the fallibility of human beings (Worthington & Wade, 1999). Emotional forgiveness is the replacement of negative, unforgiving emotions with positive emotions toward the offender (Worthington, 2005, 2006). Thus, one can be extrinsically motivated to forgive and control one's behaviors, but must experience changes in feelings toward the offender in order to experience emotional forgiveness.

While both decisional and emotional forgiveness are hypothesized to be related to positive health benefits, they may use quite different pathways. Decisional forgiveness is thought to relate to positive health through reconciliatory processes, improved relationships, and better social support (Worthington, Witvliet, Pietrini, & Miller, 2007). Stating one's intention to forgive may help soothe interpersonal relations and begin to repair relationships (Worthington & Scherer, 2004). Such improved relationships might indirectly affect health through improved social support, as a relational buffer against stress, and by increasing self-soothing responses. Additionally, deciding to forgive may well reduce rumination. Decisional forgiveness has been defined as the behavioral intention to resist an unforgiving stance (Worthington et al., 2007). As such, it involves intentionally acting toward the transgressor as though the transgression had not occurred. Accordingly, one might intentionally suppress negative, ruminative thoughts in order to be consistent with one's stated intentions, which may reduce the number of times stressful cognitions are re-experienced. In their 2007 study, McCullough, Orsulak, Brandon, and Akers confirmed that rumination about even moderate interpersonal offenses is linked with greater salivary cortisol levels.

On the other hand, emotional forgiveness is thought to relate to better health through more direct reductions of the stress response and increases in positive affect (Worthington et al., 2007). For example, when students were directed to take an empathic mindset toward a transgressor, they were shown to have reductions in heart rate, skin conductance, and other measures of autonomic nervous system arousal when compared to those who felt unforgiving (Witvliet, Ludwig, & Vander Laan, 2001). Additionally, when blood-pressure levels were compared between those who were motivated to forgive by obligation versus those who forgave due to "unconditional love", those who held the latter (more akin to emotional forgiveness) were found to have both lower systolic and diastolic rates (Huang & Enright, 2000). With respect to positive emotionality, positive affect itself has been shown to relate to mortality rates through increases in endogenous opioids, improved health practices, and better immune functioning (Pressman & Cohen, 2005).

Another key distinction regarding the "types" of forgiveness is the difference between increasing forgiveness and reducing *unforgiveness*. Unforgiveness is separate but related to forgiveness, and, like forgiveness, may occur along continua at dispositional or contextual levels. The definition of trait unforgiveness generally includes the consistent presence of negative emotions such as bitterness, hostility, anger, fearfulness, and depression (Worthington, 2005; Worthington & Wade, 1999). Wade and Worthington (2003) defined unforgiveness specifically as the delayed emotions of resentment, anger, and bitterness that arise after ruminating about a particular interpersonal hurt. The development of unforgiveness is hypothesized to involve rumination about the nature of a hurt or offense, its consequences for the victim or the relationship, and the perceived motivations of the transgressor (Berry, Worthington, Parrott, O'Connor, & Wade, 2001; Wade & Worthington, 2003). Researchers argue that it is usually experienced as an unpleasant emotional state that people are generally motivated to reduce, though a reduction of this state does not in itself constitute forgiveness (Worthington, 2001). Instead, the reduction of unforgiveness is related to forgiveness but not reciprocal to it. In their 2003 study, Wade and Worthington found only a moderate correlation between forgiveness and unforgiveness ($r = -.56$), and demonstrated that, while those who were high in forgiveness frequently showed small amounts of unforgiveness, those low in forgiveness showed a wide range of levels of unforgiveness. Thus, increasing forgiveness (prosocial cognitions, affect, and behavioral dispositions) and decreasing unforgiveness (resentment, anger, and bitterness) have been hypothesized to be supported by different and to differently relate to health outcomes (Harris & Thoresen, 2005). While increases in forgiveness implicate systems implied in both decisional and emotional forgiveness, decreases in unforgiveness primarily assume decreases in negative affect (distress, hostility, anger, etc.). Negative affect has been shown to be highly correlated with psychosomatic complaints and self-reported health, which have been found to predict mortality above and beyond objective health risks. In fact, those who report their health as "poor" are at a twofold increase in risk of mortality when compared to those who rate their health as "excellent".

This is true even after controlling for factors such as depression, income, cognitive impairment, and comorbidity (DeSalvo, Bloser, Reynolds, He, & Muntner, 2006).

The Process of Forgiveness

Another way to operationalize forgiveness is to understand it as a *process*. Instead of seeking to explain when and why forgiveness occurs, these models seek to describe the sequence of stages of forgiveness. Stage models describe a series of interdependent but not necessarily linear phases. Although such models may have been derived from theoretical perspectives (e.g. Worthington's (1998) use of the empathy-altruism hypothesis) or moral imperatives (e.g. Enright's (1996) focus on moral identity development), process models are defined by their focus on a specific sequence of changes in cognitive, affective, and/or behavioral processes (Stelan & Covic, 2006). Most process models assume that the progression through each stage is dependent upon resolution of prior stages.

There appears to be some general agreement amongst theorists on the stages involved in the process of forgiveness. These include the five steps of (a) a recognition that an offense has occurred (McCullough & Worthington, 1994) along with associated feelings of anger and hurt (Enright, 1996), (b) continued negative thoughts and emotions in response to the offense (Stelan & Covic, 2006),(c) a recognition that previous strategies of dealing with the hurt are not working, (d) a freely-chosen decision to forgive (McCullough & Worthington, 1994), and finally (e) affective, cognitive, and/or behavioral changes in the person's response to the offender (Enright, 1996; McCullough & Worthington, 1994).

Understanding the numerous processes involved in forgiveness is important in that it points out that forgiveness is not a single event (Stelan & Covic, 2006) and in that it indicates that forgiveness is a multi-dimensional construct. It is less clear, however, that forgiveness must necessarily occur in the order suggested by such models. For example, although some authors suggest that the decision to forgive must precede cognitive and affective changes (Enright, 1996), others suggest that empathic attunement with the offender precedes the decision to forgive (Worthington, 1998) or can occur at any time (Worthington, 2006). Additionally, it is not clear that all of the stages or processes are necessary to forgiveness. In particular, many models disagree about the true "endpoint" of forgiveness (Stelan & Covic, 2006). While early models saw the endpoint of forgiveness as changes in interpersonal motivations and behaviors (e.g., Nelson, 1992), more recent models have focused only on intrapsychic processes on the side of the victim, including affective states and cognitive changes (Worthington et al., 2003).

Understanding what a given researcher conceptualizes to be the endpoint of forgiveness, as well as which components they emphasize, is crucial to understanding the forgiveness-health link. Whereas intra-psychic definitions may link changes in affective states and related physiological alterations to health outcomes, interpersonal definitions likely link improvements in social functioning to health outcomes (Toussaint & Webb, 2005; Worthington & Scherer, 2004). Frequently, those who study strangers or unwanted relationships emphasize the elimination of negative affect and intra-psychic changes alone, whereas those who study ongoing relationships (e.g. one's partner or close relative) often include motivational changes and behaviors toward the offending party (Worthington, 2005). Thus, those who emphasize interpersonal changes are much more likely to focus on the indirect relationships of improved social relations and health, whereas those who focus on cognitive and affective change will look at within-person physiological links to health outcomes.

With respect to emphasizing cognitive or emotional changes, those who hold onto a specific process model of forgiveness may be blinded to changes at one or the other level if they occur out of sequence in accordance with their model. For example, if someone proposes that the decision to forgive must precede the emotional experience of forgiveness, one may miss possible improvements in health that arise from earlier, spontaneous feelings of empathy for a transgressor. Research into the process of forgiveness has found that both emotional and cognitive changes can occur dynamically as individuals move backward and forward in both positive and negative responses to an event (Enright & Fitzgibbons, 2000).

Dispositional Antecedents of Forgiveness

Another key aspect in understanding the relationship between forgiveness and health is that forgiveness occurs at both dispositional and situational levels. Those who support dispositional forgiveness suggest that forgiving attitudes and behaviors are extensions of an individual's temperament or personality. Conversely, proponents of situational forgiveness perspectives understand forgiveness as a distinct state-specific phenomenon that occurs as a result of interpersonal interactions and circumstances. The primary distinction between these perspectives is that forgiveness is either defined as a relatively stable component of an individual's personality, or as an acute reaction specific to a transgressor or situation. Though different, both perspectives may have merit. Prior research has found significant evidence to support differences in both individuals' dispositional capacities and state responses when coping with offenses (Sandage & Crabtree, 2012).

At the dispositional level, forgiveness is often referred to in the literature as "forgivingness." Forgivingness is defined as a tendency to forgive interpersonal transgressions across time and situations (Berry et al., 2001). Dispositional forgivingness is strongly linked to mental health, such that increased trait forgiveness is associated with decreased anxiety and depression (Berry & Worthington, 2001; Lawler et al., 2005). Personality traits correlated with an individual's tendency to forgive are also linked to various health outcomes. More specifically, different personality traits have been found to be associated with different health related quality of life (HRQL) dimensions. In a study by van Straten et al. (2007), researchers concluded that higher agreeableness was associated with better social and physical wellbeing. Researchers hypothesized that individuals higher in agreeableness were likely more social and relaxed. As a result, these individuals paid less attention to physical discomfort or pain. Additionally, extraversion was found to be positively correlated with improved HRQL. Researchers postulated that the external focus of extraversion may lead individuals to be less focused on their own problems (van Straten et al., 2007). In addition to personality variables, forgivingness has also been linked to empathy, religiousness, spirituality, and self-esteem, all of which are often related to positive health outcomes (Lawler et al., 2005; Wade & Worthington, 2003). Finally, a study conducted by Berry and Worthington (2001) found that high dispositional forgivingness and low trait anger predicted both mental and physical health. Thus, it can be argued that variables associated with an individual's tendency to be forgiving are also related to health outcomes. Although the exact relationship remains unclear, research in this area consistently demonstrates a link between trait forgivingness and mental health.

Although scarce, research exists that has directly examined the relationship between forgivingness and physical health. Seybold, Hill, Neumann, and Chi (2001) examined psychophysiological variables and self-report measures of the tendency to forgive others and oneself. In their study, these researchers found associations with poor health habits such as alcohol use and smoking. Additionally, individuals who scored higher on forgivingness measures exhibited lower levels of anxiety, anger, and depression, as well as lower white blood cell counts (Lawler et al., 2005; Seybold et al., 2001). Additionally, Lawler et al. (2003) found that higher trait forgiveness was negatively associated with lower resting blood pressure levels and improved post-stress recovery. Although evidence is limited, it appears trait forgiveness is associated with better physical and mental health outcomes.

Situational Correlates of Forgiveness

Researchers who adopt a more situational perspective of forgiveness have found forgiveness to be linked to a variety of contextual variables that may also be associated with psychological and physical health outcomes. These include state forgiveness itself, as well as forgiveness-related emotions, cognitions, and relational aspects of offenses. State forgiveness, or the state-specific phenomenon that occurs as a result of interpersonal interactions and situations, has been found to be linked with health outcomes such as self-reported illness, hostility, and stress. One example of situational emotions linked to health outcomes is state empathy; a time-limited, other-oriented emotion encompassing feelings of compassion and goodwill. Numerous studies have implicated empathy in pro-social interactions. Interactions commonly facilitated by empathy include cooperation, altruism, and feelings of unity between the self and others, which have been found to affect both physical and mental health (Fehr, Gelfand, & Nag, 2010). Emotion regulation has also been found to be a buffer against post-offense responses that can have adverse physiological and psychological effects such as sympathetic nervous system arousal, stress, hostility, rumination, and suppression. It has been demonstrated that emotion regulation can aid in the positive reappraisal of past events, increased positive emotions, and a reduction in physiological indicators of affect (Worthington et al., 2007).

Like affective states, state-specific mental processes seem to be correlated with forgiveness and health. A significant body of research has demonstrated that state-specific rumination is harmful to the person engaging in the rumination (Berry et al., 2001). Rumination inhibits forgiveness by triggering repetitive negative thoughts and feelings associated with the initial offense. When victims repeatedly relive an offense through rumination, the negative psychological consequences that were originally inflicted may be maintained or exacerbated. Thus, it is not surprising that rumination has been linked to both psychological and physiological consequences such as physiological activation of the stress responses, depression, sadness, and aggression (Worthington & Wade, 1999).

Relationship variables such as closeness, commitment, and satisfaction have also been found to positively relate to forgiveness. McCullough & Worthington, (1994) argued that relationship closeness fosters motivation to preserve relationships after an offense has occurred, which promotes forgiveness as a form of conflict resolution. Commitment within relationships promotes the same trend, as victims are often more cognizant of the potential consequences of continuing the conflict with offenders (Fehr et al., 2010; McCullough & Worthington, 1994). As with commitment, perceived relationship satisfaction plays an important role in the dynamics of forgiveness such that it aids in a victim's motivation to forgive. Research shows that individuals in committed relationships forgive each other in an effort to remain in the relationship (Fehr et al., 2010). Severity of the offense, repeated offenses, and the type of offense have also been found to respectively influence whether forgiveness leads to beneficial health consequences (Lawler et al., 2005).

After the offense, behaviors such as offender apologies can also impact the forgiveness process. Similar to the attribution perspective described above, apologies can be understood as "offender-initiated repair tactics" (Fehr et al., 2010). Goffman (1967) argued that apologies decouple an offender from the offensive actions he or she committed. As such, apologies often encourage victims to see their offenders as more remorseful, concerned for their well-being, and ultimately more deserving of the victim's forgiveness, thereby making it easier for the victim to forgive an offender. This process can aid in the development of positive and prosocial emotions (Witvliet et al., 2001), ultimately mitigating sympathetic nervous system activation and reducing negative emotions.

In sum, dispositional perspectives may capture personality traits that predispose persons to healthy behaviors (e.g., refraining from alcohol or tobacco use, church attendance, seeking social support) whereas situational variables may influence social support factors that impact both physical and mental health outcomes. Although the evidence for the connection between forgiveness and health is steadily expanding, future research must continue to refine and clarify our understanding of the dynamics between forgiveness and wellbeing.

Conclusion

What is quite apparent from the present review is the numerous ways in which forgiveness can be conceptualized, as well as the variety of factors influencing forgiveness that may or may not be accounted for in a given researcher's definition. Having a single conceptual definition of forgiveness may not then be as important as clarifying which definition of forgiveness is being utilized. In particular, this includes (a) identifying the theoretical or theological background of the researchers, (b) specifying if forgiveness or reductions in unforgiveness are being measured, (c) making clear distinctions between emotional and decisional forgiveness, (d) outlining the specific processes involved in forgiveness, (e) and specifying whether and which dispositional or situational variables are being emphasized.

Ultimately, researchers interested in understanding the relationship between health and forgiveness must be careful to examine the way in which forgiveness is being defined. While it is difficult to find a single definition of forgiveness that that can be wielded in all contexts, it may be equally advantageous to simply be clear as to which variables and processes are being captured in our definitions. This will allow, as Worthington (2005) suggests, for research to move away from the "shotgun" (p. 5) approach of seeking a common-core and to a more focused and nuanced understanding of the relationship between forgiveness and better health.

References

Berry, J. W., & Worthington, E. L. (2001). Forgiveness, relationship quality, stress while imagining relationship events, and physical and mental health. *Journal of Counseling Psychology, 48*, 447–455.

Berry, J. W., Worthington, E. L., Jr., Parrott, L., O'Connor, L. E., & Wade, N. G. (2001). Dispositional forgivingness: Development and construct validity of the Transgression Narrative Test of Forgivingness (TNTF). *Personality and Social Psychology Bulletin, 27*, 1277–1290.

Bhikkhu, T. (2006). *Purity of heart*. Valley Center, CA: Metta Forest Monastery.

DeSalvo, K. B., Bloser, N., Reynolds, K., He, J., & Muntner, P. (2006). Mortality prediction with a single general self-rated health question: A meta-analysis. *Journal of General Internal Medicine, 21*, 267–275.

Enright, R. D., & Fitzgibbons, R. P. (2000). *Helping clients forgive: An empirical guide for resolving anger and restoring hope*. Washington, DC: American Psychological Association.

Enright, R. D., Gassin, E. A., & Wu, C. (1992). Forgiveness: A developmental view. *Journal of Moral Education, 21*, 99–114.

Enright, R. D., & The Human Development Study Group. (1996). Counseling within the forgiveness triad: On forgiving, receiving forgiveness, and self–forgiveness. *Counseling and Values, 40*, 107–126.

Exline, J. J., Worthington, E. L., Hill, P., & McCullough, M. E. (2003). Forgiveness and justice: A research agenda for social and personality psychology. *Personality and Social Psychology Review, 7*(4), 337–348.

Fehr, R., Gelfand, M. J., & Nag, M. (2010). The road to forgiveness: A meta-analytic synthesis of its situational and dispositional correlates. *Psychological Bulletin, 136*(5), 894–914.

Freedman, S. R., & Enright, R. D. (1996). Forgiveness as an intervention goal with incest survivors. *Journal of Consulting and Clinical Psychology, 64*(5), 983–992.

Goffman, E. (1967). *Interaction ritual*. Chicago, IL: Aldine.

Harris, A. H. S., & Thoresen, C. E. (2005). Forgiveness, unforgiveness, health, and disease. In E. L. Worthington Jr. (Ed.), *Handbook of forgiveness* (pp. 321–334). New York, NY: Brunner-Routledge.

Hebl, J., & Enright, R. D. (1993). Forgiveness as a psychotherapeutic goal with elderly females. *Psychotherapy: Theory, Research, Practice, Training, 30*(4), 658–667.

Holeman, V. T., Dean, J. B., DeShea, L., & Duba, J. D. (2011). The multidimensional nature of the quest construct forgiveness, spiritual perception, and differentiation of self. *Journal of Psychology and Theology, 39*(1), 31.

Huang, S. T., & Enright, R. D. (2000). Forgiveness and anger-related emotions in Taiwan: Implications for therapy. *Psychotherapy, 37*, 71–79.

Hunter, A. (2007). Forgiveness: Hindu and Western perspectives. *Journal of Hindu-Christian Studies, 20*(1), 35–42.

Islam Awareness. (2013). *Forgiveness in Islam*. Retrieved from http://www.islamawareness.net/Salvation/forgiveness.html

Janoff-Bulman, R. (1979). Characterological versus behavioral self-blame: Inquiries into depression and rape. *Journal of Personality and Social Psychology, 37*, 1798–1809. doi:10.1037/0022-3514.37.10.1798.

Johansson, D. (2011). Who can forgive sins but god alone? Human and angelic agents, and divine forgiveness in early Judaism. *Journal for the Study of the New Testament, 33*(4), 351–374.

Kaplan, B. (1992). Social health and the forgiving heart: The Type B story. *Journal of Behavioral Medicine, 15*, 3–14.

Kearns, J. N., & Fincham, F. D. (2004). A prototype analysis of forgiveness. *Personality and Social Psychology Bulletin, 30*(7), 838–855.

Lawler, K. A., Younger, J. W., Piferi, R. L., Billington, E., Jobe, R., Edmondson, K., et al. (2003). A change of heart: Cardiovascular correlates of forgiveness in response to interpersonal conflict. *Journal of Behavioral Medicine, 26*(5), 373–393.

Lawler, K. A., Younger, J. W., Piferi, R. L., Jobe, R. L., Edmondson, K. A., & Jones, W. H. (2005). The unique effects of forgiveness on health: An exploration of pathways. *Journal of Behavioral Medicine, 28*(2), 157–167.

Lawler-Row, K. A., Scott, C. A., Raines, R. L., Edlis-Matityahou, M., & Moore, E. W. (2007). The varieties of forgiveness experience: Working toward a comprehensive definition of forgiveness. *Journal of Religion and Health, 46*(2), 233–248.

Lutjen, L., Silton, N., & Flannelly, K. (2012). Religion, forgiveness, hostility and health: A structural equation analysis. *Journal of Religion and Health, 51*(2), 468–478. doi:10.1007/s10943-011-9511-7.

McCullough, M. E., Fincham, F. D., & Tsang, J. A. (2003). Forgiveness, forbearance, and time: The temporal unfolding of transgression-related interpersonal motivations. *Journal of Personality and Social Psychology, 84*(3), 540.

McCullough, M. E., Orsulak, P., Brandon, A., & Akers, L. (2007). Rumination, fear, and cortisol: An in vivo study of interpersonal transgressions. *Health Psychology, 26*, 126–132.

McCullough, M. E., Pargament, K. I., & Thoresen, C. E. (2000). The psychology of forgiveness: History, conceptual issues, and overview. In M. E. McCullough, K. I. Pargament, & C. E. Thoresen (Eds.), *Forgiveness: Theory, research, and practice* (pp. 1–14). New York, NY: Guildford Press.

McCullough, M. E., & Worthington, E. L. (1994). Encouraging clients to forgive people who have hurt them: Review, critique, and research prospectus. *Journal of Psychology and Theology, 22*, 3–20.

McMinn, M. R., Meek, K. R., Dominguez, A. W., Ryan, J. G., & Novotny, K. A. (1999). Forgiveness motives among evangelical Christians: Implications for Christian marriage and family therapists. *Marriage and Family: A Christian Journal, 2*, 189–199.

Nelson, M. K. (1992). *A new theory of forgiveness* (Doctoral dissertation). Retrieved from ETD Collection for Purdue University (AA19229170).

Newberg, A., d'Aquili, E., Newberg, S., & deMarici, V. (2000). The neuropsychological correlates of forgiveness. In M. E. McCullough, K. I. Pargament, & C. E. Thoresen (Eds.), *Forgiveness: Theory, research, and practice* (pp. 91–110). New York, NY: Guilford.

Nietzsche, F. W. (1887). *The genealogy of morals*. New York, NY: Boni and Liveright.

Pressman, S. D., & Cohen, S. (2005). Does positive affect influence health? *Psychological Bulletin, 131*, 925–971. doi:10.1037/0033-2909.131.6.925.

Rye, M. S., Pargament, K. I., Ali, M. A., Beck, G. L., Dorff, E. N., Hallisey, C., ... Williams, J. G. (2000). Religious perspectives on forgiveness. In M. E. McCullough, K. I. Pargament, & C. E. Thoresen (Eds.), *Forgiveness: Theory, research, and practice* (pp. 17–40). New York, NY: Guilford.

Sandage, S. J., & Crabtree, S. (2012). Spiritual pathology and religious coping as predictors of forgiveness. *Mental Health, Religion and Culture, 15*(7), 689–707.

Seybold, K. S., Hill, P. C., Neumann, J. K., & Chi, D. S. (2001). Physiological and psychological correlates of forgiveness. *Journal of Psychology and Christianity, 20*, 250–259.

Stelan, P., & Covic, T. (2006). A review of forgiveness process models and a coping framework to guide future research. *Journal of Social and Clinical Psychology, 25*(10), 1059–1085.

Thoresen, C. E., Oman, D., & Harris, A. H. (2005). The *effects* of religious practices: A focus on health. In W. R. Miller & H. D. Delaney (Eds.), *Judeo-Christian perspectives on psychology: Human nature, motivation, and change* (pp. 205–226). Washington, DC: American Psychological Association.

Toussaint, L., & Friedman, P. (2009). Forgiveness, gratitude, and well-being: The mediating role of affect and beliefs. *Journal of Happiness Studies, 10*(6), 635–654.

Toussaint, L., & Webb, J. R. (2005). Gender differences in the relationship between empathy and forgiveness. *The Journal of Social Psychology, 145*(6), 673–685.

Van Straten, A., Cuijpers, P., Van Zuuren, F., Smits, N., & Donker, M. (2007). Personality traits and health-related quality of life in patients with mood and anxiety disorders. *Quality of Life Research, 16*, 1–8.

Wade, N. G., Meyer, J. E., Goldman, D., & Post, B. C. (2009). Predicting forgiveness for a difficult offense before and after treatment: The role of religious commitment, offender regret, and trait forgivingness. *Journal of Psychology and Christianity, 27*, 358–367.

Wade, N. G., Tucker, J. R., & Cornish, M. A. (2014). Forgiveness interventions and the promotion of resilience following interpersonal stress and trauma. In M. Kent, M. C. Davis, & J. W. Reich (Eds.), *The resilience handbook: Approaches to stress and trauma*. New York, NY: Routledge.

Wade, N. G., & Worthington, E. L., Jr. (2003). Overcoming interpersonal offenses: Is forgiveness the only way to deal with unforgiveness? *Journal of Counseling and Development, 81*(3), 343–353.

Walsh-Frank, P. (1996). Compassion: An East-West comparison. *Asian Philosophy, 6*(1), 5–19.

Witvliet, C. V. O., Ludwig, T. E., & Vander Laan, K. L. (2001). Granting forgiveness or harboring grudges: Implications for emotion, physiology, and health. *Psychological Science, 121*, 117–123.

Worthington, E. L., Jr. (1998). The pyramid model of forgiveness: Some interdisciplinary speculations about unforgiveness and the promotion of forgiveness. In *Dimensions of forgiveness: Psychological research and theological perspectives* (pp. 107–137). Philadelphia, PA: Templeton Foundation Press.

Worthington, E. L., Jr. (2001). Unforgiveness, forgiveness, and reconciliation in societies. In R. G. Helmick & R. L. Petersen (Eds.), *Forgiveness and reconciliation: Religion, public policy, and conflict transformation* (pp. 161–182). Philadelphia, PA: Templeton Foundation Press.

Worthington, E. L., Jr. (Ed.). (2005). *Handbook of forgiveness*. New York, NY: Brunner-Routledge.

Worthington, E. L., Jr. (2006). *Forgiveness and reconciliation*. New York, NY: Taylor & Francis Group.

Worthington, E. L., Jr., & Drinkard, D. T. (2000). Promoting reconciliation through psychoeducational and therapeutic interventions. *Journal of Marital and Family Therapy, 26*, 93–101.

Worthington, E. L., Jr., & Scherer, M. (2004). Forgiveness is an emotion-focused coping strategy that can reduce health risks and promote health resilience: Theory, review, and hypotheses. *Psychology & Health, 19*(3), 385–405.
Worthington, E. L., Jr., & Wade, N. G. (1999). The social psychology of unforgiveness and forgiveness and implications for clinical practice. *Journal of Social and Clinical Psychology, 18*, 385–418.
Worthington, E. L., Jr., Wade, N. G., Hight, T. L., Ripley, J. S., McCullough, M. E., Berry, J. W., et al. (2003). The religious commitment inventory–10: Development, refinement, and validation of a brief scale for research and counseling. *Journal of Counseling Psychology, 50*(1), 84.
Worthington, E. L., Jr., Witvliet, C. V. O., Pietrini, P., & Miller, A. J. (2007). Forgiveness, health and wellbeing: A review of evidence for emotional versus decisional forgiveness, dispositional forgivingness, and reduced unforgiveness. *Journal of Behavioral Medicine, 30*, 291–302.
Younger, J. W., Piferi, R. L., Jobe, R. L., & Lawler, K. A. (2004). Dimensions of forgiveness: The views of laypersons. *Journal of Social and Personal Relationships, 21*(6), 837–855.

Chapter 3
A Conceptual Model of Forgiveness and Health

Caroline R. Lavelock, Daniel J. Snipes, Brandon J. Griffin, Everett L. Worthington, Jr., Don E. Davis, Joshua N. Hook, Eric G. Benotsch, and James Ritter

Forgiveness has been consistently linked with physical health outcomes, including objective measures of physical health such as physiological responsiveness and recovery (Lawler et al., 2005; Lawler-Row & Piferi, 2006). For this reason, Lawler-Row, Hyatt-Edwards, Wuenssch, and Karremans (2011) argue that scholars should elucidate the theoretical connections between forgiveness and health. However, there is not yet definitive evidence regarding the mechanism for the forgiveness-health relationship (Green, DeCourville, & Sadava, 2012). In the present chapter, we describe the adverse effects of unforgiveness on physical health and develop an integrative conceptual model involving precursors as well as mechanisms that may function as a foundation for future empirical investigations on forgiveness and its influence on health.

Definitions and the Present Review

We use this definition of health: "a state of complete physical, mental and social well-being and not merely the absence of disease or infirmity" (Official Records of the World Health Organization, no. 2, p. 100). It is thus important to measure the presence of positive states (e.g., well-being) and the absence of negative states.

C.R. Lavelock (✉) • D.J. Snipes • B.J. Griffin • E.L. Worthington, Jr. (✉)
E.G. Benotsch • J. Ritter
Department of Psychology, Virginia Commonwealth University, Richmond, VA, USA
e-mail: lavelockc@vcu.edu; eworth@vcu.edu

D.E. Davis
Department of Counseling and Psychological Services, Georgia State University, Atlanta, GA, USA

J.N. Hook
Department of Psychology, University of North Texas, Denton, TX, USA

L.L. Toussaint et al. (eds.), *Forgiveness and Health*,
DOI 10.1007/978-94-017-9993-5_3

We define forgiveness as an emotion-focused coping strategy whereby victims of an offense replace negative unforgiving emotions (i.e., bitterness, anger, etc.) with positive other-oriented emotions (e.g., love, empathy, compassion; Wade, Worthington, & Meyer, 2005; Worthington & Scherer, 2004). This definition of forgiveness can expand to accommodate for a pattern of forgivingness across the lifespan (trait forgivingness); it can also include, but does not require, behavioral components often involved in related constructs, such as reconciliation. We build on this stress-and-coping model of forgiveness (Strelan & Covic, 2006; Worthington, 2006, 2013). Extending Lazarus's (1999) model of stress and coping, the offense is the initial stressor. The victim then appraises the meaning of the offense, such as the severity of injustice, or resources available to cope with the offense. To the degree that the stressor is appraised as threatening and not easily coped with, a stress response of unforgiveness manifests that may result in poor health outcomes (Worthington, Witvliet, Pietrini, & Miller, 2007). Forgiveness is one of many strategies to cope with the stress of unforgiveness. In the present review, we seek to illuminate common themes in the existing forgiveness and physical health literature and provide a research agenda based on the status of this literature.

Method of the Review

We conducted our literature search using PsycINFO through February 23rd, 2012 pairing the term "physical health" with "forgiveness." The search resulted in 99 articles. We omitted three articles due to an emphasis on sexual health, which we will not explore due to space constraints, and one article because we could not acquire an English version. A summary table and reference list of these 95 studies can be obtained from the corresponding author. Of the 95 works reviewed, 49 were correlational studies; 26, literature reviews; 6, quasi-experimental studies; 5, experimental studies; 3, case studies; 3, presentations of models or theories; 2, qualitative studies; and 1, a peer commentary. Of the 95, 48 were cross-sectional and 14 were longitudinal; 50 were peer-reviewed articles, 30 were dissertations, and 15 were book chapters.

Results

We organize the results of this review in four sections. First, we illustrate a large portion of the literature that explores unforgiveness responses and health outcomes. Then, we address person variables that serve as precursors to the forgiveness and health relationship: (1) religiousness and spirituality, (2) age, and (3) personality. Next, we focus on the theorized mechanisms that underlie the relationship between forgiveness and health: (1) change in emotions from negative to positive, (2) social support, and (3) mental and physiological responses. Finally, we address three additional questions about the association between forgiveness and health: (1) the bi-directional relationship between these two variables, (2) the effect of forgiveness interventions on health, and (3) negative aspects of forgiveness on health. Detailed results as well as operationalization of health outcomes via study measures can be found in a summary table available from the corresponding author upon request.

Unforgiveness and Health

Early research on forgiveness focused on its antithetical—the adverse effects of anger and hostility on blood pressure and cardiovascular health (for a review, see Booth-Kewley & Friedman, 1987). Accordingly, forgiveness, as a reducer of anger, became a burgeoning topic in health-related research (e.g., Berry, Worthington, O'Conner, Parrott, & Wade, 2005). Before we delve into mechanisms within the forgiveness and health relationship, we first consider the adverse effects of unforgiveness on health.

The idea of unforgiveness was fleshed out in reviews by Witvliet (2005) and Worthington, Witvliet, Pietrini, and Miller (2007); Witvliet reviewed four decades of research surrounding forgiveness and health. She posited that unforgiveness leads to rumination, avoidance, and revenge, which invites attentional, physiological, and behavioral components of emotion, causing outcomes such as anxiety, depression, hostility, and heart disease. This suggests that an emotional shift caused by components of unforgiveness is responsible for the physiological responses that lead to poor physical health. Notably, when under stress, people often respond with negative emotions like anger, resentment, anxiety, and depression. Those emotional responses are related to elevated stress responses in peripheral physiological systems. Longitudinal research on the effects of unforgiveness and its related mechanisms (e.g., unhealthy coping such as problematic drinking; Webb & Brewer, 2010) is needed to better understand how unforgiveness manifests in physical health outcomes.

Person Variables as Precursors to the Forgiveness and Health Relationship

Religiousness and Spirituality Worthington, Berry, and Parrott (2001) claimed that religion, forgiveness, and health are related to each other, involving a number of mechanisms. Forgiveness can be difficult to separate from religion due to the inherent morality of forgiveness, as well as the role of forgiveness as a religious coping mechanism. Previous research has shown the importance of religious coping in terms of improved health outcomes, even over and above the effect of non-religious coping (Pargament, Koenig, & Perez, 2000). In his 2003 review, Webb suggested that forgiveness as a spiritual coping mechanism has been tied to better health outcomes, and additional research suggests that religious coping mechanisms in general are tied to better outcomes in both mental and physical health (Pargament et al., 2000).

Personality Though personality traits such as openness and agreeableness are allied to mental and physical health, a forgiving personality potentially affects mental and physical health outcomes more than do other personality factors (Moorhead, Gill, Minton, & Myers, 2012). For example, Lawler-Row and Piferi's (2006) correlational study found that trait forgivingness was tied to well-being, stress, and depression, and was higher in women (than men), individuals over 60 (relative to younger people), and those who attend church frequently (relative to infrequent church attenders). Other studies, such as Berry and Worthington's (2001) quasi-experimental study of 39 adults in romantic relationships, found that people in happy and unhappy relationships differed in personality traits such as high forgivingness and low anger. Trait forgivingness was linked to both better mental and physical health and lower cortisol reactivity.

A victim's perception of his or her transgressor's personality has a strong impact, and this may be more important than the personality of the victim. In a longitudinal study of 39 female college students by Tabak and McCullough (2011), perceived agreeableness of the transgressor was tied to higher levels of victim forgiveness and lower levels of cortisol. This suggested that certain aspects of better cardiovascular health might result from forgiving. However, victims' levels of neuroticism and agreeableness had a small link with cortisol and forgiveness. Thus, Tabak and McCullough concluded that perceived personality of the transgressor might be more important than the victim's personality in the forgiveness-health relationship.

Age Toussaint and Webb (2005) argue that age may be another person variable affecting the relationship between forgiveness and physical health. For example, multiple correlational analyses involving 1,423 nationally representative participants suggested an association between higher forgiveness and health with old age, but not with young and middle age (Toussaint, Williams, Musick, & Everson, 2001). In addition, Turesky and Schultz (2010) conducted a qualitative review of three developmental contextual models of forgiveness. They concluded that a decline of physical health naturally occurs with increasing age. This decline in health led to increased reflection about life, which in turn led to greater striving for meaning and hence greater spirituality, as well as an increased awareness of the approach of death. The sense of impending death might stimulate review of past relationships, increasing the awareness of events that need forgiving. In combination, spirituality and a potential need for forgiveness might engender a sense of peace about the past and with death. These mental health correlates that occur as one's health deteriorates with age might contribute to higher forgiveness outcomes, illustrating a potentially bidirectional, symbiotic relationship between forgiveness and health.

Mechanisms by Which Forgiveness Might Affect Health

Change in Emotion from Negative to Positive Harris and Thoresen's (2003) model of forgiveness and health views forgiveness as functioning to reduce negative traits and increase positive traits. This combination in turn invites better health outcomes as defined by health-promoting behaviors and peak physiological condition. In effect, better health outcomes appear when a reduction of unforgiveness, an increase in positive affect, and their effects on behaviors are combined. For example, Green et al. (2012) conducted a correlational study that focused on the role of emotions in forgiveness. In 623 college freshmen, forgiveness was linked with decreased negative affect, as well as increased positive affect and social support, which were both related to better self-reported health outcomes. It appears that replacing the negative with the positive emotions and motivations, which is at the core of forgiveness, extends both the achievement of forgiveness and its relationship with health.

Social Support Forgiveness may also function to maintain one's social support network, which can influence physical health. For example, Lawler-Row and Piferi (2006) found that individuals who were more forgiving had higher levels of social support, healthy behaviors and spiritual well-being. Those variables in turn affected health outcomes such as illness presence and symptom frequency. Forgiveness and social support both involve the maintenance of relationships. In this way, forgiveness leads to greater physical health, while social isolation and other costs of unforgivingness (as previously discussed in the unforgiveness section) are historically dangerous for individuals and even groups.

Mental and Physiological Responses Forgiveness is tied to several mental health variables that may contribute to physical health outcomes. For example, Lawler et al. (2005) conducted a correlational study examining 82 adults. They concluded that, while the strongest predictor was the reduction of negative affect, both reduced negative affect and reduced stress at least partially mediated the relationship between forgiveness and physical health. In this case, physical health was defined using vital signs and self-reported physical symptoms. Trait forgivingness was also correlated with better conflict management, which fully mediated the relationship between forgiveness and health.

A number of studies have explored the role of physiological responses in explaining the association between forgiveness and physical health. Such research posits that those who forgive others tend to have stronger immune systems (Seybold, Hill, Neumann, & Chi, 2001), less physiological reactivity to stress (Witvliet, Ludwig, & Vander Laan, 2001), lower blood pressure (Lawler et al., 2005), and overall fewer physical symptoms (Toussaint et al., 2001). This research has shown the major players in physiological responses related to forgiveness to be stress-related. Forgiveness' association with lower levels of cortisol (another marker of stress) has found support in a number of studies (Berry & Worthington, 2001; Standard, 2004; Tabak & McCullough, 2011).

Taken together, many mental and physiological variables mediate between forgiveness and physical health (for reviews, see Harris & Thoresen, 2005; Lawler-Row & Reed, 2008; Thoreson, Harris, & Luskin, 2000). Friedberg, Suchday, and Srinivas (2009) conducted a correlational study of 85 cardiac inpatients. They found that by decreasing anxiety and perceived stress, the physiological responses were less and the blood cholesterol was decreased. Those decreases reduced the risk for cardiovascular problems. Thus, better health was tied to forgiveness.

Additional Questions

Could Health Influence Forgiveness? The vast majority of the studies in this review have been correlational. While usually unspoken, the implicit assumption seems to have been that changes in forgiveness cause changes in health. Few studies have shown a bidirectional impact, showing that changes in health cause changes in forgiveness. For example, a quasi-experimental study of 65 college students by Rashid (2004) examined the impact of positive psychology coursework on character strength and development. Connections between several strengths (e.g., intimate attachment, kindness, leadership) and forgiveness were mediated by self-reported peak physical health. Though further evidence is needed via true experimental designs, this study potentially suggests that forgiveness, as well as strengths in the social, religious, and personality realm, may be higher in those who are in good physical health than in poor health.

Forgiveness Interventions Several studies have explored the effects of forgiveness interventions on physical health (Baskin & Enright, 2004; Root & McCullough, 2007). For example, in a quasi-experimental study of 19 elderly individuals using Enright's therapeutic model of forgiveness, participants showed a long-term increase in forgiveness and reduced depression, and short-term improvements in self-perceived physical health (Ingersoll-Dayton, Campbell, & Ha, 2009). It makes sense that short-term health benefits might be related to enhanced state forgiveness. In a particular situation, forgiveness benefits should not be expected to be as lasting as they might be in a situation that taps into trait forgivingness. This type of conclusion can be justified by viewing the process of a forgiveness intervention, where health was found to fluctuate (Browne, 2009). According to the 11 adult participants in Browne's qualitative study, moving through forgiveness is a struggle. It can involve adverse health effects, but it often reduces health ailments in the end. Just knowing that they may reap health benefits was motivating for participants to continue.

One forgiveness intervention designed for children, targeted a very real threat to physical health—bullying. This quasi-experimental study involved 81 elementary school students. Turner (2009) found that forgiveness can stop or prevent bullying from affecting physical health as defined by physical harm. This may also prevent the victim from experiencing a stressful and physically harmful response, thus giving a potential directionality in the forgiveness and health relationship. Additionally, we see the importance of forgiveness interventions as preventative measures, not only for promoting good behavior, but for protecting mental and physical health.

When Forgiveness Is Not Healthy Not all the reviewed studies demonstrated a positive relationship between forgiveness and physical health (Edmondson, 2005; Hernandez, 2006). One correlational study of 107 adult divorcees found that forgiveness was not linked to lower depression or anxiety, let alone physical health, claiming denial was a healthier coping mechanism than forgiveness (Putnam, 2001). Denial as a substitute to forgiveness has mixed reviews. Other research suggests those who used denial as a coping response to discrimination suffered from higher blood pressure than did those who contested unfair treatment (Harrell, Hall, & Taliaferro, 2003; Krieger & Sidney, 1996).

Some studies link forgiveness to lower levels of physical health. In Toussaint and colleagues' (2001) national sample of nearly 1500 adults, those with a greater tendency to seek forgiveness were at a greater risk for psychological distress, across all age groups. The authors speculated that people who (a) take the relational risk of suggesting forgiveness, (b) may not be genuine in their search for forgiveness, or (c) are high in neuroticism or low in self-esteem, might endure poor mental health outcomes such as anxiety and rumination and the related negative health outcomes. However, it is possible that this psychological discomfort may be a short-term drawback with long term social, psychological, and physiological benefits. More research must examine forgiveness in terms of physiological ups and downs in this process. In short, it is clear that forgiveness is not always the solution for optimal outcomes.

Discussion

Several studies have now examined the links between forgiveness and physical health, and most scholars agree that there are multiple mediators that jointly explain the forgiveness-health relationship. Let us, therefore, examine what we have observed. First, we demonstrated decreased unforgiveness is related to improved physical health. Second, we identified precursors that have been studied in forgiveness and health research. Third, we illustrated that forgiveness works through a variety of mechanisms to produce positive physical health. Finally, we discussed remaining questions of directionality, intervention, and when forgiveness is not healthy. Therefore, we now integrate the above research into a tentative model of forgiveness and health. We conclude with a versatile and interdisciplinary approach to the relationship between forgiveness and physical health (see Fig. 3.1).

Three themes in the research, religiousness, personality, and age serve as precursors to forgiveness. Positive religious coping and experiences include prayer, a positive view of God, feeling forgiven by God, positive experiences with religion, and a nurturing religious culture. A forgiving personality includes high

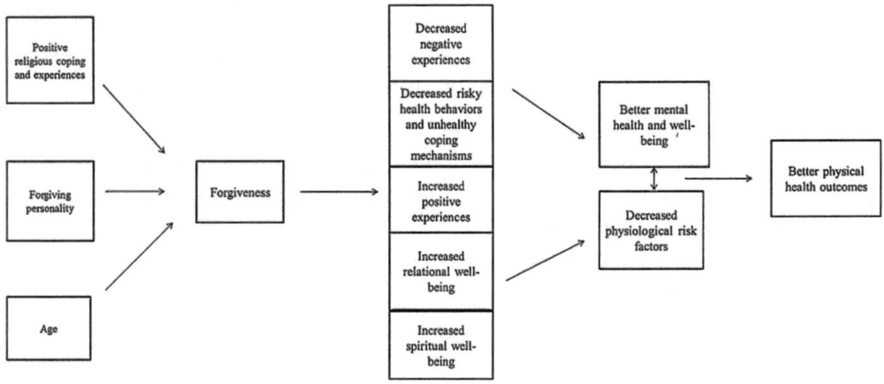

Fig. 3.1 An interdisciplinary conceptual model of forgiveness and health

agreeableness, high perceived agreeableness of a transgressor, low Type A personality tendencies, low neuroticism, and low narcissism. Age considerations include accrued life experience that tends to increase likelihood of forgiveness.

Other themes from the literature find their way into our model among our proposed mechanisms through which forgiveness impacts health. Decreased negative experiences refer to decreased guilt, anger, stress, rumination, avoidance, revenge, feelings of control, tension, anxiety, and depression. Decreased risky health behaviors and unhealthy coping mechanisms may include substance use, gambling, and risky sexual behaviors.

In addition to decreasing negative factors, our model includes increasing positive factors. Increased positive experiences include empathy, altruism, compassion, love, and virtue. Increased relational factors involve social support, high quality relationships, social skills, and conflict management. Increased spiritual well-being includes self-transcendence, inner peace, and connectedness with the sacred and with humanity (i.e., spirituality).

Importantly, this combination of mechanisms eventuates into decreased physiological risk factors and better mental health and general well-being. Decreased physiological risk factors include decreasing hypertension, fatigue, cortisol secretion, cardiovascular symptoms, and overall physical symptomology. Better immune functioning and successful aging can also be included in this category, and in combination with better mental health and general well-being, tends to describe an individual in overall good physical health.

Limitations

There are several limitations to this review. Samples used in research on forgiveness and health have over-represented female, Caucasian young adults. They are usually healthy, making it difficult to note differences in health due to forgiveness (Porter, 2004). Naturally, external validity and generalizability preclude sweeping conclusions from these findings.

Some of the earliest research in the present review noted a need for psychometrically sound measures of forgiveness (McCullough & Worthington, 1994). However, over the 20 years covered by the review, the assessment of forgiveness has improved. Notably, accurate and psychometrically sound measures have been developed and used such that forgiveness measures are useful for a number of relevant research questions (Worthington et al., 2014). Recently, physiological measures have been used to assess constructs co-occurring with unforgiveness and forgiveness. The inclusion of behavioral measures of correlates of forgiveness could offer a more objective base for forgiveness in health research. For example, requiring objective health indices (e.g., a doctor's physical) in combination with self-report health measures invites higher credibility for studies aiming to reveal changes in or associations with health.

Despite a plethora of effective interventions for forgiveness, such as Worthington's (2003) REACH Forgiveness program and Enright and Fitzgibbons's (2000) Process Model of Forgiveness, few interventions are used in this body of research on forgiveness and physical health. Both operationally and content-wise, this limits evidence on causation and directionality. Valuable content could be gleaned from interventions, yet few studies target health outcomes.

Research Agenda

There are several exciting areas for future research on the forgiveness and health relationship. Most notably, nearly every study examined in this review noted that future research must include longitudinal and experimental studies with more diverse populations.

Future Research in Religiousness Forgiveness has often been associated with religion, yet many questions remain in this context. For instance, early research noted a need for future studies to explore forgiveness and health factors of highly religious people, compared to more secular people (Coates, 1997). More research is also needed on how religious values and church rules, with an emphasis on forgiveness, affect the health of their followers (Quenstedt-Moe & Popkess, 2014). Furthermore, even if religion may be associated with the forgiveness-health link, problems might occur. It may be especially stressful when religious people, who strongly value forgiveness, have difficulty forgiving (Lawler-Row, 2010). Failing to live up to their standards for forgiveness may intensify stress. Another interesting facet of religion that warrants analysis is feeling forgiven by God. Could there be health benefits in the relief of feeling forgiven, by each other and by God?

Future Research in Personality One of the most difficult things about generalizing forgiveness research is that substantial individual differences exist in forgiveness. These differences in forgivingness and trait anger should be considered when researching and intervening (Berry & Worthington, 2001), and the forgiving person's personality should be more closely examined (Toussaint & Webb, 2005). State forgiveness and trait forgivingness need to be studied further as well (Porter, 2004); they might relate differently to health.

Future Directions in Developmental Psychology The effect of age and development on forgiveness and health has been well established (Toussaint et al., 2001). Forgiveness also aids health in decline. One might accept and forgive one's body for failing. Future studies could identify developmental changes in general and across different demographics. Might there be disparities based in gender, socioeconomic status, marital status, or race/ethnicity in forgiveness that might account for parallel disparities in health?

Future Research in Mental Health One up-and-coming avenue regarding mental health as a mediator of forgiveness and physical health is self-forgiveness. Self-forgiveness has only recently been starkly differentiated from other-forgiveness, and past studies have hinted that the two may contribute to related but distinct outcomes (Louden-Gerber, 2009). Both self and other forgiveness involve taking less offense, taking more responsibility for how one feels, and positively changing one's perception, feelings, and behavior (Luskin, 2002). These and other correlates of self and other forgiveness, including personality and religious factors, should be studied in the future as causative to the mental state, which mediates forgiveness and health.

Another important contributor to mental health is social support. Forgiveness and social support both involve the maintenance of relationships and in this way, might enable greater health. Because social support has already been established as a likely mechanism in the link between forgiveness and mental health, it may not seem worthy of extensive future investigation. However, social support should not be forgotten in the context of self-forgiveness, where little research has been conducted. For example, consider a person with strong social support in which healthy coping mechanisms like forgiveness are frequently exercised. It stands to reason that such a person could more readily practice self-forgiveness than someone who has more insecure attachments and little reference point for how to forgive.

Future Research in Physiology With few exceptions, the neuropsychological mechanisms of forgiveness have been less investigated than some other aspects of forgiveness and health (Tsuang, Eaves, Nir, Jerskey, & Lyons, 2005). Twin studies, for example, may show genetic effects on forgiveness that aid health outcomes. In a study outside of our review, Worthington and Sotoohi (2010) have reviewed the research on the physiology of forgiveness, illustrating the potential for growth in this area of study. Future studies should examine how the neurobiology of other emotions compares to that of forgiveness (Farrow & Woodruff, 2005).

Future Directions in Potential Mediators Many studies in the present review noted potential mediators to be studied in future research. Some of these include positive religious coping (Witvliet, Phipps, Feldman, & Beckham, 2004), the relationship of the victim and the transgressor, the nature of the offense (Lawler et al., 2005), cognitive flexibility (Lawler-Row & Reed, 2008), empathy, self-blame, self-doubt, poor coping skills, poor social support, and insecurity (Avery, 2008).

Future Research in Intervention and Directionality Studies that reveal the directionality of the forgiveness and health relationship have been suggested since this research began, yet few have been conducted. While it is assumed that the effect moves from forgiveness to physical health with some mediators in between, research in the opposite direction is recommended. Does physical health affect forgiveness? Only two studies in this review found results which may support that claim (Browne, 2009; Rashid, 2004).

Forgiveness interventions may reveal directionality in this relationship. The process of these interventions should be measured alongside physiological indices to see if any part of forgiveness has greater health implications (Hernandez, 2006). Such studies would offer insight into reducing negative states versus increasing positive states in terms of health outcomes.

Conclusion

Current research notes an undeniable link of forgiveness to health, but the size of the relation as well as its mechanisms remains elusive (Toussaint & Webb, 2005). In this chapter, we organize and review existing research on forgiveness and health. Major themes revealed themselves, often referring to decreasing negative experiences (stress, anger, rumination, and depression), increasing positive experiences (affect, social support, positive spiritual experiences), and physiological responses (blood pressure, cortisol). We present an interdisciplinary model which incorporates these and more themes as a way to better understand how forgiveness manifests physically. Such a model provides a bird's-eye view of the state of the field and informs future research by providing evidence from existing research and topics for further study that will aid in a more complete understanding of forgiveness.

Like anything worthwhile, one cannot rush forgiveness or it will mean nothing; it must be experienced in order to work effectively through one's pain of being hurt or offended (Fisher & Exline, 2006). This exercise of the human condition by strengthening relationships and the self through forgiveness is what brings a greater richness to the quality of life that is so intertwined with physical health.

References[1]

*Avery, C. M. (2008). The relationship between self-forgiveness and health: Mediating variables and implications for well-being. *Dissertation Abstracts International, 69*(3), 1939B.

Baskin, T. W., & Enright, R. D. (2004). Intervention studies on forgiveness: A meta analysis. *Journal of Counseling and Development, 82*, 79–90.

*Berry, J. W., & Worthington, E. L., Jr. (2001). Forgivingness, relationship quality, stress while imagining relationship events, and physical and mental health. *Journal of Counseling Psychology, 48*(4), 447–455.

Berry, J. W., Worthington, E. L., Jr., O'Connor, L. E., Parrott., L., III., & Wade, N. G. (2005). Forgivingness, vengeful rumination, and affective traits. *Journal of Personality, 73*(1), 183–225.

Booth-Kewley, S., & Friedman, H. S. (1987). Psychological predictors of heart disease: A quantitative review. *Psychological Bulletin, 101*(3), 343–362.

*Browne, P. E. (2009). Forgiveness therapy: A qualitative study of the forgiveness experience of people who have undergone forgiveness as a counseling intervention. *Dissertation Abstracts International, 70*(4), 2566B.

*Coates, D. (1997). The correlations of forgiveness of self, forgiveness of others, and hostility, depression, anxiety, self-esteem, life adaptation, and religiosity among female victims of domestic violence. *Dissertation Abstracts International, 58*(5), 2667B.

*Edmondson, K. A. (2005). Forgiveness and rumination: Their relationship and effects on psychological and physical health. *Dissertation Abstracts International, 65*(12), 6694B.

Enright, R. D., & Fitzgibbons, R. P. (2000). *Helping clients forgive: An empirical guide for resolving anger and restoring hope*. Washington, DC: American Psychological Association.

*Farrow, T. F. D., & Woodruff, P. W. R. (2005). Neuroimaging of forgivability. In E. L. Worthington, Jr. (Ed.), *Handbook of forgiveness* (pp. 259–272). New York, NY: Brunner-Routledge.

Fisher, M. L., & Exline, J. J. (2006). Self-forgiveness versus excusing: The roles of remorse, effort, and acceptance of responsibility. *Self and Identity, 5*(2), 127–146.

*Friedberg, J. P., Suchday, S., & Srinivas, V. S. (2009). Relationship between forgiveness and psychological indices in cardiac patients. *International Journal of Behavioral Medicine, 16*(3), 205–211.

*Green, M., DeCourville, N., & Sadava, S. (2012). Positive affect, negative affect, stress, and social support as mediators of the forgiveness-health relationship. *Journal of Social Psychology, 152*(3), 288–307.

Harrell, J., Hall, S., & Taliaferro, J. (2003). Physiological responses to racism and discrimination: An assessment of the evidence. *American Journal of Public Health, 93*, 243–248.

*Harris, A. H. S., & Thoresen, C. E. (2003). Strength-based health psychology: Counseling for total human health. In B. Walsh (Ed.), *Counseling psychology and optimal human functioning* (pp. 199–227). Mahwah, NJ: Lawrence Erlbaum Associates Publishers.

*Harris, A. H. S. & Thoresen, C. E. (2005). Forgiveness, unforgiveness, health, and disease. In E. L. Worthington, Jr. (Ed.), *Handbook of forgiveness* (pp. 321–334). New York, NY: Brunner-Routledge.

*Hernandez, D. H. (2006). Hostility, forgiveness, and cardiovascular reactivity to stress: Does forgiveness mediate or moderate the relation between hostility and cardiovascular reactivity to anger-eliciting laboratory experiences? *Dissertation Abstracts International, 66*(9), 5089B.

*Ingersoll-Dayton, B., Campbell, R., & Ha, J. (2009). Enhancing forgiveness: A group intervention for the elderly. *Journal of Gerontological Social Work, 52*(1), 2–16.

[1] *indicates presence of reference in Supplemental Table.

Krieger, N., & Sidney, S. (1996). Racial discrimination and blood pressure: The CARDIA study of young black and white adults. *American Journal of Public Health, 86*(10), 1370–1378.

*Lawler, K. A., Younger, J. W., Piferi, R. L., Jobe, R. L., Edmondson, K. A., & Jones, W. H. (2005). The unique effects of forgiveness on health: An exploration of pathways. *Journal of Behavioral Medicine, 28*(2), 157–167.

*Lawler-Row, K. A. (2010). Forgiveness as a mediator of the religiosity-health relationship. *Psychology of Religion and Spirituality, 2*(1), 1–16.

*Lawler-Row, K. A., Hyatt-Edwards, L., Wuenssch, K. L., & Karremans, J. C. (2011). Forgiveness and health: The role of attachment. *Personal Relationships, 18*(2), 170–183.

*Lawler-Row, K. A. & Piferi, R. L. (2006). The forgiving personality: Describing a life well lived? *Personality and Individual Differences, 41*(6), 1009–1020.

*Lawler-Row, K. A. & Reed, K. A. (2008). Forgiveness and health in women. In W. Malcolm, N. DeCourville, & K. Belicki (Eds.), *Women's reflections on the complexities of forgiveness* (pp. 75–90). New York, NY: Routledge.

Lazarus, R. S. (1999). *Stress and emotion: A new synthesis*. New York, NY: Springer.

*Louden-Gerber, G. M. (2009). A group forgiveness intervention for adult male homeless individuals: Effects on forgiveness, rumination, and social connectedness. *Dissertation Abstracts International, 69*(12), 4640A.

Luskin, F. M. (2002). *Forgive for good: A proven prescription for health and happiness*. San Francisco, CA: Harper Collins.

*McCullough, M. E., & Worthington, E. L., Jr. (1994). Encouraging clients to forgive people who have hurt them: Review, critique, and research prospectus. *Journal of Psychology and Theology, 22*(1), 3–20.

*Moorhead, H. J. H., Gill, C., Minton, C. A. B., & Myers, J. E. (2012). Forgive and forget? forgiveness, personality, and wellness among counselors-in-training. *Counseling and values, 57*(1), 81–95.

*Pargament, K. I., Koenig, H. G., & Perez, L. M. (2000). The many methods of religious coping: Development and initial validation of the R-COPE. *Journal of Clinical Psychology, 56*(4), 519–543.

*Porter, L. G. (2004). Personal narratives as reflections of identity and meaning: A study of betrayal, forgiveness, and health. *Dissertation Abstracts International, 64*(9), 4666B.

*Putnam, J. W. (2001). Revenge and forgiveness: Mutually exclusive or coexisting constructs? *Dissertation Abstracts International, 61*(8), 4424B.

*Quenstedt-Moe, G., & Popkess, S. (2014). Forgiveness and health in Christian women. *Journal of Religion and Health, 53*(1), 204–216.

*Rashid, T. (2004). Enhancing strengths through the teaching of positive psychology. *Dissertation Abstracts International, 64*(12), 6339B.

*Root, L. M., & McCullough, M. E. (2007). Low-cost interventions for promoting forgiveness. In L. L'Abate (Ed.), *Low-cost approaches to promote physical and mental health: Theory, research, and practice* (pp. 415–434). New York, NY: Springer.

Seybold, K. S., Hill, P. C., Neumann, J. K., & Chi, D. S. (2001). Physiological and psychological correlates of forgiveness. *Journal of Psychology and Christianity, 203*(3), 250–259.

*Standard, S. (2004). Effects of a forgiveness intervention on salivary cortisol, DHEA, and psychological variables. *Dissertation Abstracts International, 65*(4), 2114B.

Strelan, P., & Covic, T. (2006). A review of forgiveness process models and a coping framework to guide future research. *Journal of Social and Clinical Psychology, 25*(10), 1059–1085.

*Tabak, B. A., & McCullough, M. E. (2011). Perceived transgressor agreeableness decreases cortisol response and increases forgiveness following recent interpersonal transgressions. *Biological Psychology, 87*(3), 386–392.

*Thoreson, C. E., Harris, A. H. S., & Luskin, F. (2000). Forgiveness and health: An unanswered question. In M. E. McCullough, K. L. Pargament, & C. E. Thoreson (Eds.), *Forgiveness: Theory, research, and practice* (pp. 254–280). New York, NY: Guilford Press.

*Toussaint, L. L., & Webb, J. R. (2005). Theoretical and empirical connections between forgiveness, mental health, and well-being. In E. L. Worthington, Jr. (Ed.), *Handbook of forgiveness* (pp. 349–362). New York, NY: Brunner-Routledge.

*Toussaint, L. L., Williams, D. R., Musick, M. A., & Everson, S. A. (2001). Forgiveness and health: Age differences in a U.S. probability sample. *Journal of Adult Development, 8*(4), 249–257.

*Tsuang, M. T., Eaves, L., Nir T., Jerskey, B. A., & Lyons, M. J. (2005). Genetic influences on forgiving. In E. L. Worthington, Jr. (Ed.), *Handbook of forgiveness* (pp. 245–258). New York, NY: Brunner-Routledge.

*Turesky, D. G., & Schultz, J. M. (2010). Spirituality among older adults: An exploration of the developmental context, impact on mental and physical health, and integration into counseling. *Journal of Religion, Spirituality & Aging, 22*(3), 162–179.

*Turner, P. J. (2009). Impact of PATTS group intervention on forgiveness in children. *Dissertation Abstracts International, 70*(5), 3190B.

Wade, N. G., Worthington, E. L., Jr., & Meyer, J. E. (2005). But do they work? A meta-analysis of group interventions to promote forgiveness. In E. L. Worthington Jr. (Ed.), *Handbook of forgiveness* (pp. 423–439). New York, NY: Brunner-Routledge.

*Webb, J. R. (2003). Spiritual factors and adjustment in medical rehabilitation: Understanding forgiveness as a means of coping. *Journal of Applied Rehabilitation Counseling, 34*(3), 16–24.

*Webb, J. R., & Brewer, K. (2010). Forgiveness, health, and problematic drinking among college students in Southern Appalachia. *Journal of Health Psychology, 15*(8), 1257–1266.

*Witvliet, C. V. O. (2005). Unforgiveness, forgiveness, and justice: Scientific findings on feelings and physiology. In E. L. Worthington, Jr. (Ed.), *Handbook of forgiveness* (pp. 305–320). New York, NY: Brunner-Routledge.

Witvliet, C. V. O., Ludwig, T. E., & Vander Laan, K. L. (2001). Granting forgiveness or harboring grudges: Implications for emotions, physiology, and health. *Psychological Science, 12*, 117–123.

*Witvliet, C. V. O., Phipps, K. A., Feldman, M. E., & Beckham, J. C. (2004). Posttraumatic mental and physical health correlates of forgiveness and religious coping in military veterans. *Journal of Traumatic Stress, 17*(3), 269–273.

World Health Organization. (1948). *Definition of health. Preamble to the constitution of the World Health Organization as adopted by the International Health Conference*, New York, 19–22 June, 1946; signed on 22 July, 1946 by the representatives of 61 States (official records of the World Health Organization, no. 2, p. 100) and entered into force on 7 April 1948.

Worthington, E. L, Jr. (2003). *Forgiving and reconciling: Bridges to wholeness and hope.* Downers Grove, IL: Intervarsity Press.

Worthington, E. L., Jr. (2006). *Forgiveness and reconciliation: Theory and application*. New York, NY: Routledge.

Worthington, E. L., Jr. (2013). *Moving forward: Six steps to forgiving yourself and breaking free from the past.* Colorado Springs, CO: WaterBrook Multnomah.

Worthington, E. L., Jr., Berry, J. W., & Parrott, L., III. (2001). Unforgiveness, forgiveness, religion, and health. In T. G. Plante & A. C. Sherman (Eds.), *Faith and health: Psychological perspectives* (pp. 107–138). New York, NY: Guilford Press.

Worthington, E. L., Jr., Lavelock, C. R., Witvliet, C. V. O., Rye, M. S., Tsang, J., & Toussaint, L. (2014). Measures of forgiveness. In G. J. Boyle & D.H. Saklofske (Eds.), *Measures of personality and social psychological constructs* (pp. 474–502). New York, NY: Elsevier Academic Press.

Worthington, E. L., Jr., & Scherer, M. (2004). Forgiveness is an emotion-focused coping strategy that can reduce health risks and promote health resilience: Theory, review, and hypotheses. *Psychology & Health, 19*, 385–405.

Worthington, E. L., Jr., & Sotoohi, G. (2010). Physiological assessment of forgiveness, grudges, and revenge: Theories, research methods, and implications. *International Journal of Psychology Research, 5*(3/4), 291–316.

Worthington, E. L., Jr., Witvliet, C. V. O., Pietrini, P., & Miller, A. J. (2007). Forgiveness, health, and well-being: A review of evidence for emotional versus decisional forgiveness, dispositional forgivingness, and reduced unforgiveness. *Journal of Behavioral Medicine, 30*(4), 291–302.

Chapter 4
Measuring Forgiveness in Health-Related Contexts

Charlotte van Oyen Witvliet, Daryl R. Van Tongeren, and Lindsey Root Luna

Forgiveness has been identified as a relevant component of both physical and mental health (e.g., Webb, Toussaint, & Conway-Williams, 2012; Witvliet & McCullough, 2007). This chapter will highlight opportunities and challenges in measuring forgiveness reliably and validly within health care provision. We also offer suggestions for using forgiveness measures. In doing so, we draw from a chapter that addresses the psychometric properties of state and trait forgiveness measures (Worthington et al., 2015) and another that conceptualizes self-report and physiological assessments relevant to forgiveness and health (Witvliet & McCullough, 2007). Because medical populations face a range of challenges and health settings pose additional constraints, measures must be relevant, easy to understand, accurate, and efficient.

Conceptual Relevance of Forgiveness to Health

Our perspective on forgiveness in relation to health draws on an integrative bio-psycho-social-spiritual perspective, and we aim to promote human flourishing (see Keyes & Haidt, 2003). Our approach situates individuals within relationships with the sacred and others, while attentive to the biological underpinnings and psychological processes involved in such contextually-rich relationships. We also recognize that patients, loved ones, and health care providers will have a range of worldviews and belief systems that influence their ideas and practices related to justice and forgiveness (e.g., for a review on religion and forgiveness, see Van Tongeren et al., 2012). Despite individual differences, at its core, a transgression or

C.v.O. Witvliet (✉) • D.R. Van Tongeren • L. Root Luna
Department of Psychology, Hope College, Holland, MI, USA
e-mail: witvliet@hope.edu

L.L. Toussaint et al. (eds.), *Forgiveness and Health*,
DOI 10.1007/978-94-017-9993-5_4

offense is a moral and relational injustice that violates people's physical, psychological, relational, or spiritual boundaries. These transgressions can create a sense of unforgiveness—characterized by negative emotions (e.g., anger, resentment) toward the offender—relevant to the perceived severity of the violation and the degree of injustice suffered (see Worthington, 2005).

Forgiving involves both truth-telling and transformation. Granting forgiveness is the process whereby an individual honestly considers the wrongdoer and the wrongdoing, and then replaces destructive, negative responses toward an offender, with positive, other-oriented cognitive, behavioral, and emotional responses (e.g., empathy; McCullough, 2001; McCullough, Worthington, & Rachal, 1997; Strelan & Covic, 2006; Worthington, 2005). These changes are considered to be spiritual and embodied (Witvliet & McCullough, 2007), and they unfold over time (McCullough, Root Luna, Berry, Tabak, & Bono, 2010). Notably, although many stressors are not related to transgressions, transgressions and associated rumination prompt stress responses that are relevant to many medical conditions.

A Stress-and-Coping Model of Forgiveness

Viewed through a stress-and-coping framework (Worthington & Scherer, 2004), injustices and unforgiveness activate stress responses. Ruminating about hurtful interpersonal transgressions or harboring grudges prompts cardiovascular and sympathetic nervous system stress responses (Witvliet, Ludwig, & Vander Laan, 2001). Furthermore, offense rumination impairs parasympathetic nervous system responding, as indicated by decreased heart rate variability (Witvliet, Knoll, Hinman, & DeYoung, 2010). Forgiveness is one possible moral and relational response that can also reduce stress and promote relational repair with God, others, and oneself. This, in turn, can decrease health-eroding and increase health-promoting processes. However, there are other ways to reduce the stress associated with an injustice. For example, individuals can overlook, excuse, or trivialize the offense—responses that are distinct from forgiveness.

Evidence suggests that although forgiveness is but one of many options, it is one that can have considerable beneficial effects on one's health. Worthington and Scherer (2004) suggest that forgiveness may directly improve health by reducing hostility and cardiovascular strain, buffering the immune system (e.g., on cellular level, on a neuro-endocrine level, and through the release of antibodies), and improving central nervous system functioning (e.g., via the amygdala, hypothalamus, and the vagal nerve). Furthermore, while forgiveness does not always occur along with reconciliation, forgiveness may indirectly promote health by improving social support, reducing stress in marriages, and promoting relational skills and bonds.

Forgiving (or Receiving Forgiveness from) Whom? Self, Others, and the Sacred

In the health care context, forgiveness-relevant questions for patients, families, and medical professionals likely will address (a) whether the medical concerns have resulted from accidental or intentional injury from oneself, (b) if medical concerns were due to betrayals or failures of others (e.g., accidental or intentional acts, from a stranger, loved one, or professional), and (c) whether the person experiences anger and resentment toward God for allowing the injury or illness to occur. Thus, we see that one fruitful approach includes considering forgiveness in healthcare settings across three levels of analysis: self, others, and the Sacred.

Some reports suggest that, when relevant, assessing forgiveness within a health care setting may facilitate patient motivation to participate in treatments. This assessment, and the resulting intervention, may aid recovery following an injury caused by the self or by another. For example, a published case study explored the impact of unforgiveness toward the self, following an injury, and how this unforgiveness appeared to affect her motivation to engage in physical therapy (Bauman, 2008). Others have encouraged well-trained clinicians to implement forgiveness-related interventions (or enfold forgiveness into clinical interactions) as ways to improve the health of individuals with chronic illnesses or diseases (Elliott, 2011).

Alternatively, some medical situations are complicated by the actions or inactions of health care professionals. Allan and McKillop (2010) suggested that the increased likelihood of forgiveness serves as a strong rationale for a medical standard that requires adverse medical events to be disclosed. Clearly, intrapersonal and interpersonal unforgiveness has the potential to impact health outcomes. Furthermore, these situations may lead individuals to attribute blame to God for allowing (or causing) these events to occur, or could cause one to question one's relationship to the Sacred in the wake of existentially-unsettling medical events.

The relationship between the self and the Divine, God, or the Sacred provides an additional framework for considering the impact of forgiveness on health. Fitchett, Rybarczyk, DeMarco, and Nicolas (1999) found that incorporating spiritual and religious variables when engaged in rehabilitation may be welcomed by patients, as the patients were more likely to endorse that psychological treatment was very helpful if it addressed spiritual issues. How these issues are addressed matters: Ken Pargament has found that religious coping can include both positive and negative responses, with negative religious coping (measured by three items assessing feelings that God abandoned them, questioning God's love, and the viewing the Devil as a causal agent in one's negative life events) associated with greater risk for mortality (Pargament, Koenig, Tarakeshwar, & Hahn, 2001). Similarly, Exline, Yali, and Lobel (1999) found that people who felt alienated from God, were angry at God, and viewed God as responsible for a negative situation, reported greater anxiety and depression. Fitchett et al. (1999) found that anger at God (assessed by the Brief R-COPE item, "I express anger at God for letting this happen") predicted poorer

Table 4.1 Assessing forgiveness in healthcare

Possible situations where forgiveness may be relevant	Assessment suggestions and case examples
Granting Forgiveness for Actions or the Failure to Act	*(1) Do you blame anyone for wrongs or hurts in your life?(Y/N)*
	(2) Do you want to address this as part of your health care?(Y/N)
Interpersonal	*If addressing blame toward others, use the TRIM −18 state measure of benevolence, avoidance, and revenge* (McCullough et al., 2006)
Close Relationships	A patient contracts HIV from a partner
Strangers	A car accident caused by a stranger leaves a patient with a spinal cord injury
Medical professionals	Medical malpractice results in a medical condition
Intrapersonal	*If addressing self-blame, use State Self-Forgiveness Scale* (Wohl et al., 2008)*; add questions about responsibility-taking and reparative behaviors* (*based on* Exline et al., 2011; Fisher & Exline, 2006)
Self	A patient's nicotine addiction and smoking behavior leads to a stroke and extensive rehabilitation
Sacred	*If addressing blame toward God, use Attitudes Toward God Scale* (Wood et al., 2010)
Resolving Anger at God	A patient with cancer is alienated from and angry at God for allowing this to happen
Receiving Forgiveness for Actions or the Failure to Act	*(1) Do you feel blamed by anyone for wrongs or hurts in life?(Y/N)*
	(2) Do you want to address this as part of your health care?(Y/N)
Interpersonal	*Note: Scales are needed*
Close Relationships	A patient facing death seeks or receives forgiveness from a child or spouse for past wrongs
Intrapersonal	*Note: Scales are needed*
Resolving Self-Condemnation	A person who has gone through all AA steps continues to be burdened by guilt and shame even though others have granted forgiveness
Sacred	*Note: Scales are needed*
Receiving Forgiveness from God	Confession one's previous moral shortcomings, embracing grace and forgiveness, and living out of a renewed identity (e.g., religious conversion)

recovery of their activities of daily living 4 months later. Given the extant evidence, we agree with Webb (2003), that addressing forgiveness and other spiritual factors is important in holistic treatment.

When deciding what forgiveness aspects to assess and address, it is important to consider each of the three features or levels of analysis of forgiveness discussed above (see Table 4.1 for a summary). One can assess granting and receiving forgiveness interpersonally, receiving forgiveness from God and resolving anger at God, and self-forgiveness or resolving self-condemnation (while avoiding self-justifications that overlook one's responsibility toward those harmed). When considering measures, healthcare professionals will also need to attend to whether it is most relevant to measure dispositional traits or states related to forgiveness. Even people who normally score high on trait forgivingness can be in an unforgiving state. Whether this state response of forgiveness becomes a dispositional trait pattern is important. The sequelae of unforgiving or forgiving responses, particularly when a pattern or trait, can involve physical health (for a review, see Worthington, Witvliet, Pietrini, & Miller, 2007), and mental health (for a review, see Toussaint & Webb, 2005).

It is also important to consider views about justice and forgiveness. Both are important and can co-occur in responses to an offense (Worthington, 2009), although justice and forgiveness involve different moral responses from victims. Responses to unjust relational breaches often call for offenders to own responsibility and repair relational harm through confession, apology, restitution, and repentance; this is important to assess for offenses generally, and perhaps especially in self-forgiveness (Exline, Root, Yadavalli, Martin, & Fisher, 2011). When handled well interpersonally, reparative responses may naturally evoke interpersonal forgiveness. Yet, these perpetrator responses are not always present, and when they are, they can be handled poorly, sometimes adding further injury. Whereas some people will consider interpersonal forgiveness conditional on the justice-oriented actions of perpetrators, others will be unconditionally forgiving (as measured by Toussaint, Owen, & Cheadle, 2012). Even with altruistic forgiveness, victims can set boundaries to prevent additional harm, and sometimes receiving a gift of mercy will evoke repentance in perpetrators. Furthermore, forgiveness may be a decision or an emotionally heartfelt response that unfolds over time partially or fully (see Worthington, 2005).

Healthcare Settings

Settings for health care provision vary widely. Examples include primary care medical offices, ambulatory care walk-in clinics, public and private hospitals (including nonprofit and for profit facilities), rehabilitation hospitals for physical injuries and diseases, rehabilitation programs for substance disorders in which patients may be receiving additional medical intervention for organ damage (e.g., heart, kidneys, liver), home health care, and palliative care such as hospice. Within these types of settings, the specialties of health care providers and services will vary in ways that influence how they assess, study, or address forgiveness. As a result, each of these settings presents opportunities and limitations regarding the accessibility of forgiveness assessment and intervention due to time, expertise, or relevance to overall patient care.

For example, parish nursing programs in churches may offer blood pressure clinics. In such a setting, a nurse and elder or pastor might be able to address issues related to forgiveness holistically. A brief measure of forgiveness and unforgiveness could be a springboard for self-understanding and pastoral care.

As another example, a patient in a Veterans Affairs Medical Center might receive a range of services from interdisciplinary providers (e.g., medical doctors, nurses, social workers, psychologists, and chaplains) who are aware of issues related to military training, combat, person on person violence, and the emerging area of moral injury in which aspects of confession, atonement, and forgiveness are highly relevant. Depending on the distance that patients travel for care or the regularity of appointments, some veterans could have brief assessments and conversations about forgiveness, whereas others may have ongoing therapy (individually or in groups) or pastoral care that allows for follow-up assessments that guide intervention and care.

Medical Diagnosis Characteristics

Medical patients or clients rarely present with a primary concern of unforgiveness or forgiveness. However, medical intake forms or interviews can, and perhaps should, give patients or loved ones opportunities to indicate psychosocial concerns or the desire to address relational or spiritual care. For example, medical screenings could include the following: *Sometimes people experience blame—whether blaming others or being blamed—for hurts in life. Right now, do you blame someone (or God) for hurtful or offensive actions or inaction? If so, do you want to address these concerns in your healthcare as part of caring for you as a whole person?*

Providers can be attentive to the presence of interpersonal conflict or guilt, suggesting the relevance of a forgiveness assessment. Given that 12-step rehabilitation programs incorporate steps of responsibility-taking, confession, and making amends relevant to forgiveness, such treatment programs ought to assess unforgiveness and forgiveness (see Chap. 10 of this volume for a complete discussion). A medical focus on the individual client or patient in these and other settings emphasizes the importance of validity and reliability dimensions of assessment tools. For example, examining the reliability of self-report instruments highlights the value of small standard errors of measurement. Additionally, cost and practical time constraints typically rule out the use of purchased forgiveness assessments, long measures, or those that need to be sent away for scoring. Finally, assessors ought to be aware of the possibility that people may be reluctant to indicate forgiveness if they fear it may alienate health care providers, decrease quality of care, or jeopardize legal pursuit of justice. Researchers and practitioners ought to consider the role of social desirability bias.

Other medical features are relevant to assessment. Some medical conditions or treatments may involve strong pain or clouded cognition, suggesting the importance of straightforward, single item forgiveness measures (e.g., a 0–10 scale could be used to ask how resolved the forgiveness issue is for domains of self, others, and the Sacred). Within the ongoing treatment of individuals, assessments that begin as single-item measures could transition to brief or longer multi-item measures if forgiveness themes are strongly relevant and pain is managed, thinking is clarified, and trust is built.

Medical treatments and healing processes can move through a variety of phases. Some of these involve remission or recovery, along with ongoing anxiety about whether the cancer will return or a cardiac event will recur. Research points to the relevance of learning how to forgive as vital for bio-psycho-social-spiritual flourishing, including reduced cardiovascular risks (e.g., Waltman et al., 2009). Specifically, veterans with documented reversible myocardial ischemia who demonstrated stress-related myocardial perfusion deficits were randomly assigned to a 10-week forgiveness or control program. Participants in the forgiveness therapy showed significant reductions in deficits, as well as increased forgiveness scores (Waltman et al., 2009). This research highlights the value of integrating forgiveness into one's holistic plan of treatment within a healthcare setting. Toward that end, we now review measurement approaches and considerations for health-related contexts.

Measures of Forgiveness

Overview of Measures

We turn toward reviewing what qualities may make measures particularly useful in health care settings. However, for more comprehensive documentation of forgiveness measures for use in a variety of settings (not limited to health-related contexts), we refer researchers to Worthington et al. (2015). They review a range of self-report, behavioral, and physiological forgiveness measures (that are also provided within the chapter). Collectively, the self-report forgiveness measures (five state and two trait interpersonal forgiveness, one state and one trait self-forgiveness) are generally strong—with considerable evidence supporting estimated reliabilities and construct validities. As we highlight in the next section, however, many researchers in health contexts have historically designed individual self-reported forgiveness questions to measure particular questions of forgiveness. While behavioral measures are useful dependent variables in experimental research laboratory studies, they are currently not valid or reliable for practical use with individuals.

Research hospital settings may assess chemical measures (e.g., cortisol and alpha amylase, or oxytocin, which are relevant to unforgiveness or forgiveness, respectively) and measures of the central nervous system and peripheral physiology (i.e., blood pressure, heart rate, heart rate variability, skin conductance, and electrical activity of facial muscles), if pertinent to the individual's health condition. Witvliet and McCullough (2007) identified stronger and weaker approaches to physiological measurement and forgiveness. Specifically, studies that measure cardiovascular and other peripheral physiology responses before, during, and after conditions in repeated measures designs have reliably distinguished unforgiving and forgiving interpersonal state responses (e.g., Witvliet et al., 2001, 2010).

Empirical Evidence Linking Forgiveness-Relevant Measures and Health

Researchers have focused on different aspects of forgiveness with a range of health issues. For example, Lee (2011) assessed older adults (65–97) without severe mental or physical health conditions and found that forgiveness of self, others, and God was correlated negatively with anxiety and depression and positively with well-being, self-control, vitality, and general health (all measured through the General Well-Being Schedule; Dupuy, 1984). They measured forgiveness using three single-items that were then collapsed together from the Brief Multidimensional Measures of Religiousness/Spirituality (Fetzer Institute & National Institute on Aging Working Group, 2003). However, when using this more global, brief measure (Cronbach's alpha = 0.78), forgiveness did not contribute uniquely to the variance in health outcomes when ethnicity, age, gender, education, loss of a spouse and driving ability, social support, financial support, and spiritual experience were considered using the model they specified (Lee, 2011).

We contend that there are three levels of analysis that are useful to consider when examining forgiveness in health-related contexts: self, others, and the sacred. Accordingly, we review empirical evidence on how forgiveness may be assessed within these domains, and we present forgiveness links to health-related outcomes.

Forgiveness of Self

Many studies that examine forgiveness of self also measure forgiveness of others. Here, we highlight health-related research with an accent on self-forgiveness variables. Self-forgiving trait attitudes – as measured by the 15 item Forgiveness of Self scale (Mauger et al., 1992); internal consistency of $\alpha = .77$ for the described study – predicted lower mood disturbance and higher quality of life (Romero et al., 2006). This particular trait measure focused more on difficulty forgiving, from which researchers inferred forgiving attitudes. Thus, this research suggests that lower unforgiveness of oneself was associated with higher quality of life.

Martin, Vosvick, and Riggs (2012) used the trait Forgiveness of Self and Forgiveness of Other subscales of the Heartland Forgiveness Scale (six items on each subscale; Thompson et al., 2005). On a bivariate level, forgiveness of *self* was related to better reported physical functioning, lower perceptions of pain, better HIV-related health perceptions, and better social functioning. Forgiveness of *others* was related to better social functioning. When examining the interaction between attachment anxiety and each of the forgiveness subscales, both forgiveness of self and forgiveness of others interacted with attachment style. For those with greater attachment anxiety, more forgiveness of self was related to better health perceptions. Similarly, participants with high attachment anxiety reported less pain when they had forgiven others than those with low anxiety. Also drawing on the distinction between forgiveness of self and others, a study of spinal-cord injury survivors indicated that trait forgiveness of self (two items; trait level) and trait forgiveness of others (five items; trait level) operate differently; each measured by adapting items specific for their population, Webb and colleagues (Webb, Toussaint, Kalpakjian, & Tate, 2010) found that whereas forgiveness of self was positively related to health behavior (i.e., acting in a health-conscious way), forgiveness of others was related to self-reported general health status (i.e., how good one reports feeling, overall). Thus, forgiveness of self and forgiveness of others are distinct processes, each with unique effects on health.

However, forgiveness of self is not unequivocally and positively related to one's health behaviors. Wohl and Thompson (2011) examined state self-forgiveness for smoking behaviors (on a 7-item scale, $\alpha = .82$) and found that forgiving oneself for smoking decreases motivation to change the unhealthy behavior. The authors suggest that self-forgiveness for *past* behaviors may have positive health outcomes, but forgiving oneself for *current* unhealthy behaviors likely undermines one's motivation to self-regulate and stop the behavior.

Forgiveness of Others

Individuals can vary in their typical tendencies to forgive (i.e., *trait-related variables*) and the degree to which they forgive a particular offender for a specific offense (i.e., *state-related variables*). We review research on forgiving traits and states as they relate to health-related contexts, below.

Trait-Related Variables In a study of older adults, Toussaint et al. (2012) found that endorsing two items measuring the trait of forgiving others conditionally ("Before I can forgive others, they must apologize to me for the things they have done" and "Before I can forgive others, they must promise not to do the same thing again"), rather than unconditionally, was associated with higher mortality rates. This may have been the case because perpetrators rarely meet the hopes of victims for adequate confessions, apologies, and amends, and thus victims may have held onto unforgiveness, with a health-hampering set of stress responses. Thus, a forgiving disposition appears to positively affect one's health.

High levels of forgiveness of others (as measured and inferred by the 15 item Forgiveness of Others Scale; FOS; Mauger et al., 1992; internal consistency of $\alpha. = .66$ in the described study) was found to predict lower levels of anxiety, depression, and perceived stress, as well as lower ratios of total cholesterol to HDL and LDL to HDL after controlling for age and gender (Friedberg, Suchday, & Srinivas, 2009). The psychological measures (anxiety, depression, perceived stress) did not mediate the relationships between forgiveness and cholesterol.

State-Related Variables Although individuals can vary in the degree to which they regularly and dispositionally offer forgiveness, variations in degree of forgiveness for specific offenses (i.e., state forgiveness) are extremely important to consider. That is, even individuals who are typically forgiving by disposition might not forgive a particularly painful offense (e.g., an egregious betrayal or spiritual desecration). However, we may be measuring people when they are in an early part of the forgiveness process. Thus, we emphasize the importance of assessing state levels of forgiveness at multiple time points in individual health care contexts.

In a study of adults suffering from chronic (lower-back) pain, Carson et al. (2005) measured state forgiveness with the 60-item Enright Forgiveness Inventory (EFI; Subkoviak, Enright, Wu, & Gassin, 1995), and forgiveness self-efficacy regarding one's ability to engage in forgiveness-related tasks, using the 14-item Forgiveness Self Efficacy Scale (FSES; Thoresen et al., 2001). State forgiveness and forgiveness self-efficacy were related to lower sensory pain, less anger, and less psychological distress (Carson et al., 2005). That is, individuals who were more forgiving of a recent offender and who felt more confident in their ability to forgive, reported experiencing less sensory pain, anger, and distress. Moreover, additional analyses revealed that anger mediated the relationship between forgiveness and sensory pain, as well as the relationship between forgiveness and psychological distress, suggesting that forgiveness helps reduce anger, which can, in turn, lead to lower pain and less distress. Finally, it is worth noting that both the EFI ($\alpha = .98$ in the chronic pain sample) and the FSES ($\alpha = .93$ in the chronic pain sample) demonstrated acceptable estimated internal consistency in the chronic pain sample, suggesting that longer, established self-reported measures may be appropriate with some patients in certain settings.

Within a palliative care population, forgiveness has also been measured using the EFI. The Enright process model was used in four individual sessions (Hansen, Enright, Baskin, & Klatt, 2009). Participants were randomly assigned to the intervention or a wait-list control. Participants in the experimental condition experienced increases in forgiveness, hope, and quality of life, as well as decreases in anger, as compared to the waitlist control. However, once people in the wait-list control condition worked through the intervention, there were no significant differences between conditions on these variables.

Trait and State Variables Some research has examined both trait and state forgiveness-related variables in parallel. Lawler et al. (2003) examined the relationship between both state and trait forgiveness with physiological reactivity and recovery. State responses were measured by the TRIM-12 (12 items; McCullough et al., 1998) and the Acts of Forgiveness scale (AFS, 45 items; Drinnon & Jones, 1999). Both state measures were correlated with lower blood pressure, heart rate, and rate pressure product. During a discussion of a transgressor, diastolic blood pressure, mean arterial pressure and rate pressure product were also correlated with state forgiveness. Trait forgiveness was assessed with the Forgiving Personality Inventory (FPI, 33 items; Drinnon, Jones, & Lawler, 2000) and was associated with greater reductions in diastolic blood pressure and mean arterial pressure. Lawler et al. (2003) posited that forgiveness may reduce allostatic load as well as perceptions of stress, indirectly influencing health.

More recently, Lawler-Row, Hyatt-Edwards, Wuensch, and Karremans (2011) found that in healthy young adults forgiveness (using the AFS and FPI [described above] in an SEM path model) had a strong direct effect on health-related problems, conceptualized as loneliness, perceived stress, and physical symptoms. Physiologically, only trait forgiveness was linked with systolic blood pressure, but trait and state forgiveness were associated with heart rate; those participants who reported higher state forgiveness experienced greater increases in heart rate as they recalled a hurt, but they also had quicker recovery.

Assessing Views of God Another important consideration in health-related settings is assessing one's view of the Divine. In a longitudinal study of disease progression among patients with HIV, Ironson et al. (2011) assessed a positive view of God and negative view of God; each scale included six items that asked about general and personal beliefs. Overall, positive views of God (i.e., as forgiving and benevolent; total subscale score, including both general and personal items) predicted improved health and slower disease progression, whereas negative views of God (i.e., as punishing and judgmental; total subscale score, including both general and personal items) predicted accelerated disease progression (Ironson et al., 2011). Importantly, one's perceptions of God, including whether or not God is forgiving, has significant associations with how rapidly or slowly HIV-related disease may progress over time.

Conversely, other research has linked responses to a single-item measure of unconditional forgiveness from God with mortality. Toussaint et al. (2012) found that the belief that God forgives unconditionally (i.e., "God forgives me right away for things I have done; there is nothing I must do first") was associated with higher mortality rates in a study of 1200 adults over age 66. The authors posited that if people believe God will forgive them anyway, they may engage in behaviors that might otherwise prohibited by their religion, and which are also health-endangering.

Such research (not the only research to do so) demonstrates that forgiveness is not a panacea, nor is it unilaterally beneficial. Operational definitions of forgiveness matter greatly. We encourage researchers to be clear when reporting their forgiveness items and measures, and assessors should carefully select items with adequate specificity and sufficient precision to accurately measure their particular (forgiveness) construct of interest. Finally, although a complete review is beyond the scope of this chapter, we encourage readers to examine the extensive work on forgiveness and health-related outcomes among aging populations by Krause and colleagues (e.g., Krause & Ellison, 2003).

Limitations of Current Measures and Future Research Directions

Despite the quality of the research in this area, the current state of assessment has limitations. For example, one limitation is that, whereas some measures focus positively on the distinctive characteristics of forgiveness, others infer forgiveness from low endorsement of unforgiving responses. However, reducing difficulty forgiving or reducing unforgiveness is not necessarily the same thing as increasing forgiveness. For example, the Mauger et al. (1992) scales seem to measure difficulty forgiving self and others. The earlier TRIM measured Avoidance and Revenge (McCullough et al., 1998), and later added a Benevolence subscale to measure more positive aspects of state forgiveness (McCullough et al., 2006), which we recommend for state-level assessments of interpersonal unforgiveness and forgiveness.

In addition, many health findings are linked to single-item or few-item forgiveness measures that researchers designed or used from other sources, which is a potential limitation that might hinder future research. To date, publications with brief measures have had adequate psychometrics, but it will be important to more systematically develop very brief measures that can address the many states and traits associated with forgiveness processes across contexts and with various populations. One brief trait forgiveness measure that incorporates a balanced suite of emotional changes in forgiveness is the 10 item Trait Forgivingness Scale (TFS; Berry, Worthington, O'Connor, Parrott, & Wade, 2005). The TFS has strong psychometric properties commending it for trait interpersonal forgiveness and health research.

Toward that end, in healthcare settings, measures used need to appropriately address people's responses to transgressions in a way that respects them as integrated physical, psychological, relational, and spiritual beings. There is a need for brief state measures that address all facets related to responding both as transgressors and as those transgressed against, dealing with aspects of responsible confession and relational repair, overcoming unforgiveness and granting forgiveness, and addressing human relationships with God, others, and within oneself. Professionals need measures that are brief, appropriately calibrated to patient reading levels, seem relevant for patients and providers, are responsive to religious and cultural dimensions, and receive timely and sensitive follow-up with appropriate referrals as needed.

Open-ended questions or a modification of the visual analogue pain scale (e.g., 1–10 scale) could be used to expediently assess pain related to interpersonal hurts alongside physical ones. A follow-up question could ask whether patients want to address forgiveness of self, other, or God in their care. If so, we propose using state assessments with the following brief, psychometrically sound scales. For example, we suggest using state (rather than trait) measures to assess state self-forgiveness (Wohl, DeShea, & Wahkinney, 2008), along with questions about the degree to which people own responsibility for their offense and the types of reparative actions they have made (per Exline et al., 2011; Fisher & Exline, 2006), state forgiveness and unforgiveness of another person (18-item TRIM; McCullough et al., 2006), and state responses to the Sacred (the 4-item Attitude Toward God Scale; Wood et al., 2010) (see Table 4.1). These measures can be administered pre-, post-, and at follow-up to determine the effectiveness of forgiveness interventions from a chaplain or clergyperson, psychologist or social worker as part of holistic patient care.

Potential risks may occur in measuring forgiveness. Some people who experience unforgiving hurt, angry, vengeful, or avoidant responses, will conclude on their own that forgiveness is a possible response, and some will want to forgive, but not know how. For them, we recommend state assessments of forgiveness relevant to self, others, and God that are brief, relevant, and as reliable and valid as possible. This measurement needs to be linked with appropriate psychosocial and/or spiritual care. It is vital to have genuine assurance of safety or justice that holds wrongdoers accountable for their actions along with the pursuit of forgiveness. Others may experience assessments of forgiveness as pressure to forgive, rather than an invitation to consider the journey of forgiveness as one relevant to spiritual, interpersonal, psychological, and embodied flourishing. Patients will benefit from integrating their theology, values, and faith-related practices (if they are persons of faith) with what we have also learned through scientific studies.

Conclusions

Inevitably, measures are related to underlying presuppositions and worldviews, so assessments in health care provision must be sensitive to patient perspectives. It may be wise to invite patients and families to reflect on the measures used, and consider whether they fit well or poorly with their belief systems. Moreover, some methods and measures are more likely to be suitable in health care. Veterans Affairs Medical Centers and university research hospitals may have post-doctoral and faculty researchers who are able to incorporate physiological measures such as heart rate variability, blood pressure, cholesterol, cortisol, oxytocin, or other stress or emotion-relevant measures, particularly when treating people with stress-related disorders.

Although forgiveness is a topic of relevance to patients, families and loved ones, as well as medical providers, it does not always need to be assessed or addressed in the health care setting. Forgiveness is a vital moral response to the injustices and relational breaches caused by transgressions, and while it has restoring and healing dimensions, it cannot be viewed as a cure-all or reduced to serving a self-soothing function. Rather, forgiveness is a robust response to a relational violation that has implications for one's health. As research in this area accelerates, we suspect that appropriate measures will play central role in catalyzing such work.

References

Allan, A., & McKillop, D. (2010). The health implications of apologizing after an adverse event. *International Journal for Quality in Health Care, 2*(2), 126–131.

Bauman, J. (2008). The role of forgiveness in rehabilitation. *Journal of Health Care Chaplaincy, 14*(2), 75–82. doi: 10.1080/08854720802129018.

Berry, J. W., Worthington, E. L., Jr., O'Connor, L., Parrott, L., III, & Wade, N. G. (2005). Forgiveness, vengeful rumination, and affective traits. *Journal of Personality, 73*, 1–43.

Carson, J. W., Keefe, F. J., Goli, V., Fras, A. M., Lynch, T. R., Thorp, S. R., et al. (2005). Forgiveness and chronic low back pain: A preliminary study examining the relationship of forgiveness to pain, anger, and psychological distress. *The Journal of Pain, 6*, 84–91.

Drinnon, J. R., & Jones, W. H. (1999). *Measuring an act of forgiveness*. Paper presented at Southeastern Psychological Association, Mobile, AL.

Drinnon, J. R., Jones, W. H., & Lawler, K. A. (2000). *Measurement of forgiveness*. Paper presented at Society of Personality and Social Psychology, Nashville, TN.

Dupuy, H. (1984). The psychological well-being schedule. In N. Wenger, M. Mattson, C. Furberg, & J. Elinson (Eds.), *Assessment of quality of life in clinical trials of cardiovascular therapies* (pp. 353–356). New York, NY: Le Jacq Publishing.

Elliott, B. (2011). Forgiveness therapy: A clinical intervention for chronic disease. *Journal of Religion and Health, 50*, 240–247.

Exline, J. J., Root, B. L., Yadavalli, S., Martin, A. M., & Fisher, M. L. (2011). Reparative behaviors and self-forgiveness: Effects of a laboratory-based exercise. *Self and Identity, 10*, 101–126.

Exline, J. J., Yali, A. M., & Lobel, M. (1999). When God disappoints: Difficulty forgiving God and its role in negative emotion. *Journal of Health Psychology, 4*, 365–379.

Fetzer Institute & National Institute on Aging Working Group. (2003). *Multidimensional measurement of religiousness/spirituality for use in health research: A report of the Fetzer Institute National Institute on Aging Working Group*. Kalamazoo, MI: Fetzer Institute.

Fisher, M. L., & Exline, J. J. (2006). Self-Forgiveness versus excusing: The roles of remorse, effort, and acceptance of responsibility. *Self and Identity, 5*, 127–146.

Fitchett, G., Rybarczyk, B. D., DeMarco, G. A., & Nicolas, J. J. (1999). The role of religion in medical rehabilitation outcomes: A longitudinal study. *Rehabilitation Psychology, 44*(4), 333–353.

Friedberg, J. P., Suchday, S., & Srinivas, V. S. (2009). Relationship between forgiveness and psychological and physiological indices in cardiac patients. *International Journal of Behavioral Medicine, 16*, 205–211. doi: 10.1007/s12529-008-9016-2.

Hansen, M. J., Enright, R. D., Baskin, T. W., & Klatt, J. (2009). A palliative care intervention in forgiveness therapy for elderly terminally ill cancer patients. *Journal of Palliative Care, 25*(1), 51–60.

Ironson, G., Stuetzle, R., Ironson, D., Balbin, E., Kremer, H., George, A., et al. (2011). View of God as benevolent and forgiving or punishing and judgmental predicts HIV disease progression. *Journal of Behavioral Medicine, 34*, 414–425.

Keyes, C. M., & Haidt, J. (2003). *Flourishing: Positive psychology and the life well-lived.* Washington, DC: American Psychological Association.

Krause, N., & Ellison, C. G. (2003). Forgiveness by God, forgiveness of others, and psychological well-being in late life. *Journal for the Scientific Study of Religion, 42*, 77–93.

Lawler, K. A., Younger, J. W., Piferi, R. L., Billington, E., Jobe, R., Edmondson, K., & Jones, W. (2003). A change of heart: Cardiovascular correlates of forgiveness in response to interpersonal conflict. *Journal of Behavioral Medicine, 26*(5), 373–393.

Lawler-Row, K. A., Hyatt-Edwards, L., Wuensch, K. L., & Karremans, J. C. (2011). Forgiveness and health: The role of attachment. *Personal Relationships, 18*, 170–183.

Lee, K. H. (2011). The role of spiritual experience, forgiveness, and religious support on the general well-being of older adults. *Journal of Religion, Spirituality, and Aging, 23*, 206–223.

Martin, L. A., Vosvick, M., & Riggs, S. A. (2012). Attachment, forgiveness, and physical health quality of life in HIV+ adults. *AIDS Care, 24*, 1333–1340.

Mauger, P. A., Perry, J. E., Freeman, T., Grove, D. C., McBride, A. G., & McKinney, K. E. (1992). The measurement of forgiveness: Preliminary research. *Journal of Psychology and Christianity, 11*, 170–180.

McCullough, M. E. (2001). Forgiveness: Who does it and how do they do it? *Current Directions in Psychological Science, 10*, 194–197.

McCullough, M. E., Root Luna, L. M., Berry, J. W., Tabak, B. A., & Bono, G. (2010). On the form and function of forgiving: Modeling the time-forgiveness relationship and testing the valuable relationships hypothesis. *Emotion, 10*, 358–376.

McCullough, M. E., Root, L. M., & Cohen, A. D. (2006). Writing about the benefits of an interpersonal transgression facilitates forgiveness. *Journal of Consulting and Clinical Psychology, 74*, 887–897.

McCullough, M. E., Worthington, E. L., Jr., & Rachal, K. C. (1997). Interpersonal forgiveness in close relationships. *Journal of Personality and Social Psychology, 75*, 321–326.

McCullough, M. E., Rachal, K. C., Sandage, S. J., Worthington, E. L., Jr., Brown, S. W., & Hight, T. L. (1998). Interpersonal forgiving in close relationships: II theoretical elaboration and measurement. *Journal of Personality and Social Psychology, 75*(6), 1586–1603. doi: http://dx.doi.org/10.1037/0022-3514.75.6.1586.

Pargament, K. I., Koenig, H. G., Tarakeshwar, N., & Hahn, J. (2001). Religious struggle as a predictor of mortality among medically ill elderly patients: A 2-year longitudinal study. *Archives of Internal Medicine, 161*(15), 1881–1885.

Romero, C., Kalidas, M., Elledge, R., Chang, J., Liscum, K. R., & Friedman, L. C. (2006). Self-forgiveness, spirituality and psychological adjustment in women with breast cancer. *Journal of Behavioral Medicine, 29*(1), 29–36. doi: 10.1007/s10865-005-9038-z.

Strelan, P., & Covic, T. (2006). A review of forgiveness process models and a coping framework to guide future research. *Journal of Social and Clinical Psychology, 25*, 1059–1085.

Subkoviak, M. J., Enright, R. D., Wu, C.-R., & Gassin, E. A. (1995). Measuring interpersonal forgiveness in late adolescence and middle adulthood. *Journal of Adolescence, 18*, 641–655.

Thompson, L. Y., Snyder, C. R., Hoffman, L., Michael, S. T., Rasmussen, H. N., Billings, L. S., . . . Roberts, D. E.(2005). Dispositional forgiveness of self, others, and situations. *Journal of Personality, 73*, 313–359. doi: 10.1111/j.1467-6494.2005.00311.x.

Thoresen, C. E., Luskin, F. M., Harris, A. H. S., Benisovich, S. V., Standard, S., Bruning, B., et al. (2001). Effects of forgiveness intervention on perceived stress, state and trait anger, and self-reported health. *Annals of Behavioral Medicine, 23*, S37.

Toussaint, L., Owen, A. D., & Cheadle, A. (2012). Forgive to live: Forgiveness, health, and longevity. *Journal of Behavioral Medicine, 35*, 375–386.

Toussaint, L., & Webb, J. R. (2005). Theoretical and empirical connections between forgiveness, mental health, and well-being. In E. L. Worthington Jr. (Ed.), *Handbook of forgiveness* (pp. 349–362). New York, NY: Routledge.

Van Tongeren, D. R., Worthington, E. L., Jr., Davis, D. E., Hook, J. N., Gartner, A. L., Jennings, D. J., II, . . . Greer, T. W.(2012). Forgiveness and religion: Update and current status. In M. R. Maarmi (Ed.), *Mapping forgiveness* (pp. 53–70). Oxford, England: Interdisciplinary Press.

Waltman, M. A., Russell, D. C., Coyle, C. T., Enright, R. D., Holter, A. C., & Swoboda, C. M. (2009). The effects of a forgiveness intervention on patients with coronary artery disease. *Psychology and Health, 24*(1), 11–27. doi: 10.1080/08870440801975127.

Webb, J. R. (2003). Spiritual factors and adjustment in rehabilitation: Understanding forgiveness as a means of coping. *Journal of Applied Rehabilitation Counseling, 34*(3), 16–24.

Webb, J. R., Toussaint, L., & Conway-Williams, E. (2012). Forgiveness and health: Psycho-spiritual integration and the promotion of better healthcare. *Journal of Health Care Chaplaincy, 18*, 57–73.

Webb, J. R., Toussaint, L., Kalpakjian, C. Z., & Tate, D. G. (2010). Forgiveness and health-related outcomes among people with spinal cord injury. *Disability and Rehabilitation, 32*, 360–366.

Witvliet, C. V. O., Knoll, R. W., Hinman, N. G., & DeYoung, P. A. (2010). Compassion-focused reappraisal, benefit-focused reappraisal, and rumination after an interpersonal offense: Emotion regulation implications for subjective emotion, linguistic responses, and physiology. *The Journal of Positive Psychology, 5*, 226–242.

Witvliet, C. V. O., Ludwig, T. E., & Vander Laan, K. L. (2001). Granting forgiveness or harboring grudges: Implications for emotions, physiology, and health. *Psychological Science, 12*, 117–123.

Witvliet, C. V. O., & McCullough, M. E. (2007). Forgiveness and health: A review and theoretical exploration of emotion pathways. In S. Post (Ed.), *Altruism and health: Perspectives from empirical research* (pp. 258–276). New York, NY: Oxford University Press.

Wohl, M. J. A., DeShea, L., & Wahkinney, R. L. (2008). Looking within: Measuring state self-forgiveness and its relationship to psychological well-being. *Canadian Journal of Behavioural Science, 40*, 1–10.

Wohl, M. J. A., & Thompson, A. (2011). A dark side to self-forgiveness: Forgiving the self and its association with chronic unhealthy behaviour. *British Journal of Social Psychology, 50*, 354–364.

Wood, B. T., Worthington, E. L., Jr., Exline, J. J., Yali, A. M., Aten, J. D., & McMinn, M. R. (2010). Development, refinement, and psychometric properties of the attitudes toward God scale (ATGS-9). *Psychology of Religion and Spirituality, 2*, 148–167.

Worthington, E. L., Jr. (Ed.). (2005). *Handbook of forgiveness*. New York, NY: Brunner-Routledge.

Worthington, E. L., Jr. (2009). *A just forgiveness: Responsible healing without excusing injustice*. Downers Grove, IL: InterVarsity Press.

Worthington, E. L., Jr., Lavelock, C., Witvliet, C. V. O., Rye, M. S., Tsang, J., & Toussaint, L. (2015). Measures of forgiveness. In G. J. Boyle & D. H. Saklofske (Eds.), *Measures of personality and social psychological constructs*. Chennai, India: Elsevier.

Worthington, E. L., Jr., & Scherer, M. (2004). Forgiveness is an emotion-focused coping strategy that can reduce health risks and promote health resilience: Theory, review, and hypotheses. *Psychology and Health, 19*, 385–405.

Worthington, E. L., Jr., Witvliet, C. V. O., Pietrini, P., & Miller, A. J. (2007). Forgiveness, health, and well-being: A review of evidence for emotional versus decisional forgiveness, dispositional forgivingness, and reduced unforgiveness. *Journal of Behavioral Medicine, 30*(4), 291–302. doi: 10.1007/s10865-007-9105-8.

Part II
Empirical Evidence of Forgiveness-Health Connections

Chapter 5
Forgiveness and Physiological Concomitants and Outcomes

Kevin T. Larkin, Carol Goulet, and Casey Cavanagh

The frequent and persistent experience of anger, depression, and anxiety has been linked to numerous negative health consequences, ranging from occurrence of cardiovascular disease (Rozanski, Blumenthal, & Kaplan, 1999) to the progression of cancer (Lutgendorf & Sood, 2011) as well as the onset of behavioral and substance use disorders. Although the exact mechanisms through which the experience of these emotional states cause cellular or organ dysfunction remains to be elucidated, considerable evidence has implicated various components of the physiological response to environmental stress, including the autonomic nervous system, the hypothalamic-pituitary-adrenal (HPA) system, and the inflammatory response mediated by the immune system (McEwen & Stellar, 1993). It is well known that the physiological actions that occur when humans detect threat in their environments (e.g., the proverbial encounter with a bear in the woods) are adaptive, but become maladaptive when they occur in situations where one's life is not in danger, when these types of situations occur too frequently, or when the responses to these situations persist long after the source of threat has disappeared. Presumably, in these incidents, the cascade of neural, hormonal, and immunological changes that occur to prepare the body to confront or escape the source of threat are not used for their intended purpose, leaving them to damage the body organs and tissues they were designed to protect.

Because unforgiveness involves the chronic experience of bitterness, resentment, anger, and fear (Worthington & Wade, 1999), it is plausible that choosing not to forgive an offender has negative health consequences. However, after reviewing the body of literature supporting an association between forgiveness and health, Thoresen, Harris, and Luskin (2000) could only conclude that "no controlled studies have demonstrated that forgiveness affects physical health outcomes either

K.T. Larkin (✉) • C. Goulet • C. Cavanagh
Department of Psychology, West Virginia University, Morgantown, WV, USA
e-mail: klarkin@mail.wvu.edu

L.L. Toussaint et al. (eds.), *Forgiveness and Health*,
DOI 10.1007/978-94-017-9993-5_5

positively or negatively" (p. 254). Fortunately, many investigators considered this conclusion as a challenge to examine whether the physiological stress response was moderated by forgiveness, and we are in better position to evaluate this empirical question today. The aim of this chapter is to provide a comprehensive overview of empirical work that has examined relations between forgiveness and the various physiological parameters comprising the human stress response. Accepting the risk of oversimplifying human physiology, we chose to present study findings according to the primary organ systems (i.e., central nervous system, peripheral nervous system, HPA system) being measured in each study. We do not mean to ignore the complexity of the feedback systems that connect organ systems and the underlying physiological processes, but we have chosen this approach for ease of presentation and to acknowledge that most research has yet to employ more sophisticated multi-system measurement methods. It should be noted that most of the studies that comprise this literature also involve measurement of non-physiological parameters, including both self-report measures of affect and symptoms as well as observable behaviors. Because the purpose of this chapter is to review the relation between forgiveness and physiological functioning, only results pertaining to parameters that contribute to this purpose are considered.

Forgiveness and Central Nervous System Functioning

Because resentment, rumination, and worry represent cognitive phenomena, it is likely that engaging in them chronically, as an unforgiving person does, influences cortical functioning. The most common method for this approach involves use of functional brain imaging devices including functional magnetic resonance imaging (fMRI) and positron emission tomography (PET). Research has identified several brain regions activated during social cognition and making moral judgments, including "the medial prefrontal cortex (MPFC), temporo-parietal junction, precuneus/posterior cingulate, amygdala, superior temporal sulcus, and temporal poles" (Mitchell, 2008, p. 142). Based upon these findings, these brain regions have been the logical areas of interest for explorations of cortical activity associated with forgiveness.

In the first neuroimaging study to examine forgiveness, Farrow et al. (2001) contrasted cortical responses associated with making judgments in scenarios involving forgiveness (e.g., "which crime was more forgivable?") with scenarios involving either social reasoning or experiencing empathy. Although some common brain regions were activated while making forgiveness and empathy judgments, differential activation in other cortical areas (e.g., left superior frontal area and posterior cingulate) provided evidence that making empathy and forgiveness judgments reflected distinctive cortical activity. Farrow et al. (2005) replicated these findings by showing comparable activations in the posterior cingulate in response to forgiveness judgments among patients being treated for PTSD. Using the same methodology, Lee et al. (2006) examined neural activity during forgiveness and empathic judgments among patients with schizophrenia and healthy controls. Controls exhibited increased activation in brain regions associated with social cognition in response to forgiveness judgments (e.g., MPFC) in comparison to patients with schizophrenia, a finding attributed to the reduced social awareness that occurs during acute phases of this disorder. Increased activation of brain regions associated with social cognition was observed for patients following treatment, reflecting their improved ability to make social judgments, including those that involve forgiveness.

Using a sample of healthy adults who imagined a hurtful event with either instructions to forgive the offender or not, Pietrini and colleagues (2004) reported cortical differences between forgiveness and unforgiveness using fMRI. In this regard, this study involved exposure to an actual hurtful event rather than fictional scenarios used in the studies described above. Findings revealed that forgiveness was associated with activation of brain regions involved in emotion regulation and moral judgment, including the MPFC, amygdala, anterior cingulate, and striatum.

In another fMRI study, Young and Saxe (2009) asked healthy adults to make moral judgments to scenarios of a protagonist who harmed another person. Results revealed that greater activation of the right temporo-parietal junction (RTPJ) was related to lower ratings of moral blame (i.e., greater forgiveness) during accidental harm conditions when compared to participants assigning high ratings of moral blame. No associations were observed between moral blame ratings and measures obtained from any other cortical region examined.

Using PET, Hayashi et al. (2010) examined willingness to forgive perpetrators using scenarios in which either serious or minor transgressions were committed by honest or dishonest persons. Ratings of willingness to forgive, an abstract judgment process, were lowest in situations in which serious transgressions were committed by dishonest persons. Results revealed increased activation during minor transgressions in the right medial frontal gyrus, right caudate nucleus, right cerebellum, and the left MPFC. Correlations between ratings of forgiveness and cortical activation in all brain regions, however, were not significant.

Cumulatively, studies examining cortical responses to forgiveness have implicated several brain regions, typically those associated with social awareness, attentional processing, and social cognition. Only one study (i.e., Pietrini et al., 2004) showed an association between forgiveness and amygdala response, which may not be that surprising since this study was the only one of its type to expose participants to recollections of actual hurtful events. Cortical responses to making forgiveness judgments about fictional perpetrators are likely different from responses associated with personally-relevant forgiveness scenes. It is noteworthy that no study examining cortical activation associated with forgiveness measured physiological responses occurring outside of the central nervous system; these responses are discussed in the next section.

Forgiveness and Peripheral Nervous System Functioning

There is over a century's worth of data showing that the experience of emotion influences organs other than the brain, presumably through the autonomic and somatic nervous systems. It is well established that upon exposure to stress, heart rate (HR) and blood pressure (BP) increases, pupils dilate, and sweating occurs on the palms and feet. Alterations in somatic nervous system activity occur as well in response to stress, as evidenced by increased muscle tension and rate of respiration. If forgiveness possesses beneficial physiological effects, one would expect it to be linked with attenuated responses of the autonomic and somatic nervous systems. We now have some empirical support that this may indeed be the case. Although far from conclusive, many investigations from multiple laboratories using a variety of experimental methods have provided support for an association between forgiveness and dampened peripheral nervous system responses to stress. Foremost among these efforts is the programmatic empirical work involving exposure to imaginal scenes of forgiveness and unforgiveness conducted by Witvliet and colleagues and the betrayal recall studies done by Lawler-Row and her laboratory.

Exposure to Imaginal Scenes of Forgiveness – Findings from Witvliet's Laboratory

Using a within-subjects methodology in which college student participants are instructed to imagine several brief scenarios during a single laboratory session, Witvliet has conducted several investigations exploring the physiology of forgiveness. Although she has examined numerous physiological parameters, the staples of her protocol involve assessing cardiovascular indices like HR and the electrical activity [via electromyogram (EMG)] of three different facial muscle groups: *corrugator* (brow), *orbicularis oculi* (under the eye), and *zygomatic* (cheek). Muscle activity in the forehead and around the eyes is associated with expression of anger (i.e., expected during unforgiveness), but muscle activity in the cheek is associated with smiling or acceptance (i.e., expected during forgiveness). Her pioneering effort (Witvliet, Ludwig, & Vander Laan, 2001) contrasted physiological responses to imagining an actual interpersonal offense using either unforgiving (holding a grudge and reliving the hurt) or forgiving scripts (granting forgiveness and empathizing with the offender). Results revealed that *corrugator* and *orbicularis oculi* EMG, HR, BP, and skin conductance levels were all higher during imagination of the unforgiving scripts than during imagination of the forgiving scripts.

Using scripts of an actual interpersonal offense in which the participant hurt another person, Wivliet, Ludwig, and Bauer (2002) showed that reliving the incident was associated with greater *corrugator* EMG than seeking forgiveness, but no differences were observed among the other EMG measures, HR, or skin conductance. Three additional scenes were generated based on the victim's response: the victim held a grudge, granted forgiveness, or engaged in reconciliation. In contrast to the grudge scene, reduced *corrugator* EMG was observed during the reconciliation and being forgiven outcome scripts. *Zygomatic* EMG was higher following the being forgiven script, supporting the hypothesis that forgiving was associated with increased positive emotion. Skin conductance, in contrast to expectations, showed slower habituation during recovery from the reconciliation outcome script than the grudge script, suggesting that reconciliation may involve emotional processing.

Acknowledging that forgiveness, apology, and restitution all attenuate physiological responses that occur while imagining an injustice, Witvliet et al. (2008) designed a study to compare the physiological effects of forgiveness with the effects of using other methods of obtaining justice. Using a burglary scenario, participants imagined either forgiving or not forgiving the offender with each of three different justice outcomes: (a) no justice (the offender was not caught), (b) retributive justice (the offender was caught and punished), and (c) restorative justice (the offender expressed remorse and replaced the stolen objects). Exposure to all forgiveness scripts, regardless of justice outcomes, resulted in lower HR and *corrugator* EMG than exposure to scripts without forgiveness. *Orbicularis oculi* EMG was also lower during forgiveness scripts, but only during the no justice condition. In the no forgiveness scenes, retributive justice resulted in reduced rate pressure product [RPP; HR X systolic blood pressure (SBP)], an indicator of autonomic arousal, and restorative justice resulted in reduced skin conductance. Although restorative and retributive justice resulted in beneficial physiological effects, they were not as prominent as reductions observed for forgiveness.

In an effort to examine two distinct modes of reappraisal for coping with interpersonal offenses, Witvliet, Knoll, Hinman, and DeYoung (2010) instructed participants to imagine an actual offense in which participants (a) ruminated over the incident, (b) engaged in compassion-focused reappraisal (forgiveness), and (c) engaged in benefit-focused reappraisal (gratitude). Like their prior work, the rumination script was associated with greater *corrugator* EMG than either reappraisal script conditions. The forgiveness script was associated with lower *orbicularis oculi* EMG and HR than rumination. Interestingly, the gratitude script was associated with increased *zygomatic* EMG and HR variability (greater parasympathetic activation), which reflected increased positive affect. In a similar study, participants imagined an actual offense and were instructed to (a) ruminate over the incident, (b) engage in compassion-focused reappraisal (forgiveness), and (c) engage in emotional suppression (Witvliet, DeYoung, Hofelich, & DeYoung, 2011). Replicating their prior work, the rumination script was associated with greater *orbicularis oculi* EMG than forgiveness reappraisal or emotion suppression. Emotion suppression was associated with lower *corrugator* EMG and HR than rumination and lower *zygomatic* EMG than both forgiveness and rumination. No differences in HR variability were observed.

Across these studies, Witvliet and colleagues have consistently demonstrated differences in physiological response to imagining instances of forgiveness and unforgiveness. Although imagining forgiveness was always associated with reduced physiological responses when compared with imaging scenes without forgiveness, other strategies (e.g., receiving an apology, seeking and obtaining restitution) also resulted in attenuated physiological responses, but not as prominent as the reductions observed for forgiveness. When measuring *corrugator* and *orbicularis oculi* EMG activity, findings were relatively uniform across studies. Some support existed for associations between forgiveness and reductions in HR, and measures of BP and skin conductance have produced the least consistent associations with imagining forgiveness.

Exposure to Betrayal Recall – Findings from the Lawler-Row Laboratory

Paralleling the decade of work by Witvliet, Lawler-Row and colleagues conducted five studies examining the physiological responses associated with forgiveness of actual betrayal events that participants experienced. Lawler-Row was also interested in examining individual difference characteristics of forgivingness (trait forgiveness) and whether participants forgave the betrayal event they reported (state forgiveness) or still held a grudge. In the first study from her laboratory, young adults' physiological responses to two interviews were assessed, one focusing on a betrayal by a parent and the other focusing on a betrayal by a friend or partner (Lawler et al., 2003). Trait forgivingness was negatively correlated with BP taken during the entire session and state measures of forgiveness were negatively correlated with all measures of BP as well as HR. Analysis of reactivity to the interviews revealed that higher forgiveness was associated with lower BP and *corrugator* EMG response and faster recovery from the parent interview, but not the friend/partner interview. Analysis of RPP revealed that participants low in both trait and state forgiveness exhibited the largest RPPs during the interview. Neither skin conductance nor HR reactivity was associated with trait or state forgiveness.

Using a similar methodology, Lawler et al. (2005) attempted to replicate their findings on a sample of community-dwelling adults. Although no significant differences were observed among high and low forgivingness groups on BP and HR, low trait forgivers exhibited higher RPP responses to the initial part of the interview than high trait forgivers. Because significant inverse associations were observed between both trait and state forgiveness and self-reported health symptoms, mediation by RPP reactivity was tested, but not found to be significant. In Edmondson's (2005) dissertation, which was conducted in the laboratory of Lawler, the experimental protocol was modified slightly to examine rumination following the betrayal interview. State forgiveness was associated with reductions in BP reactivity during the interview.

Acknowledging the inverse relation between forgiveness and the experience of anger, Lawler-Row, Karremans, Scott, Edlis-Matityahou, and Edwards (2008) tested whether the beneficial physiological effects of forgiveness observed in previous work were due to reductions in anger that occurs when one person forgives another. Replicating previous findings, high state and trait forgivers exhibited lower cardiovascular responses to a remembered offense than did low trait forgivers. Although some of these relations were partly mediated by anger, relations between forgiveness and cardiovascular responses remained significant controlling for anger, suggesting that the positive physiological effects associated with forgiveness were not simply due to a reduction in the experience of anger.

In their most recent empirical work, Lawler-Row, Hyatt-Edwards, Wuensch, and Karremans (2011) explored how attachment relates both to forgiveness and to physiological responses to reliving interpersonal stress. A significant interaction was observed; reduced HRs were observed among participants who exhibited both high state forgiveness and high attachment scores. In this regard, the beneficial effect of forgiveness during reliving of betrayal events was only detected among participants with secure attachments.

In sum, the five studies from Lawler-Row's laboratory confirmed that forgiveness was associated with reduced cardiovascular reactions during exposure to betrayal recollections. Although relations were observed between trait forgivingness and reduced physiology in some of this work, relations between state measures of forgiveness and attenuated physiological responses were more consistently observed. These studies also demonstrated the importance of exposing experimental participants to recollections of events that have personally impacted them, and confirmed that the physiological phenomena observed in Witvliet's laboratory could be replicated when participants confronted meaningful events from their lives.

Exposure to Betrayal Recall – Findings from Other Researchers

Although the Witvliet and Lawler-Row laboratories have demonstrated consistently that forgiveness dampens physiological responses of the peripheral nervous system, several other investigators have contributed to this literature. An early effort of this type was conducted by Huang and Enright (2000), who interviewed adults in Taiwan about an interpersonal conflict that was forgiven. Although no BP differences were observed during a control interview, results revealed that Level 4 forgivers (those who saw forgiveness as a duty) exhibited higher BPs during the first minute of the conflict interview than Level 6 forgivers (those who saw forgiveness as an act of love), but no differences in BP were observed during the remainder of the interview.

In Hall's (2006) dissertation, college students visualized a past hurtful situation using two different outcomes: getting revenge and forgiving the other person. Consistent with prior work, SBPs were elevated during the revenge imagery in comparison to the forgiveness imagery, although the extent to which these findings could be attributed to order of task presentation (revenge imagery was always presented first) is unclear. In another dissertation, Semenec (2009) showed no relation between measures of trait forgivingness and either HR or BP response during interviews in which they described either being hurt or hurting others.

In a study of transgressions in marital relationships, Hannon, Finkel, Kumashiro, and Rusbult (2012) asked couples to discuss a recent conflict in which one spouse was identified as the "victim" and the other as the "perpetrator." Among "victims," high trait forgivingness was associated with lower BPs; however, no association between forgivingness and BP was observed among "perpetrators." Higher victim conciliatory behavior (i.e., consistent with having forgiven the perpetrator) was related to lower BP of victims as well as perpetrators; no association was observed between perpetrator conciliatory behavior and BPs of either victim or perpetrator.

Using a between-subjects design, Larsen et al. (2012) contrasted recollections of a recent interpersonal betrayal using one of three instructional sets: (a) forgiving the offender; (b) ruminating about the incident; and (c) distraction. Participants assigned to both forgiveness and distraction conditions had lower BP responses than those in rumination condition, regardless of level of trait forgivingness. Although distraction yielded short-term benefits in terms of reduced cardiovascular responding, BP increased during recovery. Only forgiveness was associated with attenuated BPs during both imaginal exposure and recovery periods.

Exposure to Anger Recall and Other Cognitive Stressors

Given the central importance of anger among persons who have been exposed to betrayal, several investigators have used anger recall or exposure to laboratory tasks that evoke anger as experimental stimuli instead of personal betrayal recollections. In Olson's dissertation (2004), psychiatric patients discussed recent events that provoked anger. Although state forgiveness was associated with lower self-reported anger, no significant relations were observed between forgiveness and any physiological measure (HR, BP, and skin conductance).

Friedberg, Suchday, and Shelov (2007) examined hemodynamic responses (i.e., stroke volume, cardiac output, and total peripheral resistance) to an anger recall task and serial subtraction using impedance cardiography. Trait forgivingness was associated with faster DBP recovery from tasks, but no differences were observed between high versus low forgivingness and cardiovascular responses to the two tasks. Similarly, Tartaro, Luecken, and Gunn (2005) failed to find an association between forgiveness and measures of BP and HR reactivity to a Stroop interference task. In sum, investigations employing anger recall or mental stress tasks have not shown cardiovascular responses to stress to be associated with measures of forgiveness.

Exposure to Standardized Interpersonal Stressors

One issue that has not been addressed satisfactorily among researchers who expose study participants to recollections of actual betrayal events is the broad range of events selected by study participants. Certainly, forgiving someone for forgetting to pick you up from work on a rainy day reflects a less intense transgression than forgiving a spouse for cheating on you for years. Recalling events that were partially forgiven is likely different than recalling those that have not been forgiven, and recalling events that happened decades ago is likely different than recalling recent events. This same problem applies to anger recall tasks, where the intensity of the situations described by participants varies widely. In the interest of demonstrating experimental control, it behooves researchers to either standardize types of events or at the very least, rate them in terms of intensity. Some researchers have addressed this problem by using standard live "betrayals" during laboratory sessions, typically involving harassment during task completion.

Hernandez, Larkin, and Whited (2009) and Whited, Wheat, and Larkin (2010) have employed this type of experimental method for examining the physiological effects of forgiveness. Results of the former study showed that forgiving the confederate was associated with reduced SBP response to the standardized harassment. Results from the latter study revealed that high trait forgivingness participants exhibited faster DBP recovery from stress than low trait forgiveness participants, but no differences were observed for SBP, HR, or HR variability during recovery. Although few in number, findings from the two studies exposing participants to standard laboratory-induced transgressions complement findings from studies using methods where participants imagined or discussed personally-relevant betrayal events.

Forgiveness and Resting Physiological States

Studies described so far have examined relations between forgiveness and physiological parameters by exposing individuals to betrayal episodes, recollection of incidents that provoked anger, or standardized laboratory manipulations. However, a few studies have examined relations between forgiveness and physiological parameters during periods of rest. Many studies described in the previous sections measured resting physiological states even though their aims were to examine changes in response to recollections of betrayal. Some of these studies showed evidence that increased forgiveness was associated with dampened resting states (e.g., Friedberg et al., 2007; Lawler et al., 2003; Lawler-Row et al., 2011, 2008), but others have not (e.g., Edmondson, 2005; Huang & Enright, 2000; Lawler et al., 2005; Whited et al., 2010). Semenec (2009) reported mixed findings in this regard, with forgiveness of self being associated with lower resting DBP but forgiveness of others being associated with *higher* resting SBP. Of course, forgiveness of self and others are quite different experiences, with the former more focused on overcoming self-condemnation and guilt and the latter overcoming the hurt and betrayal.

Seybold, Hill, Neumann, and Chi (2001) measured resting measures of peripheral nervous system functioning and found no relations between forgiveness and resting HR, BP, or *corrugator* EMG. In contrast, Toussaint and Williams (2003) found a significant inverse association between trait forgivingness and resting DBP in a sample of diverse, community-dwelling adults. Buck, Williams, Musick, and Sternthal (2009) conducted a similar study that examined associations between forgiveness and resting BPs. By assessing multiple parameters associated with religious behaviors, they identified two variables associated with lower DBP: finding meaning in life and forgiveness of self. In contrast, in a study of clergymen undergoing treatment, Brenneis (2001) found an inverse relation between resting BP and forgiveness.

In contrast to studies examining physiological response to images or discussions of transgressions, anger recall interviews, or standardized interpersonal stressors, findings from studies examining relations between forgiveness and resting physiological states have been inconsistent. Some studies have shown that forgiveness was associated with dampened physiological resting states, some have shown no association between forgiveness and physiological tone, and others have shown forgiveness was associated with increased physiological arousal during periods of rest.

Forgiveness and Endocrine System Functioning

Parallel to the peripheral nervous system, numerous hormonal effects are observed when organisms are exposed to stress, including increased cortisol and various hormonal releasing factors circulating in the blood. In contrast, higher levels of oxytocin are detected when organisms engage in nurturing behaviors. Like peripheral nervous system activity, forgiveness has been hypothesized to be associated with lower cortisol levels and responses.

Forgiveness and Neuroendocrine Responses to Stress

Several investigators have explored the association between forgiveness and neuroendocrine responses to stress. In an early study of this type, Berry and Worthington (2001) showed that cortisol reactions to imagery about a current relationship were lower among high trait forgiving individuals. In studies previously described, Edmondson (2005) reported that state forgiveness was associated with diminished cortisol during rumination of a betrayal event, and Tartaro et al. (2005) reported results supporting an association between forgiveness and lower cortisol reactivity to a Stroop task. However, in an attempt to replicate these findings, Ward (2010) found that forgiveness was not related to cortisol reactivity to the Stroop task.

Tabak and McCullough (2011) measured cortisol before and after delivery of a video-recorded speech directed at the perpetrator of a recent transgression. Although significant cortisol reactions were observed following the task, measures of forgiveness were not related to cortisol during task recovery. In another article, no association between forgiveness and cortisol was again observed, but oxytocin reactivity to the speech was associated with less forgiveness (Tabak, McCullough, Szeto, Mendez, & McCabe, 2011). Because oxytocin is considered to be a marker for attention to relationships, the inverse relation between oxytocin reactivity and forgiveness suggests that the magnitude of this neuroendrine reaction may be a marker of relational distress.

Forgiveness and Resting Neuroendocrine State

Like measures of peripheral nervous system functioning, some investigators have examined the relation between dispositional forgiveness and resting neuroendocrine states. In most of these studies, no relation between trait forgivingness and resting cortisol or oxytocin has been observed (e.g., Berry & Worthington, 2001; Gregory, 2005; Seybold et al., 2001; Tabak & McCullough, 2011; Tabak et al., 2011; Ward, 2010), with the sole exception being a significant inverse relation between forgiveness and resting cortisol observed by Toussaint and Williams (2003).

Although inconsistent findings have been reported in studies examining the relation between forgiveness and neuroendocrine activity, there is some evidence that cortisol reactivity is lower among forgiving individuals and higher among those who ruminate about transgressions (Berry & Worthington, 2001; Edmondson, 2005; Tartaro et al., 2005). The only study that has been conducted on oxytocin illuminated an interesting association that warrants replication and further investigation (Tabak et al., 2011).

Forgiveness and Immune System Functioning

Because organisms respond to threat by preparing their bodies to resist invasions by viruses and bacteria, immune system functioning is also influenced by stress. In particular, specific cytokines (e.g., IL-6) and other immune system parameters [e.g., natural killer (NK) cell activity] have been shown to increase during acute stress presentations, but then become less responsive under chronic stress. Unfortunately, not many studies have examined the relation between forgiveness and immune system functioning. By analyzing blood from community-dwelling adults at rest, Seybold et al. (2001) reported that greater forgiveness was correlated with a few markers of improved immune system functioning; however, no relation with forgiveness was observed for the other measures of lymphocyte functioning assessed (e.g., NK cells). After controlling for relevant demographic and health factors, Owen, Hayward, and Toussaint (2011) reported that CD4 cell percentage was significantly higher among individuals with HIV/AIDS who endorsed greater forgiveness. Although results from both studies that have examined the relation between forgiveness and immune system functioning support an association, more empirical work is needed in this area.

Physiological Alterations Occurring During the Forgiveness Process

Although a range of experimental methods have been devised to examine the physiological effects of forgiveness, only a few have prospectively followed individuals who have decided to forgive another person. Given the duration the process of forgiveness often takes, this is understandable. Although intervention studies have yet to be devised to examine physiological mechanisms of therapeutic change, if forgiveness is associated with reduced stress responses, we would expect to observe attenuated physiological stress responses among participants as they engage in the process of forgiveness, especially those who report completely forgiving the offender.

Standard (2004) and Gregory (2005) conducted dissertations that compared physiological changes during participation in a forgiveness intervention with controls receiving no intervention. Standard found that cortisol was reduced among treatment participants at post-treatment in contrast to controls, and a trend toward improved glucocorticoid functioning was observed among treatment participants. In contrast, Gregory showed no differences in HR, BP, or cortisol from pre- to post-treatment between participants in forgiveness intervention and controls. Similarly, Tibbits, Ellis, Piramelli, Luskin, and Lukman (2006) reported no significant change in BP following completion of a forgiveness intervention by patients with essential hypertension in contrast to controls. It should be noted that each of these studies only examined resting physiological states and did not expose participants to any betrayal-related stimuli either before or after treatment.

Using fMRI, Farrow et al. (2005) assessed cortical activity of PTSD patients before and after undergoing a forgiveness-based intervention. Changes in cortical activation occurred following treatment in brain regions involved in social cognition (i.e., increased posterior cingulate gyrus and precuneus activation). It should be noted, however, that no control group was used in this study and the extent to which these changes could be attributed to forgiveness was unclear. In the most recent intervention study, Waltman et al. (2009) compared coronary blood flow (via radionuclide imaging) during recall of a hurtful event among cardiac patients participating in either a forgiveness intervention or coping skills control group. Blood flow perfusion defects occurring during anger recall declined among the intervention group relative to the control condition during a ten-week follow up assessment.

Summary and Conclusions

Fifteen years have passed since Thoreson and colleagues (2000) issued their challenge to the field to address the paucity of research examining the relation between forgiveness and health. Almost all of the studies described in this chapter were conducted since this challenge was issued, and we are in a far better place to address whether forgiveness is associated with health benefits as a consequence. Although the relation between forgiveness and health outcomes is covered extensively in the chapters that follow, this chapter focused on the relation between forgiveness and physiological responses to stress, including recollection of incidents of betrayal and injustice. In brief, almost all studies described in this chapter found that forgiveness in some way was associated with attenuated physiological stress responses. Significant relations have been much less consistently observed when study methods only examine resting physiological states.

Much work needs to be done to elucidate fully how forgiveness alters the body's physiological response. It is unclear, for example, why significant findings are observed in a given physiological parameter in one study but not another. Even among studies conducted in the same laboratories, patterns of findings differ across studies using fairly equivalent methodologies. It also appears that significant findings are more consistently observed when the stimuli presented pertain to an interpersonal transgression. Studies that have used typical laboratory stress stimuli (e.g., anger recall; mental arithmetic) have not shown relations between physiological measures of the stress response and forgiveness. Among studies directly exposing participants to betrayal events, numerous methods have been used, ranging from those that interview participants on personally-relevant events to those that involve making judgments about the behaviors of hypothetical persons in standard vignettes. It is quite likely that emotional responses and their associated physiological responses would differ depending upon the personal relevance of the experimental stimuli. It is also clear that a preponderance of studies examining the physiology of forgiveness has been conducted on college students. Although it can easily be argued that betrayal and forgiveness reflect important social phenomena to which young adults are exposed, generalizing these findings to persons of other ages and health conditions are important avenues for future investigations to consider. Finally, given the rapid advances in technology occurring in the experimental community, it will be important for the field to begin to explore how central and peripheral nervous system functioning in conjunction with neuroendocrine system functioning concurrently respond to betrayal and forgiveness. Given the promising findings that have occurred over the past fifteen years, we are sure to learn more as we continue to address these unresolved questions and issues.

References

Berry, J. W., & Worthington, E. L., Jr. (2001). Forgivingness, relationship quality, stress while imagining relationship events, and physical and mental health. *Journal of Counseling Psychology, 48*, 447–455.

Brenneis, M. J. (2001). The relationship between forgiveness and physical health indicators in recovering members of the clergy. *Journal of Ministry in Addiction & Recovery, 7*, 43–59.

Buck, A. C., Williams, D. R., Musick, M. A., & Sternthal, M. J. (2009). An examination of the relationship between multiple dimensions of religiosity. *Social Science & Medicine, 68*, 314–322.

Edmondson, K. A. (2005). Forgiveness and rumination: Their relationship and effects on psychological and physical health. *Dissertation Abstracts International: Section B: The Sciences and Engineering, 65*(12-B), 6694.

Farrow, T. F. D., Hunter, M. D., Wilkinson, I. D., Gouneea, C., Fawbert, D., Smith, … Woodruff, P. W. R. (2005). Quantifiable change in functional brain response to empathic and forgivability judgments with resolution of posttraumatic stress disorder. *Psychiatry Research: Neuroimaging, 140*, 45–53.

Farrow, T. F. D., Zheng, Y., Wilkinson, I. D., Spence, S. A., Deakin, J. F. W., Tarrier, N., … Woodruff, P. W. R. (2001). Investigating the functional anatomy of empathy and forgiveness. *NeuroReport, 12*, 2433–2438.

Friedberg, J. P., Suchday, S., & Shelov, D. V. (2007). The impact of forgiveness on cardiovascular reactivity and recovery. *International Journal of Psychophysiology, 65*, 87–94.

Gregory, J. C. (2005). Comparing forgiveness interventions: An extended group versus a brief expressive writing exercise. *Dissertation Abstracts International: Section B: The Sciences and Engineering, 66*(6-B), 3409.

Hall, L. R. (2006). Neuroticism, forgiveness of others, and blood pressure. *Dissertation Abstracts International: Section B: The Sciences and Engineering, 67*(2-B), 1149.

Hannon, P. A., Finkel, E. J., Kumashiro, M., & Rusbult, C. E. (2012). The soothing effects of forgiveness on victims' and perpetrators' blood pressure. *Personal Relationships, 19*, 279–289.

Hayashi, A., Abe, N., Ueno, A., Shigemune, Y., Mori, E., Tashiro, M., & Fuji, T. (2010). Neural correlates of forgiveness for moral transgressions involving deception. *Brain Research, 1332*, 90–99.

Hernandez, D. H., Larkin, K. T., & Whited, M. C. (2009). Cardiovascular response to interpersonal provocation and mental arithmetic among high and low hostile young adult males. *Applied Psychophysiology and Biofeedback, 34*, 27–35.

Huang, S. T., & Enright, R. D. (2000). Forgiveness and anger-related emotions in Taiwan: Implications for therapy. *Psychotherapy, 37*, 71–79.

Larsen, B. A., Darby, R. S., Harris, C. R., Nelkin, D. K., Milam, P., & Christenfeld, N. J. S. (2012). The immediate and delayed cardiovascular benefits of forgiving. *Psychosomatic Medicine, 74*, 745–750.

Lawler, K. A., Younger, J., Piferi, R. A., Billington, E., Jobe, R., Edmondson, K., & Jones, W. H. (2003). A change of heart: Cardiovascular correlates of forgiveness in response to interpersonal conflict. *Journal of Behavioral Medicine, 26*, 373–393.

Lawler, K. A., Younger, J. W., Piferi, R. L., Jobe, R. L., Edmundson, K. A., & Jones, W. H. (2005). The unique effects of forgiveness on health: An exploration of pathways. *Journal of Behavioral Medicine, 28*, 157–167.

Lawler-Row, K. A., Hyatt-Edwards, L., Wuensch, K. L., & Karremans, J. C. (2011). Forgiveness and health: The role of attachment. *Personal Relationships, 18*, 170–183.

Lawler-Row, K. A., Karremans, J. C., Scott, C., Edlis-Matityahou, M., & Edwards, L. (2008). Forgiveness, physiological reactivity and health: The role of anger. *International Journal of Psychophysiology, 68*, 51–58.

Lee, K., Brown, W. H., Egleston, P. N., Green, R. D. G., Farrow, T. F. D., Hunter, M. D., … Woodruff, P. W. R. (2006). A functional magnetic resonance imaging study of social cognition in schizophrenia during an acute episode and after recovery. *American Journal of Psychiatry, 163*, 1926–1933.

Lutgendorf, S. K., & Sood, A. K. (2011). Biobehavioral factors and cancer progression: Physiological pathways and mechanism. *Psychosomatic Medicine, 73*, 724–730.

McEwen, B. S., & Stellar, E. (1993). Stress and the individual: Mechanisms leading to disease. *Archives of Internal Medicine, 153*, 2093–2101.

Mitchell, J. P. (2008). Contributions of functional neuroimaging to the study of social cognition. *Current Directions in Psychological Science, 17*(2), 142–146.

Olson, C. B. (2004). Emotions and psychophysiological response in post traumatic stress disorder. *Dissertation Abstracts International: Section B: The Sciences and Engineering, 65*(10-B), 5417.

Owen, A. D., Hayward, R. D., & Toussaint, L. L. (2011). *Forgiveness and immune functioning in people living with HIV-AIDS*. Paper presented at the 32nd annual meeting of the Society for Behavioral Medicine, Washington, DC.

Pietrini, P., Ricciardi, E., Gentili, C., Vanello, N., Sani, L., & Guazzelli, M. (2004). How the brain responds to hurtful events: Neural activity elicited by aggressive versus forgiving behavior in humans. *International Journal of Psychophysiology, 54*, 26. [Abstract]

Rozanski, A., Blumenthal, J. A., & Kaplan, J. (1999). Impact of psychological factors on the pathogenesis of cardiovascular disease and implications for therapy. *Circulation, 99*, 2192–2217.

Semenec, S. C. (2009). The relationship of self and other-forgiveness to interpersonal stress reactivity and recovery. *Dissertation Abstracts International: Section B: The Sciences and Engineering, 69*(10-B), 6435.

Seybold, K. S., Hill, P. C., Neumann, J. K., & Chi, D. S. (2001). Physiological and psychological correlates of forgiveness. *Journal of Psychology and Christianity, 20*, 250–259.

Standard, S. (2004). Effects of a forgiveness intervention on salivary cortisol, DHEA, and psychological variables. *Dissertation Abstracts International: Section B: The Sciences and Engineering, 65*(4-B), 2114.

Tabak, B. A., & McCullough, M. E. (2011). Perceived transgressor agreeableness decreases cortisol response and increases forgiveness following recent interpersonal transgressions. *Biological Psychology, 87*, 386–392.

Tabak, B. A., McCullough, M. E., Szeto, A., Mendez, A., & McCabe, P. M. (2011). Oxytocin indexes relational distress following interpersonal harms in women. *Psychoneuroendocrinology, 36*, 115–122.

Tartaro, J., Luecken, L. J., & Gunn, H. E. (2005). Exploring heart and soul: Effects of religiosity/spirituality and gender on blood pressure and cortisol stress responses. *Journal of Health Psychology, 10*, 753–766.

Thoresen, C. E., Harris, A. H. S., & Luskin, F. (2000). Forgiveness and health: An unanswered question. In M. E. McCullough, K. I. Pargament, & C. E. Thoresen (Eds.), *Forgiveness: Theory, research, and practice* (pp. 254–280). New York, NY: Guilford Press.

Tibbits, D., Ellis, G., Piramelli, C., Luskin, F., & Lukman, R. (2006). Hypertension reduction through forgiveness training. *Journal of Pastoral Care & Counseling, 60*, 27–34.

Toussaint, L. L., & Williams, D. R. (2003). *Physiological correlates of forgiveness: Findings from a racially and socio-economically diverse sample of community residents*. Paper presented at scientific findings about forgiveness conference, Atlanta, GA.

Waltman, M. A., Russell, D. C., Coyle, C. T., Enright, R. D., Holter, A. C., & Swoboda, C. M. (2009). The effects of a forgiveness intervention on patients with coronary artery disease. *Psychology and Health, 24*, 11–27.

Ward, A. M. (2010). The relationship between religiosity and religious coping to stress reactivity and psychological well-being. *Dissertation Abstracts International: Section B: The Sciences and Engineering, 71*(12-B), 7744.

Whited, M. C., Wheat, A. L., & Larkin, K. T. (2010). The influence of forgiveness and apology on cardiovascular reactivity and recovery in response to mental stress. *Journal of Behavioral Medicine, 33*, 293–304.

Witvliet, C. V., DeYoung, N. J., Hofelich, A. J., & DeYoung, P. A. (2011). Compassionate reappraisal and emotion suppression as alternatives to offense-focused rumination: Implications for forgiveness and psychophysiological well-being. *Journal of Positive Psychology, 6*, 286–299.

Witvliet, C. V., Knoll, R. W., Hinman, N. G., & DeYoung, P. A. (2010). Compassion-focused reappraisal, benefit-focused reappraisal, and rumination after an interpersonal offense: Emotion-regulation implications for subjective emotion, linguistic responses, and physiology. *Journal of Positive Psychology, 5*, 226–242.

Witvliet, C. V., Ludwig, T. E., & Vander Laan, K. L. (2001). Granting forgiveness or harboring grudges: Implications for emotion, physiology, and health. *Psychological Science, 121*, 117–123.

Wivliet, C. V., Ludwig, T. E., & Bauer, D. J. (2002). Please forgive me: Transgressors' emotions and physiology during imagery of seeking forgiveness and victim responses. *Journal of Psychology and Christianity, 21*, 219–233.

Witvliet, C. V. O., Worthington, E. L., Root, L. M., Sato, A. F., Ludwig, T. E., & Exline, J. J. (2008). Retributive justice, restorative justice, and forgiveness: An experimental psychophysiology analysis. *Journal of Experimental Social Psychology, 44*, 10–25.

Worthington, E. L., & Wade, N. G. (1999). The social psychology of unforgiveness and forgiveness and implications for clinical practice. *Journal of Social and Clinical Psychology, 18*, 385–418.

Young, L., & Saxe, R. (2009). Innocent intentions: A correlation between forgiveness for accidental harm and neural activity. *Neuropsychologia, 47*, 2065–2072.

Chapter 6
Forgiveness and Mental Health

Brandon J. Griffin, Everett L. Worthington, Jr., Caroline R. Lavelock, Nathaniel G. Wade, and William T. Hoyt

Investigations of the effects of forgiveness on positive and poor mental health proliferated during the last decade. In the present chapter, we build upon a prior review by Toussaint and Webb (2005) in which a mediation model was described to illustrate how five primary mediators—social support, interpersonal functioning, health behaviors, personal control, and rumination—connect unforgiveness and mental health. While Toussaint and Webb's empirical foundation consisted of only 13 correlational studies, research on forgiveness and mental health has accelerated since the time of their analysis. In this chapter, we report a decade review.

The scope of the current project is broad for several reasons. First, scholars assess different types of forgiveness (e.g., forgiveness of oneself and others, seeking and receiving forgiveness, etc.) rather than a single ubiquitous phenomenon (Fehr, Gelfand, & Nag, 2010). Also, forgiveness may be categorized as either decisional (e.g., a volitional act) or emotional (i.e., an embodied experience; Worthington, Hook, Utsey, Williams, & Neil, 2007) as well as either state forgiveness (i.e., a situation-specific response) or trait forgivingness (i.e., a disposition to forgive that is stable across circumstances and over long portions of the lifespan). Second, definitions of mental health are equally multifarious, considering both positive and

B.J. Griffin (✉) • E.L. Worthington, Jr. (✉) • C.R. Lavelock
Department of Psychology, Virginia Commonwealth University, Richmond, VA, USA
e-mail: griffinb2@mymail.vcu.edu; eworth@vcu.edu

N.G. Wade
Department of Psychology, W117 Lagomarcino Hall, Iowa State University, Ames, IA, USA
e-mail: nwade@iastate.edu

W.T. Hoyt
Department of Counseling Psychology, University of Wisconsin – Madison, Madison, WI, USA

L.L. Toussaint et al. (eds.), *Forgiveness and Health*,
DOI 10.1007/978-94-017-9993-5_6

poor outcomes as well as differences between diagnosable mental disorders and non-clinical levels of psychological symptoms.

Stress-and-Coping Model of Forgiveness

A stress-and-coping model provides a paradigm to explore the effects of forgiveness on health. Proponents of the model suggest that emotion-focused health outcomes emerge when individuals encounter stressors, form appraisals, endure stress reactions, and attempt to cope (Lazarus, 1999). According to the forgiveness-adapted model, offenses that are committed by or against oneself may serve as initial stressors, such that being either the victim or perpetrator of an offense might initiate the coping process (Strelan & Covic, 2006; Worthington, 2006, 2013).

Proponents of the forgiveness-adapted stress-and-coping model argue that transgressions function as stressors. One then appraises the severity of the transgression (called the injustice gap; Worthington, 2006), whether the transgression poses a threat, and the resources that may enable one to manage the injustice. Appraisals are followed by a stress-response, which might include maladaptive emotional and motivational responses, critical and punitive behavioral reactions, and faulty patterns of thinking. In fact, two stress responses that are of particular interest to the forgiveness-adapted model are *unforgiveness* toward others and *self-condemnation* toward oneself. Both unforgiveness and self-condemnation are comprised of a complex amalgamation of chronic negative emotions, which is subsequently believed to engender physical and mental health problems. Yet, negative emotion might be adaptive if one is motivated to attempt to constructively cope with the offense. Although one might attempt to use a variety of coping strategies (e.g., excusing, seeking revenge, pursuing legal justice, accepting, forbearing, etc.), we focus on one particular coping response: forgiveness.

Method of the Review

We searched the PsycINFO database during September, 2012. Searches were performed by pairing forgiv* and unforgiv* with terms such as mental health, disorder, affect, well-being, and satisfaction. Retained studies included quantitative measures of forgiveness and at least one indicator of positive or poor mental health. Because the purpose of this chapter is to build upon the foundation of previous reviewers (Toussaint & Webb, 2005), articles published before the year 2003 were excluded. We also examined the reference sections of articles. Fifty-five articles are reviewed below—a fourfold increase over the number of empirical studies available at the time of the 2005 review. We created a supplemental summary table of the 54 articles, which is available from the second author upon request.

Mental Health Outcomes of Forgiveness in Victims of Offense

We organize investigations of the forgiveness-mental health relationship among victims of offense according to four propositions (See Table 6.1). Propositions 1 and 2 provide evidence of the mental health effects experienced by victims who harbor unforgiveness toward and who forgive offenders. Propositions 3 and 4 respectively examine individual differences and psychological states that influence the relationship between forgiveness and mental health for victims of harm.

Proposition 1: Unforgiveness Is a Stress-Reaction Related to Poor Mental Health

Ten empirical studies support our first proposition. For example, Worthington and Scherer (2004) reviewed the literature and suggested that physiological indicators, including brain, hormonal, and sympathetic nervous system activity, as well as changes in blood chemistry, all imply that physical indicators of stress accompany higher levels of unforgiveness toward others. The target of one's unforgiveness, however, might be more than solely other people. In a correlational study of 160 religious adults, Strelan, Acton, and Patrick (2009) found that unforgiveness toward a higher power (i.e., God, nature, or humanity) is associated with increased levels of stress ($r = .33$) and depression ($r = .38$).

Chronic negative emotion comprises the core of unforgiveness (Harris & Thoresen, 2005; Worthington, Witvliet, Pietrini, & Miller, 2007). Indeed, Green, DeCourville, and Sadava (2012) found that negative affect ($r = -.61$), stress ($r = -.55$), and positive affect ($r = .49$) were each associated with mental health and mediated the forgivingness-health relationship among undergraduates ($N = 623$). Yet, one's emotions are influenced by critical cognitions and punitive behaviors. Maltby, Day, and Barber (2005) examined the effects of unforgiving affect, cognition, and behavior among undergraduates ($N = 224$) and found that unforgiving cognitions uniquely predicted decreased subjective well-being (i.e., short-term imbalance between positive and negative affect; $r = -.35$); whereas, forgiving affect ($r = .35$) and behavior ($r = .34$) predicted increased psychological health (i.e., long-term development and growth).

Table 6.1 Forgiveness and mental health in victims of offense

Propositions
Proposition 1: Unforgiveness Is a Stress-Reaction Related to Poor Mental Health
Proposition 2: Forgiveness is a Coping Strategy Related to Improved Mental Health
Proposition 3: Individual Differences Moderate the Impact of Forgiveness on Health
Proposition 4: Psychological States Mediate the Impact of Forgiveness on Health

Hartwig Moorhead, Gill, Barrio Minton, and Myers (2012) examined the effects of unforgiveness on the well-being of counselors-in-training ($N = 115$), reporting that unforgiving motivation, especially instance-specific revenge ($r = -.35$), was negatively related to total well-being. In addition, Macaskill (2012) found that the tendency to withhold forgiveness from others was positively linked to trait anger ($N = 295$, $r = .36$; $N = 233$, $r = .52$), trait anxiety ($N = 233$, $r = .26$) and life dissatisfaction ($N = 233$, $r = .19$) among undergraduates. Summarily, research continues to affirm Toussaint and Webb's (2005) assertion that a direct effect of forgiveness on mental health results from reducing unforgiveness, especially negative emotions such as bitterness, fear, and anger.

Proposition 2: Forgiveness Is a Coping Strategy Related to Improved Mental Health

The relationship between forgiveness and mental health can be (and has been) studied in different ways. First, forgiveness can be examined in light of its relationships to psychological symptoms as well as to diagnoses of mental disorders. Put another way, what is the relationship between forgiveness and mental illness? Twenty-seven empirical studies reviewed herein pertain to this question.

Findings indicate that state forgiveness (i.e., forgiveness of a specific offense and offender) and trait forgivingness (i.e., a general disposition to forgive) are both inversely related to psychological symptoms (Lawler-Row, 2010; Maltby, Day, & Barber, 2004), although examinations of trait forgivingness occur far more frequently in the literature. In one correlational study, Messay, Dixon, and Rye (2012) found that trait forgivingness and situational (i.e., state) forgiveness were respectively related to lower levels of depression ($r = -.14$, $r = -.30$), anxiety ($r = -.21$, $r = -.24$), and stress ($r = -.27$, $r = -.29$) among undergraduates ($N = 242$). Likewise, trait forgivingness was associated with lower levels of trait anger (r = −.49), neuroticism (r = −.49), rumination (r = −.69), fear (r = −.44), and hostility (r = −.35) among undergraduates ($N = 233$; Berry, Worthington, O'Connor, Parrott, & Wade, 2005) as well as post-traumatic stress disorder (r = −.25) among students who endured interpersonal trauma ($N = 229$; Orcutt, Pickett, & Pope, 2005).

The general relationship between forgiveness and reduced mental illness is also present in older adults. In a national survey of Americans who were 66 years of age or older ($N = 1500$), those who expressed a disposition to forgive others reported less depressed affect ($\beta = -.18$), somatic symptoms ($\beta = -.181$), and death anxiety ($\beta = -.194$; Krause & Ellison, 2003). However, this relationship attenuated if victims required acts of contrition from offenders, and conditional forgiveness was further related to an increased risk of mortality ($B = .346$) among older adults ($N = 1{,}232$) according to Toussaint, Owen, and Cheadle (2012).

Another way that the relationship between forgiveness and mental health can be examined is through associations with indicators of well-being, or healthy psychological functioning. Fourteen empirical studies suggest that forgiveness promotes positive mental health outcomes. For example, among Swiss citizens ($N = 962$), trait forgivingness was positively associated with life satisfaction (r = .23), positive affect (r = .25), and optimism (r = .26; Allemand, Hill, Ghaemmaghami, & Martin, 2012). Forgivingness has also been correlated with social support network size (r = .17), satisfaction with one's support network (r = .18), and vitality (r = .30) among undergraduates ($N = 623$; Green et al., 2012). In addition, Webb, Toussaint, Kalpakjian, and Tate (2010) studied forgivingness among a clinical sample of people diagnosed with spinal cord injuries ($N = 140$) and found that forgivingness of others was a positively linked to self-rated health ($r = .20$) and life satisfaction (r = .26).

Although many studies relate forgiveness to improved mental health outcomes, most studies are correlational and most are cross-sectional. This leaves uncertainty regarding the direction of the causal effects. Certainly, theories have been proposed in support of the longitudinal impact of forgiveness on mental health (Worthington, Witvliet et al., 2007). However, the opposite might also be true; people who are more psychologically healthy might be in a better position to forgive. People with less depression or a larger social network, for example, might have more psychological and social resources to achieve forgiveness or to be more dispositionally forgiving. One longitudinal study provides evidence for this hypothesis by showing that earlier ratings of psychological adjustment (i.e., depression and rumination) predicted changes in forgiveness of an interpersonal offense (Orth, Berking, Walker, Meier, & Znoj, 2008). In contrast, earlier ratings of forgiveness did not predict improvement in depression or rumination. Therefore, although the relationship between forgiveness and mental health is a strong and robust finding, much work remains to be done in order to determine the directions of these effects.

Proposition 3: Individual Differences Moderate the Impact of Forgiveness on Health

Having established the overall relationship between forgiveness and health, we now consider differences between people that make one person more or less likely to reap the mental health benefits associated with forgiveness. Fourteen empirical studies pertain to the third proposition. In the present chapter, we consider differences with regard to age, sex, and motivation to forgive others.

Toussaint, Williams, Musick, and Everson (2001) first observed that forgiveness of others more strongly predicted improved physical and mental health in middle and old-aged adults than in young adults ($N = 1{,}423$). More recently, using a sample of 962 adults, Allemand et al. (2012) sought to provide an explanation of these age-related differences and concluded that one's perspective of the future – the extent to which one believes their time remaining is open-ended or limited in duration – moderated the relationship between dispositional forgivingness and positive mental health outcomes (positive affect, life satisfaction and optimism). Hill and Allemand (2010) argued further that forgiving others may be crucial to the health of victims who perceive time as limited and value a few quality experiences rather than a large quantity of novel experiences.

Sex also has been shown to qualify the forgiveness-mental health relationship, especially with regard to some dimensions of forgiveness. For example, Toussaint, Williams, Musick, and Everson-Rose (2008a) compared men and women in a national sample of 1,423 adults. Results revealed that forgiveness of self was associated with lower levels of depression in men. But, among women, forgiveness of self, others, and feeling forgiven by God each predicted reduced depression. This study demonstrates the heterogeneity in the association between forgiveness and mental health that depends upon an individual's sex.

A victim's motivation for forgiving an offender might also influence the relation between forgiveness on mental health. In a correlational study of people in the workplace ($N = 420$), Cox, Bennett, Tripp, and Aquino (2012) examined the influence of why a victim forgave on the forgiveness-health relationship. The benefits of forgiveness could not be consistently assumed across various motivations to forgive (i.e., moral, relational, apologetic, religious, and lack of alternatives). In fact, participants who forgave due to lack of alternatives or the requirement of a higher power reported higher levels of stress, but victims who forgave for moral reasons experienced lower levels of stress.

Proposition 4: Psychological States Mediate the Impact of Forgiveness on Health

Mediator variables explain how a predictor variable (such as forgiveness) may be causally related to an outcome variable (such as mental health). Five empirical studies pertain to the fourth proposition and describe mediators of the forgiveness-health relationship. While the knowledge of variables that mediate the forgiveness-health relationship is beginning to develop, it is evident that mediating variables cannot be assumed to play a consistent role across types of forgiveness and for both positive and poor mental health outcomes.

First, rumination mediates the effects of forgiveness on mental health and may also mediate the effects of unforgiveness on mental health. Nolen-Hoeksema, Wisco, and Lyubomirsky (2008) define rumination as a response pattern in which one repeatedly focuses on the undesirable symptoms of distress without making an effort toward change. Specifically, Ysseldyk, Matheson, and Anisman (2007) found that ruminative brooding mediated the relationships between forgiveness and depressive affect as well as life satisfaction among undergraduates ($N = 183$).

Second, hopelessness has been shown to mediate the relationship between forgiveness and 12-month prevalence of a major depressive episode. Among respondents to a nationally representative telephone survey ($N = 1,423$), Toussaint,

Williams, Musick, and Everson-Rose (2008b) found that hopelessness partially mediated the relationships between depression and forgiveness of others and self. In contrast, hopelessness did not mediate the relationships between depression and feeling forgiven by God or seeking forgiveness, which was possibly due to the weaker relationships between these types of forgiveness and depressive outcomes that were observed.

Third, in a series of correlational studies, Karremans, Lange, Paul, Ouwerkerk, and Kluwer (2003) described a mediated moderation effect between forgiveness and mental health outcomes (i.e., state self-esteem and negative affect). Interpersonal commitment between a perpetrator and victim of harm moderated the impact of forgiving (or not forgiving) one's offender, such that in situations involving high commitment the effects of forgiving (or not forgiving) were stronger. Furthermore, the mediating variable, psychological tension, was greatest when pre-offense relationship commitment was strong, and it nearly disappeared in the context of weak relational commitment. Such an effect might also explain investigations of forgiveness and mental health in the context of romantic relationships (Miller & Worthington, 2010; Paleari, Regalia, & Fincham, 2011).

Mental Health Outcomes of Forgiveness in Perpetrators of Offense

A growing interest in perpetrators of offense now pervades investigations of the relationship between forgiveness and mental health. In fact, Worthington (2013) maintains that perpetrators who (1) commit wrongdoing against others or (2) fail to live according to one's own standards or expectations might experience *self-condemnation*, a blend of negative emotions (i.e., guilt, shame, and regret) that is similar to unforgiveness, except that is directed toward oneself. In the present chapter, we examine mental health outcomes reported by perpetrators who seek and feel forgiveness, and those who self-forgive. Seventeen studies addressed the association between forgiveness and mental health outcomes among perpetrators of offense.

Seeking and Receiving Forgiveness is Related to Perpetrators' Mental Health

Investigations of seeking forgiveness emerged around the beginning of the twenty-first century (Sandage, Worthington, Hight, & Berry, 2000). In a recent correlational study, Toussaint, Williams, Musick and Everson-Rose (2008a) surveyed adults and found that women more often sought forgiveness than did men and that seeking forgiveness was related to a greater likelihood of depression in women (OR = 1.71,

$N = 709$) but unrelated in men (OR = 1.38, $N = 563$). Likewise, people who were affiliated with Catholic or Protestant Christian traditions were observed to more readily seek forgiveness than others with no religious affiliation, but this finding has yet to be connected to the forgiveness-health relationship (Toussaint & Williams, 2008).

Although further evidence is needed to support preliminary findings suggesting that seeking forgiveness is positively related to poor mental health, the study of seeking forgiveness illuminates the process by which perpetrators of harm begin to repair the spiritual, social, and psychological consequences of wrongdoing. In fact, the adapted stress-and-coping model provides a foundation for such investigations given that people who experience greater stress as a result of self-condemning emotions (i.e., guilt and shame) are hypothesized to be more likely to attempt to cope with an offense using strategies including, but not limited too, seeking forgiveness (see Riek, 2010). Moreover, Ingersoll-Dayton, Torges, and Krause (2010) found that feeling unforgiven by others was positively related to rumination ($r = .12$) and depression ($r = .12$), unforgiveness of self was positively related to rumination ($r = .19$) and depression ($r = .11$), and not feeling forgiven by God was unrelated to rumination or depression among older adults ($N = 965$).

On the other hand, feeling forgiven by others and by a higher power (e.g., God, nature, humanity in general) has been associated with improved mental health outcomes. For example, Lyons, Deane, Caputi, and Kelly (2011) investigated the mental health effects of receiving forgiveness from others and from God in a correlational study of people pursuing substance use treatment from faith-based rehabilitation centers ($N = 277$). Feeling forgiven by others was related to resentment ($r = -.33$) and purpose in life ($r = .42$), and feeling forgiven by God was related to resentment ($r = -.33$) and purpose in life ($r = .38$). Thus, perpetrators of offense who seek and receive forgiveness appear to report lower levels of poor mental health outcomes as well as higher levels of positive mental health outcomes overall.

Self-Forgiveness is Related to Improved Mental Health in Perpetrators of Harm

Most research from the perspective of offenders involves self-forgiveness. In fact, Hall and Fincham (2008) theorize that the consequences of self-condemnation and the rewards of self-forgiveness may be closely linked to mental health. Also, correlational evidence is beginning to support the claim that self-forgiveness is negatively related to dystonic symptoms (i.e., anger, anxiety, life dissatisfaction) as well as positively related to well-being (i.e., balanced affect, happiness, satisfaction with life, and gratitude) (Macaskill, 2012; Toussaint & Friedman, 2009).

Self-forgiveness may contribute to the mental health of people who are prone to feel high levels of self-condemnation (Worthington & Langberg, 2012). For example, Witvliet, Phipps, Feldman, and Beckham (2004) studied 213 male veterans in a PTSD clinic and found that self-condemnation was related to depression ($\beta = .22$), PTSD symptoms ($\beta = .19$), state anxiety ($\beta = .16$), and trait anxiety ($\beta = .28$). Self-forgiveness may also be a useful coping strategy for people who receive life-changing and chronic diagnoses such as cancer ($N = 81$; Romero et al., 2006), chronic musculoskeletal pain ($N = 144$; Rippentrop, Altmaier, Chen, Found, & Keffala, 2005), and spinal cord injuries ($N = 144$; Webb et al., 2010). Research is needed to examine the origin of self-condemnation in clinical populations.

Overall, investigations of the forgiveness-health relationship from the perspective of perpetrators are beginning to accrue. Evidence suggests that forgiveness is one coping method that alleviates unforgiving and self-condemning stress-related emotions and that promotes better mental health among both victims and perpetrators of offense.

Directions for Further Inquiry

In the past decade, substantial knowledge has been gained about the association between forgiveness and mental health. The forgiveness-health literature, however, continues to evolve. We therefore offer the following directions for future inquiries of the relationship between forgiveness and mental health among both victims and perpetrators of offense. First, further research is required to examine the forgiveness-health relationship among victims of offense with respect to each aforementioned proposition. According to Proposition 1, unforgiveness is a stress-reaction related to deleterious mental health outcomes. But, forgiveness is not the only way to cope with unforgiveness toward a perpetrator (Worthington, 2006). It is unknown how forgiveness might compare to other coping strategies such as excusing an offense, forbearing harm, or pursuing legal justice. Proposition 2 provides two perspectives (connections to mental illness and well-being) by which the forgiveness-mental health relationship might be examined. Yet, more is known about the attenuation of negative outcomes (i.e., depression, anxiety, and hostility) as opposed to the augmentation of positive outcomes (i.e., life satisfaction, gratitude, optimism, etc.). Proposition 3 discusses demographic variables that moderate the forgiveness-health relationship and suggests that the literature is primed for investigations of personality and related processes that might influence the effect of forgiveness on mental health (e.g., religiousness). Finally, as demonstrated in Proposition 4, the effects of psychological states that mediate the forgiveness-mental health relationship have only begun to be studied. Further research is required to examine the indirect effects of forgiveness on mental health, especially with respect to different types of forgiveness as well as to both poor and positive mental health outcomes.

Second, research is needed to examine forgiveness from the perspective of offenders. The mental health sequelae of feeling forgiven (or not) by God, by others, and by oneself—under a variety of personality and situational conditions—have hardly been addressed, especially with respect to the interplay of the three (see Ingersoll-Dayton et al., 2010). For example, does feeling forgiven by others or by God affect feelings of self-forgiveness? Or, might a perpetrator of harm seek forgiveness from others by "paying it forward" if making amends with the actual victim of offense is impossible?

Third, of the 54 studies in the present review, 40 assessed populations other than college students. This represents commendable attention to the association between forgiveness and mental health among diverse samples. Further research might assess populations at high risk to develop mental health disorders as a result of unforgiveness and to those inclined to flourish by learning to forgive (i.e., veterans, victims of trauma and abuse, etc.). Even so, psychometrically sound instruments and measurement strategies are needed to accurately assess the types of forgiveness discussed herein. For example, it is unclear to what extent instruments that purport to measure self-forgiveness are confounded by simply letting oneself off the hook and if this problem might attenuate or inflate the impact of self-forgiveness on health.

Fourth, investigations that lend themselves to causal research designs—experimental and longitudinal designs—are desperately needed to untangle sequences of influential conditions. Time sequenced inquiries might investigate the links between attempts to seek divine forgiveness, seek forgiveness of others (which includes the variety of their responses), and attempts to forgive oneself. We need to understand the differences between forgiving and unforgiving over time, especially considering the long-term effects of stress on health.

Fifth, although the majority of evidence in support of the forgiveness-mental health relationship is associative in nature, some researchers have developed interventions to improve mental health by promoting forgiveness (for a review, see Wade, Hoyt, & Worthington Jr, 2014). Priority should be given to interventions that may be adapted to various modes of delivery (i.e., group therapy, self-directed workbook, community intervention) in order to effectively disseminate treatment. Applications of these interventions have not been often addressed—and have not been a focus of the present review. Yet, some intervention researchers (Reed & Enright, 2006) have assessed whether forgiveness interventions result in reductions of mental health symptoms and improvements in well-being. We note, however, that interventions can produce mental health improvements for many reasons other than the content of the intervention. Thus, basic psychological researchers need to lay a solid causal groundwork that interventionists can draw upon.

Conclusion

During the recent decade, the literature seems to indicate an impending shift in forgiveness research. The first wave of research on the relationship between forgiveness and mental health that dominated until recently sought to answer the question "Is forgiveness an effective predictor of mental health outcomes?" The literature reviewed herein could return a tentative "Yes," citing an overall moderate effect size between forgiveness and mental health. Yet, a new wave of forgiveness research seeks to discover "Why is forgiveness a successful coping strategy?" and "In what context is the forgiveness-health relationship strongest?" Whereas we were once concerned with general mental health outcomes, we now focus on the differences between people that might qualify the effects of forgiveness on mental health outcomes as well as mechanisms through which forgiveness may help improve these outcomes among a variety of types of forgiveness among both victims and perpetrators of offense.

References[1]

*Allemand, M., Hill, P. L., Ghaemmaghami, P., & Martin, M. (2012). Forgivingness and subjective well-being in adulthood: The moderating role of future time perspective. *Journal of Research in Personality, 46*, 32–39.

**Barber, L., Maltby, J., & Macaskill, A. (2005). Angry memories Appears in Chapter and in Summary Table; ** Appears only in Summary Table.} ?> and thoughts of revenge: The relationship between forgiveness and anger rumination. *Personality and Individual Differences, 39*, 253–262.

*Berry, J. W., Worthington, E. L., Jr., O'Connor, L. E., Parrott, L., III, & Wade, N. G. (2005). Forgivingness, vengeful rumination, and affective traits. *Journal of Personality, 73*(1), 183–225. doi:10.1111/j.1467-6494.2004.00308.x.

**Bono, G., McCullough, M. E., & Root, L. M. (2008). Forgiveness, feeling connected to others, and well-being: Two longitudinal studies. *Personality and Social Psychology Bulletin, 34*(2), 182–195. doi:10.1177/0146167207310025.

**Brown, R. P., & Phillips, A. (2005). Letting bygones be bygones: Further evidence for the validity of the tendency to forgive scale. *Personality and Individual Differences, 38*(3), 627–638. doi:10.1016/j.paid.2004.05.017

**Burnette, J. L., Davis, D. E., Green, J. D., Worthington, E. L., Jr., & Bradfield, E. (2009). Insecure attachment and depressive symptoms: The mediating role of rumination empathy and forgiveness. *Personality and Individual Differences, 46*(3), 276–280.

*Cox, S. S., Bennett, R. J., Tripp, T. M., & Aquino, K. (2012). An empirical test of forgiveness motives' effects on employees' health and well-being. *Journal of Occupational Health Psychology, 17*(3), 330–340. doi:10.1037/a0028314.

Fehr, R., Gelfand, M. H., & Nag, M. (2010). The road to forgiveness: A meta-analytic synthesis of its situation and dispositional correlates. *Psychological Bulletin, 136*(5), 894–914.

*Green, M., DeCourville, N., & Sadava, S. (2012). Positive affect, negative affect, stress, and social support as mediators of the forgiveness-health relationship. *Journal of Social Psychology, 152*(3), 288–307.

Hall, J. H., & Fincham, F. D. (2008). The temporal course of self-forgiveness. *Journal of Social and Clinical Psychology, 27*(2), 174–202.

Harris, A. H. S., & Thoresen, C. E. (2005). Forgiveness, unforgiveness, health, and disease. In E. L. Worthington Jr. (Ed.), *Handbook of forgiveness*. New York, NY: Routledge.

*Hartwig Moorhead, H. J., Gill, C., Barrio Minton, C. A., & Myers, J. E. (2012). Forgive and forget? Forgiveness, personality, and wellness among counselors-in-training. *Counseling and Values, 57*, 81–95.

[1]*Appears in Chapter and in Summary Table; **Appears only in Summary Table.

*Hill, P. L., & Allemand, M. (2010). Forgivingness and adult patterns of individual differences in environmental mastery and personal growth. *Journal of Research in Personality, 44*(2), 245–250. doi:10.1016/j.jrp.2010.01.006.

**Hill, P. L., & Allemand, M. (2011). Gratitude, forgivingness, and well-being in adulthood: Tests of moderation and incremental prediction. *Journal of Positive Psychology, 6*(5), 397–407.

**Hirsch, J. K., Webb, J. R., & Jeglic, E. L. (2011). Forgiveness, depression, and suicidal behavior among a diverse sample of college students. *Journal of Clinical Psychology, 67*(9), 896–906.

**Hirsch, J. K., Webb, J. R., & Jeglic, E. L. (2012). Forgiveness as a moderator of the association between anger expression and suicidal behaviour. *Mental Health, Religion & Culture, 15*(3), 279–300. doi:10.1080/13674676.2011.571666.

*Ingersoll-Dayton, B., Torges, C., & Krause, N. (2010). Unforgiveness, rumination, and depressive symptoms among older adults. *Aging & Mental Health, 14*(4), 439–449.

**Jacinto, G. A. (2009). The self-forgiveness process of caregivers after the death of care-receivers diagnosed with Alzheimer's disease. *Journal of Social Service Research, 36*(1), 24–36.

*Karremans, J. C., Lange, V., Paul, A. M., Ouwerkerk, J. W., & Kluwer, E. S. (2003). When forgiving enhances psychological well-being: The role of interpersonal commitment. *Journal of Personality and Social Psychology, 84*(5), 1011–1026.

**Kira, I. A., Lewandowski, L. A., Temlin, T. N., Ramaswamy, V., Ozkan, B., & Mohanesh, J. (2009). The effects of post-retribution inter-group forgiveness: The case of Iraqi refugees. *Peace and Conflict, 15*, 385–413.

*Krause, N., & Ellison, C. G. (2003). Forgiveness by god, forgiveness of others, and psychological well-being in late life. *Journal for the Scientific Study of Religion, 42*(1), 77–93. doi:10.1111/1468-5906.00162.

*Lawler-Row, K. (2010). Forgiveness as a mediator of the religiosity—Health relationship. *Psychology of Religion and Spirituality, 2*(1), 1–16. doi:10.1037/a0017584.

**Lawler-Row, K., & Piferi, R. L. (2006). The forgiving personality: Describing a life well lived? *Personality and Individual Differences, 41*(6), 1009–1020.

Lazarus, R. S. (1999). *Stress and emotion: A new synthesis*. New York, NY: Springer.

*Lyons, G. C. B., Deane, F. P., Caputi, P., & Kelly, P. (2011). Spirituality and the treatment of substance use disorders: An exploration of forgiveness, resentment and purpose in life. *Addiction Research and Theory, 19*(5), 459–469.

*Macaskill, A. (2012). Differentiating dispositional self-forgiveness from other-forgiveness: Associations with mental health and life satisfaction. *Journal of Social and Clinical Psychology, 31*(1), 28–50.

**Maltby, J., Day, L., & Barber, L. (2004). Forgiveness and mental health variables: Interpreting the relationship using an adaptational-continuum model of personality and coping. *Personality and Individual Differences, 37*(8), 1629–1641.

*Maltby, J., Day, L., & Barber, L. (2005). Forgiveness and happiness: The differing contexts of forgiveness using the distinction between hedonic and eudaimonic happiness. *Journal of Happiness Studies, 6*, 1–13.

*Messay, B., Dixon, L. J., & Rye, M. S. (2012). The relationship between quest religious orientation, forgiveness, and mental health. *Mental Health, Religion & Culture, 15*(3), 315–333. doi:10.1080/13674676.2011.574271.

*Miller, A. J., & Worthington, E. L., Jr. (2010). Sex differences in forgiveness and mental health in recently married couples. *Journal of Positive Psychology, 5*(1), 12–23.

Nolen-Hoeksema, S., Wisco, B. E., & Lyubomirsky, S. (2008). Rethinking rumination. *Perspectives in Psychological Science, 3*(5), 400–424.

*Orcutt, J. K., Pickett, S. M., & Pope, B. (2005). Experiential avoidance and forgiveness as mediators in the relation between traumatic interpersonal events and posttraumatic stress disorder symptoms. *Journal of Social and Clinical Psychology, 24*(7), 1003–1029.

Orth, U., Berking, M., Walker, N., Meier, L. L., & Znoj, H. (2008). Forgiveness and psychological adjustment following interpersonal transgressions: A longitudinal analysis. *Journal of Research in Personality, 42*(2), 365–385. doi:http://dx.doi.org/10.1016/j.jrp.2007.07.003

**Paleari, F. G., Regalia, C., & Fincham, F. D. (2011). Inequity in forgiveness: Implications for personal and relational well-being. *Journal of Social and Clinical Psychology, 30*(3), 297–324. doi:10.1521/jscp.2011.30.3.297.

**Peterson, C., Park, N., & Seligman, M. E. P. (2006). Greater strengths of character and recovery from illness. *Journal of Positive Psychology, 1*(1), 17–26.

Reed, G. L., & Enright, R. D. (2006). The effects of forgiveness therapy on depression, anxiety, and posttraumatic stress for women after spousal emotional abuse. *Journal of Consulting and Clinical Psychology, 74*(5), 920–929.

**Rhode-Brown, J., & Rudestam, K. E. (2011). The role of forgiveness in divorce adjustment and the impact of affect. *Journal of Divorce & Remarriage, 52*(2), 109–124.

Riek, B. M. (2010). Transgressions, guilt, and forgiveness: A model of seeking forgiveness. *Journal of Psychology and Theology, 38*(4), 246–254.

*Rippentrop, A. E., Altmaier, E. M., Chen, J. J., Found, E. M., & Keffala, V. J. (2005). The relationship between religion/spirituality and physical health, mental health, and pain in a chronic pain population. *Pain, 116*(3), 311–321.

*Romero, C., Kalidas, M., Elledge, R., Chang, J., Liscum, K. R., & Friedman, L. C. (2006). Self-forgiveness, spirituality, and psychological adjustment in women with breast cancer. *Journal of Behavioral Medicine, 29*(1), 29–36.

**Rye, M. S., Folck, C. D., Heim, T. A., Olszewski, B. T., & Traina, E. (2004). Forgiveness of an ex-spouse: How does it relate to mental health following a divorce? *Journal of Divorce & Remarriage, 41*(3–4), 31–51. doi:10.1300/J087v41n03_02.

**Sandage, S. J., & Jankowski, P. J. (2010). Forgiveness, spiritual instability, mental health symptoms, and well-being: Mediator effects of differentiation of self. *Psychology of Religion and Spirituality, 2*(3), 168–180.

*Sandage, S. J., Worthington, E. L., Jr., Hight, T. L., & Berry, J. W. (2000). Seeking forgiveness: Theoretical context and an initial empirical study. *Journal of Psychology and Theology, 28*, 21–35.

**Stoia-Caraballo, R., Rye, M. S., Pan, W., Brown Kirschman, K. J., Lutz-Zois, C., & Lyons, A. M. (2008). Negative affect and anger rumination as mediators between forgiveness and sleep quality. *Journal of Behavioral Medicine, 31*, 478–488.

*Strelan, P., Acton, C., & Patrick, K. (2009). Disappointment with God and well-being: The mediating influence of relationship quality and dispositional forgivingness. *Counseling and Values, 53*(3), 202–213.

Strelan, P., & Covic, T. (2006). A review of forgiveness process models and a coping framework to guide future research. *Journal of Social and Clinical Psychology, 25*(10), 1059–1085. doi:10.1521/jscp.2006.25.10.1059.

**Suchday, S., Friedberg, J. P., & Almeida, M. (2006). Forgiveness and rumination: A cross-cultural perspective comparing India and the US. *Stress and Health, 22*, 81–89. doi:10.1002/smi.1082.

*Toussaint, L., & Friedman, P. (2009). Forgiveness, gratitude, and well-being: The mediating role of affect and beliefs. *Journal of Happiness Studies, 10*(6), 635–654.

*Toussaint, L., Owen, A. D., & Cheadle, A. (2012). Forgive to live: Forgiveness, health, and longevity. *Journal of Behavioral Medicine, 35*(4), 375–386.

Toussaint, L., & Webb, J. R. (2005). Theoretical and empirical connections between forgiveness, mental health, and well-being. In E. L. Worthington (Ed.), *Handbook of forgiveness* (pp. 349–362). New York, NY: Brunner-Routledge.

Toussaint, L., Williams, D. R., Musick, M. A., & Everson, S. A. (2001). Forgiveness and health: Age differences in a U.S. probability sample. *Journal of Adult Development, 8*(4), 249–257. doi:10.1023/A:1011394629736.

*Toussaint, L., Williams, D. R., Musick, M. A., & Everson-Rose, S. A. (2008a). The association of forgiveness and 12-month prevalence of major depressive episode: Gender differences in a probability sample of U.S. adults. *Mental Health, Religion & Culture, 11*(5), 485–500.

*Toussaint, L., Williams, D. R., Musick, M. A., & Everson-Rose, S. A. (2008b). Why forgiveness may protect against depression: Hopelessness as an explanatory mechanism. *Personality and Mental Health, 2*(2), 89–103.

Toussaint, L. L., & Williams, D. R. (2008). National survey results for protestant, catholic, and nonreligious experiences of seeking forgiveness and of forgiveness of self, of others, and by God. *Journal of Psychology and Christianity, 27*(2), 120–130.

**Tse, W. S., & Yip, T. H. J. (2009). Relationship among dispositional forgiveness of others, interpersonal adjustment and psychological well-being: Implication for interpersonal theory of depression. *Personality and Individual Differences, 46*, 365–368.

**Unterrainer, H., Ladenhauf, K. H., Moazedi, M. L., Wallner-Liebmann, S., & Fink, A. (2010). Dimensions of religious/spiritual well-being and their relation to personality and psychological well-being. *Personality and Individual Differences, 49*(3), 192–197. doi:10.1016/j.paid.2010.03.032.

Wade, N. G., Hoyt, W. T., Kidwell, J. E. M., & Worthington, E. L. (2014). Efficacy of psychotherapeutic interventions to promote forgiveness: A meta-analysis. *Journal of Consulting and Clinical Psychology, 82*, 154–170.

**Watson, M. J., Lydecker, J. A., Jobe, R. L., Enright, R. D., Gartner, A., Mazzeo, S. E., et al. (2011). Self-forgiveness in anorexia nervosa and bulimia nervosa. *Eating Disorders: The Journal of Treatment & Prevention, 20*(1), 31–41.

**Webb, J. R., Robinson, E. A. R., & Brower, K. J. (2009). Forgiveness and mental health among people entering outpatient treatment with alcohol problems. *Alcoholism Treatment Quarterly, 27*(4), 368–388. doi:10.1080/07347320903209822.

**Webb, J. R., Robinson, E. A. R., & Brower, K. J. (2011). Mental health, not social support, mediates the forgiveness-alcohol outcome relationship. *Psychology of Addictive Behaviors, 25*(3), 462–473.

**Webb, J. R., Robinson, E. A., Brower, K. J., & Zucker, R. A. (2006). Forgiveness and alcohol problems among people entering substance abuse treatment. *Journal of Addictive Diseases, 25*(3), 55–67.

*Webb, J. R., Toussaint, L., Kalpakjian, C. Z., & Tate, D. G. (2010). Forgiveness and health-related outcomes among people with spinal cord injury. *Disability and Rehabilitation, 32*(5), 360–366.

*Witvliet, C. V. O., Phipps, K. A., Feldman, M. E., & Beckham, J. C. (2004). Posttraumatic mental and physical health correlates of forgiveness and religious coping in military veterans. *Journal of Traumatic Stress, 17*(3), 269–273.

Worthington, E. L., Jr. (2006). *Forgiveness and reconciliation: Theory and application*. New York, NY: Brunner-Routledge.

Worthington, E. L., Jr. (2013). *Moving forward: Six steps to forgiving yourself and breaking free from the past*. Colorado Springs, CO: WaterBrook Multnomah.

Worthington, E. L., Jr., Hook, J. N., Utsey, S. O., Williams, J. K., & Neil, R. L. (2007). *Decisional and emotional forgiveness*. Washington, DC: International Positive Psychology Summit.

Worthington, E. L., Jr., & Langberg, D. (2012). Self-forgiveness in treating complex trauma and moral injury in present and former soldiers. *Journal of Psychology and Theology, 40*, 274–288.

Worthington, E. L., Jr., & Scherer, M. (2004). Forgiveness is an emotion-focused coping strategy that can reduce health risks and promote health resilience: Theory, review, and hypotheses. *Psychology & Health, 19*(3), 385–405.

Worthington, E. L., Jr., Witvliet, C. V. O., Pietrini, P., & Miller, A. J. (2007). Forgiveness, health, and well-being: A review of evidence for emotional versus decisional forgiveness, dispositional forgivingness, and reduced unforgiveness. *Journal of Behavioral Medicine, 30*(4), 291–302.

*Ysseldyk, R., Matheson, K., & Anisman, H. (2007). Rumination: Bridging a gap between forgivingness, vengefulness, and psychological health. *Personality and Individual Differences, 42*, 1573–1584.

Chapter 7
Forgiveness and Physical Health in Healthy Populations

Alyssa C.D. Cheadle and Loren L. Toussaint

Forgiveness occurs when a person lets go of negative emotions, thoughts, or behaviors about a transgression or a transgressor and attempts to develop a response of kindness, generosity, or compassion (Enright & Fitzgibbons, 2000; Enright, Freedman, & Rique, 1998). Over the last 30 years, significant research has linked forgiveness and related constructs to physical health.

Various types of forgiveness and related constructs have been studied to assess their unique associations with physical health including unforgiveness. Whereas forgiveness is letting go of negative and embracing of positive thoughts and behaviors, unforgivingness has been conceptualized as a response toward a transgressor consisting of multiple negative emotions that could include hatred, anger, fear, hostility, and resentment (Worthington, Sandage, & Berry, 2000; Worthington & Wade, 1999). Though forgiveness and unforgiveness are related, they are conceptually distinct.

Both forgiveness and unforgiveness can be further categorized by when forgiving occurs and who is being forgiven by whom. Forgiveness and unforgiveness may refer to responses to specific offenses which is called state forgiveness or state unforgiveness. More commonly studied is the tendency to be forgiving or unforgiving, called trait or dispositional forgivingness or unforgivingness. Furthermore, forgiveness of a specific offense may be conditional or unconditional. Conditional forgiveness of others is characterized by requirements made of the transgressor by the victim before forgiveness is granted; these requirements may be an apology, act of contrition, display of remorse, etc. (Merolla, 2008; Walrond-Skinner, 1998).

A.C.D. Cheadle, M.A., MTS (✉)
Department of Psychology, University of California, Los Angeles, CA 90095, USA
e-mail: cheadle@ucla.edu

L.L. Toussaint, Ph.D. (✉)
Department of Psychology, Luther College, Decorah, IA, USA
e-mail: touslo01@luther.edu

L.L. Toussaint et al. (eds.), *Forgiveness and Health*,
DOI 10.1007/978-94-017-9993-5_7

In addition to state and trait forgivingness and unforgivingness and conditional forgiveness, forgiveness and unforgiveness can be characterized by who is doing the forgiving and who is being forgiven.

Though much research has focused on forgiveness of others or the tendency to forgive others, many studies have also examined forgiveness of the self and feeling forgiven by God. Whereas forgivingness and unforgivingness of others are inherently experiences and traits of victims of transgressions, forgivingness of the self and feeling forgiven by God are experiences of the transgressor. Thus, forgivingness of others and forgivingness of the self or forgiveness by God likely differ in the feelings that accompany or motivate these states and traits. Forgiveness [and unforgiveness] of others occurs because one has been transgressed against and is likely accompanied or motivated by feelings of hurt, anger, and resentment, among others. Forgiveness of the self or by God occurs, or is called for, because one has transgressed and is likely to be accompanied or motivated by feelings of guilt, regret, and shame (Worthington, 2013; Worthington & Langberg, 2012). Forgiveness of the self is often assessed as a trait, or the tendency to forgive the self. Similarly, feeling forgiven by God is often assessed as the tendency to feel forgiven by God. Much extant research considers multiple forgiveness-related constructs in one study. Though these constructs are related, they are distinct and thus should be hypothesized to be associated with physical health in unique ways or via unique pathways. Other researchers have investigated the health associations of constructs related to forgivingness, like anger and hostility, and made theoretical arguments about the implications of these findings for the forgivingness-health relationship (e.g. Hernandez, Larkin, & Whited, 2009; see also Harris & Thoresen, 2005).

Theoretical Models of Associations of Forgivingness and Health

Forgivingness is theorized to be related to health for a number of reasons. Most significantly, forgivingness is hypothesized to promote health by reducing stress (Strelan & Covic, 2006; Worthington & Scherer, 2004). Unforgivingness could be expected to be related to poor health because it causes interpersonal stress as well as stress through related negative emotions like hostility, anger, and rumination (Harris & Thoresen, 2005). Interpersonal transgressions are social stressors. Transgressions engender negative emotions like anger, hostility, and unforgiveness. Hostility has been associated with a myriad of poor health outcomes including coronary heart disease and mortality (Miller, Smith, Turner, Guijarro, & Hallet, 1996). Unforgiveness itself is hypothesized to contribute to negative physiological states in the short term and some empirical evidence supports this (see Worthington & Scherer, 2004; see also Chap. 5, in this volume).

The way in which unforgiveness functions as a stressor likely depends on the characteristics of the unforgiveness. Unforgiving emotions that are triggered by interpersonal transgressions are likely to be intermittent stressors (Harris & Thoresen, 2005; Worthington, 2006). If one is repeatedly unforgiving in response to interpersonal transgressions, this may have a cumulative negative effect on health outcomes. However, even repeatedly unforgiving individuals are not likely to be unforgiving at every opportunity. Furthermore, social situations that occasion forgiveness or unforgiveness are not continually occurring. Thus, it is unlikely that unforgivingness would cause stress at the level of chronicity thought to lead to significant, long-term health consequences. However, if unforgiveness becomes a pattern of thought, like rumination, it may constantly generate physiological reactivity which may have negative consequences for health in the long term (Brosschot, Gerin, & Thayer, 2006). Furthermore, unforgiveness may function as a stress generator in social contexts, leading to social situations that become chronically stressful (see Hammen, 2006 for a conceptual review of stress generation within the context of depression). A more nuanced theoretical approach to the conceptualization of forgiveness and unforgiveness within the stress and coping framework and corresponding empirical research is warranted. Other theories and pathways of the forgivingness-health association have been proposed and are reviewed in Chap. 3, in this volume.

Acts of forgiveness may reduce the negative emotions and/or reduce the negative effects associated with the social stress of unforgiveness. To the extent it does so, forgivingness could prevent or assuage the expected negative health consequences of stress. However, forgiveness is not the only way to reduce unforgiveness. Unforgiveness can be reduced by receiving an apology, experiencing restitution or justice, distracting oneself from thoughts about the transgression, or accepting that the transgression occurred and moving on, among other strategies (see Worthington, 2001). Because unforgiveness can be reduced by experiences other than forgiveness, it is clear that unforgiveness and forgiveness are not opposites, but are conceptually distinct constructs.

The emotional replacement hypothesis of forgiveness suggests that emotional forgiveness occurs when unforgiveness and negative emotions associated with it are replaced by positive, prosocial emotions like empathy, compassion, and love (Worthington, 2006; Worthington & Wade, 1999). Thus, forgiveness would not be expected to have its sole benefit through reducing unforgiveness. It would have the additional benefits associated with the positive emotions that replace unforgiveness. This is similar to arguments made by positive psychologists about positive emotions in general: they have benefits above and beyond their displacement of, or simply the lack of, negative emotions (Lyubomirsky, King, & Diener, 2005). Furthermore, the positive emotions that commonly replace unforgiveness are hypothesized to have health benefits (Fredrickson, 2001). Positive affect, composed of many different positive emotions, has been associated with beneficial immune and neuroendocrine functioning as well as longevity and self-reports of global health, physical symptoms, and visits to health centers (Fredrickson & Losada, 2005; Lyubomirsky et al., 2005). It could be hypothesized that forgiveness would be associated with similar health outcomes because it facilitates these positive emotions. Furthermore, forgiveness is a prosocial act that likely facilitates greater social support above and beyond simply the lack of unforgiveness in a social setting (Fredrickson, 2001). Social support is known to have associations with positive health (see Uchino, 2009 for a review). Thus, the associations of forgiveness and health would be hypothesized to be distinct from the associations of health to other strategies that simply reduce unforgiveness as well as distinct from simply the lack of the negative effects of unforgiveness.

The negative health effects of unforgivingness and related constructs have received much more research attention than the direct, positive health effects of forgivingness. This may reflect differences in the chronology or strength of these effects (Berry & Worthington, 2001) or simply the historical focus on negative emotions in the social sciences (Seligman & Csikszentmihalyi, 2000). However, in the last 10 years, more research has begun to show that forgiveness is associated with better health.

Physical health can be conceptualized and measured in multiple ways as well. While much early research focused on associations of forgivingness and general physical health as measured by self-rated health, other research has assessed associations between forgivingness and symptomatic markers of physical health. In the early 2000s, many researchers began to study associations of forgivingness and physiological and biological markers of health and disease. Other researchers have focused on the associations of forgivingness to health outcomes including mortality and disease. The results of this research suggest that, in general, forgivingness is related to positive physical health and unforgivingness is related to poor health.

While much of this research has been conducted with clinical populations or people suffering from a common medical condition, it is important to consider forgivingness among healthy populations because one's health status may affect the association of forgivingness to health in a number of ways. Firstly, in a healthy population, forgivingness may be hypothesized to relate to indicators of general health rather than disease-specific markers and outcomes. Furthermore, the health correlates and consequences may be hypothesized to differ in strength in persons who are generally healthy rather than compromised. Relatedly, the time frame of health consequences of forgivingness and unforgivingness may be longer in healthy individuals than in individuals who are already experiencing poor health. Secondly, health status may affect the importance of forgiveness. On one hand, healthy persons may have access to more health-promoting resources, and thus, forgivingness may play a smaller role in their well-being. Alternatively, healthy persons may have more social contact, and thus, have greater need or opportunity for forgivingness. For these reasons, it is important to consider findings on associations of forgiveness and related constructs to health among healthy populations separate from disease populations.

Empirical Findings of Associations of Forgivingness, Unforgivingness, and Health

As forgivingness and unforgivingness are conceptually distinct, it is expected that these constructs are differentially associated with health. Similarly, forgivingness with different actors, targets, or conditional status would be expected to be differentially associated with health. Extant research provides some evidence of differential associations. Because researchers often consider many types of forgiveness in one study without explicit hypotheses for each construct, it can be difficult to untangle these differential associations. Below, findings on different types of forgivingness in the same studies are discussed together, though, in general, the discussions of forgivingness and unforgivingness are separate.

Forgivingness and Self-Rated Physical Health Many studies have linked forgivingness to self-rated health. Often, self-rated health is assessed with a single measure that simply asks respondents to rate their current overall physical health. Though this measure may seem crude, evidence suggests that it is strongly associated with objective measures of health (Idler, 1992; Idler & Benyamini, 1997). In a large telephone study of 1,423 adult respondents, Toussaint and colleagues (2001) assessed associations of forgivingness of others and unforgivingness of self to self-rated health. They found that the tendency to forgive others was related to better self-reported physical health for older adults (65 years of age and older). The tendency to be less unforgiving of the self was related to better self-rated health for young and middle age adults (18–44, 45–64 years of age respectively; Toussaint, Williams, Musick, & Everson, 2001).

Studies of associations between forgivingness and self-rated health have also been assessed with more sophisticated measures of self-reports of aspects of physical health. In a laboratory study of 39 undergraduates, Berry and Worthington (2001) examined personality traits associated with both forgivingness and unforgivingness. Using an imagery task, they elicited stress responses specific to the participants' romantic relationships. Physical health was measured by the SF-36 Health Survey which assesses four physical health domains: physical functioning, bodily pain, role limitations due to physical health, and general health. They found that neither trait forgivingness nor transgression-specific forgiveness were related to physical health. However, in a regression analysis of these data, a composite of both forgivingness scales and a trait anger scale was significantly associated with physical health status, suggesting that a combination of qualities of forgivingness are associated with physical health. In contrast, in another small study of undergraduates, researchers found that the tendency to forgive others did not significantly predict perceived physical health. In contrast, the tendency to forgive the self uniquely predicted almost seven percent of perceived physical health measured by the Medical Outcomes Study Short Form (Wilson, Milosevic, Carroll, Hart, & Hibbard, 2008). Likewise, a recent study of potential mediators of the forgivingness-health link failed to find a direct relationship between trait forgivingness and physical health, as measured by the

SF-36 Health Survey, in a large sample of 623 undergraduates (Green, Decourville, & Sadava, 2013).

Associations of self-rated health and forgivingness may be dependent on the measure of physical health used. Single item ratings are reliably associated with aspects of forgivingness while more detailed measures of self-reports of aspects of physical health are not reliably related to forgivingness. To some extent measurement may be confounded with quality of sample, however, so a word of caution is in order here. Forgivingness and health associations vary by both measurement approach and sample characteristics (i.e., student vs. general population). Nonetheless, another line of research indicates that forgivingness is consistently related to a different type of self-report measure of health: physical health symptoms.

Forgivingness and Physical Health Symptoms Going beyond self-ratings of physical health, some research has linked forgivingness to symptomatic markers of physical health ranging from checklists of health symptoms to medication use. Many studies have used multiple symptomatic markers and thus evidence will be presented by study rather than by marker.

A number of these studies have been conducted by Kathleen Lawler-Row and her colleagues. In a laboratory study of 108 undergraduates, Lawler and colleagues (2003) examined associations of trait forgivingness and state forgiveness and self-reported illness symptoms. They found that self-reports of illness symptoms were negatively correlated with state forgiveness. Furthermore, path analysis examining associations of trait forgivingness and state forgiveness, stress, and health suggested that forgivingness has an indirect effect on health by reducing perceived stress. In this study, self-reports of illness were measured by items of the Cohen-Hoberman Physical Symptoms (CHIPS) checklist that assessed physical health (excluding items on the checklist that assess psychological symptoms of distress). In two separate samples, Lawler and colleagues found that CHIPS scores were significantly correlated with actual visits to the student health clinic (Lawler et al., 2003). Building on these findings, a 2008 study by Lawler-Row and colleagues examined associations of trait forgivingness and state forgiveness and physiological markers as well as symptomatic markers of physical health in a laboratory study of 114 undergraduates. Findings on symptomatic markers are reviewed here. As part of the paradigm, participants were interviewed about a time they were upset by their parents. In this sample, individuals who described an event that they struggled to forgive had more physical symptoms. Additionally, researchers found that trait forgivingness was related to using fewer medications, and less alcohol (for a full review of associations between forgiveness and substance use, see Chap. 10, in this volume). State forgiveness was significantly associated with endorsing fewer physical symptoms experienced in the past month on the CHIPS scale (Lawler-Row, Karremans, Scott, Edlis-Matityahou, & Edwards, 2008). In a similar laboratory study of 81 community adults (27–82 years of age) by the same research team, researchers found that both state forgiveness and trait forgivingness were negatively correlated with physical symptoms experienced in the past month and with medication use, poor sleep quality, fatigue, and somatic complaints measured by the Recovery Stress Questionnaire (REST-Q; Lawler et al., 2005).

In a series of studies testing the hypothesis that forgivingness mediates the religion-health relationship, Lawler-Row (2010) found the following support for the forgivingness-physical health symptoms connection: In a study of 605 older adults (50–92 years of age) self-reported history of the tendency to forgive others was related to fewer physical symptoms experienced in the past month on the CHIPS scale. History of tendency to forgive the self was also inversely related to this measure of physical symptoms. In a study of 253 older adults (52–87 years of age), trait forgivingness was related to experiencing fewer somatic illness symptoms. In a study of 80 middle-aged persons (27–60 years of age), state forgiveness of a particular transgression and transgressor was related to physical symptoms experienced in the last month on the CHIPS scale, medication use, and sleep quality. Trait forgivingness was also related to sleep quality (Lawler-Row, 2010).

The substantial research by Lawler-Row and colleagues indicates that there are robust links between both state forgiveness and trait forgivingness of others, as well as trait forgiveness of the self, and physical health as measured by illness symptoms and behaviors (i.e. medication use). However, some evidence does not support this association for unforgivingness. In a cross-sectional questionnaire study of 324 undergraduates, Maltby and colleagues (2001) found that failure to forgive others as well as failure to forgive oneself were not associated with somatic symptoms as measured by the General Health Questionnaire-28 (GHQ; Maltby, Macaskill, & Day, 2001). The authors of this study did not suggest interpretations of this unexpected finding. However, the items on the General Health Questionnaire pertaining to physical symptoms are fewer than on the CHIPS checklist and they pertain mostly to somatic symptoms that might accompany psychological distress (Goldberg & Hillier, 1979). It may be that some of the physical symptoms represented on the CHIPS are more reliably associated with forgivingness and are responsible for observed relationships.

Forgivingness and Somatic Symptoms A large body of research has assessed links between forgivingness and mental health. This research is reviewed in Chap. 6, in this volume. Some research has assessed associations of forgivingness to somatic symptoms of poor mental health and depression. These somatic symptoms are at the intersection of mental and physical health (Webb, Toussaint, & Conway-Williams, 2012). Items measuring somatic symptoms may include fatigue and sleep issues and poor appetite. As these symptoms are measures of physical health as well, exemplary findings are reviewed here. In a study of over a thousand African American and White American older adults from the Medicare Beneficiary Eligibility List, Krause and Ellison (2003) found that the tendency to forgive others was associated with fewer somatic symptoms of depression including difficulty sleeping, poor appetite, and little energy as measured by the Center for Epidemiologic Studies-Depression scale. Belief in forgiveness by God was not significantly associated with these somatic symptoms. Conditional forgivingness, which may functionally represent unforgivingness, was associated with more somatic symptoms (Krause & Ellison, 2003).

Overall, this research shows that forgivingness is related to symptomatic markers of physical health including medication use, somatic symptoms of depression like fatigue and appetite, sleep quality, and endorsement of a variety of symptoms of poor health in multiple domains. It could be hypothesized that these symptoms are representative of or lead to disease.

A robust program of research conducted by a number of researchers has sought to connect forgivingness to biomarkers associated with health and disease. Forgivingness has been related to markers of cardiovascular functioning, immune functioning, and endocrine functioning. This research has been conducted with healthy samples as well as clinical and disease samples. For a full review of this research, see Chap. 5, in this volume.

Unforgivingness and Physical Health To better understand the associations of forgivingness and physical health, some researchers have investigated links between forgivingness and health outcomes that are more long-term than physiological markers. This research is based on the theoretical assertion that effects of stress and thus, the stress of unforgivingness, may take years to accumulate, showing up as chronic disease conditions that ultimately lead to death.

Two studies have assessed unforgiveness and cross-sectional indicators of physical health. A study by Toussaint and Cheadle (2010) investigated associations between unforgivingness and physical health in a sample of 1,024 older adults (over 66 years of age) drawn from the Centers for Medicare and Medicaid Services Beneficiary Eligibility List. We found that in this sample, the tendency to be unforgiving of others was negatively associated with self-rated physical health. However, as reviewed earlier, Maltby and colleagues (2001) found that failure to forgive others as well as failure to forgive oneself were not associated with the physical health indicator of somatic symptoms (Maltby et al., 2001).

Two studies have assessed associations of unforgiveness and long term health outcomes. One study has focused on cardiovascular health outcomes. In a study using data from the National Epidemiological Survey on Alcohol and Related Conditions (NESARC), a nationally representative sample of 49,093 U.S. adults, Toussaint and Cheadle (2009) investigated associations of unforgivingness and cardiovascular incidents. We found that a tendency to experience unforgivingness was related to a significantly greater likelihood of experiencing a cardiovascular incident, including arteriosclerosis, hypertension, angina pectoris (chest pain), tachycardia, and heart attack within the past year. Specifically, those who reported both that there are many people they cannot forgive and that it generally takes them a long time to forgive were 2.12 times more likely to report having experienced a cardiovascular incident within the past year compared to those who reported neither problem with forgiveness. Similarly, those who reported only that there are many people that they cannot forgive were 1.94 times more likely, and those who reported only that it takes them a long time to forgive were 1.51 times more likely to have experienced a cardiovascular incident in the past year. Odds were similar, though slightly lower, for physician-diagnosed cardiovascular disease incidents. These relationships remained robust after controlling for sociodemographic variables, anger, and major depression (Toussaint & Cheadle, 2009). Though much research has connected forgivingness and cardiovascular functioning (see Chap. 5, in this volume), this was the first study to link unforgivingness to chronic cardiovascular health conditions.

Another study by the same research team assessed associations between forgivingness and mortality (Toussaint, Owen, & Cheadle, 2012). As forgivingness is hypothesized to have cumulative effects on health, it was hypothesized that forgivingness would be related to chronic health conditions, and ultimately, mortality. In a sample of 1,232 Christian and non-religious older adults from the Religion, Aging, and Health longitudinal survey, seven types of forgiveness were assessed: unforgivingness of others, conditional and unconditional forgivingness of others, feeling forgiven by others, forgivingness of self, and believing in conditional and unconditional forgiveness from God. We found that conditional forgivingness of others and belief in God's unconditional forgiveness predicted greater mortality risk over a 12-month period. After controlling for sociodemographic variables, religious factors, and health behaviors, only conditional forgivingness of others remained significant. Analyses suggested that this association was mediated by physical health status, though not by psychological variables including depressive affect, depressive somatic symptoms, life satisfaction, or perceived control nor by organizational religiousness, current smoking, or drinking behaviors. Conditional forgivingness is thought to be related to poor health because requiring acts from another person likely constrains the instances of forgiveness an individual experiences. Thus, the association of conditional forgivingness to poor health may reflect the observed link between unforgivingness and poor health. This hypothesis is supported by the Krause and Ellison (2003) finding that conditional forgiveness was associated with more somatic symptoms of depression among older adults.

The study also revealed an intriguing association of believing in God's unconditional forgivingness and poor health, but this could reflect poor health behaviors, passivity, and less engagement in interpersonal forgivingness behavior, all of which are linked to poor health. Furthermore, the association was not robust to the effects of socio-demographic, religious, or health behavior controls. This study was the first to link unforgivingness to mortality outcomes.

Summary of Empirical Research A large body of research provides evidence that various types of forgivingness are related to aspects of physical health including self-rated general health, symptomatic measures of physical health, and disease and mortality outcomes. The majority of findings indicate that forgivingness is generally related to better physical health. In particular, much research has found associations between state forgiveness and trait forgivingness of others and better physical health (Lawler et al., 2003; Lawler-Row, 2010; Lawler-Row et al., 2008). Much of the research using measures of state forgiveness and trait forgivingness have examined associations with self-rated physical health, but not long-term health outcomes.

While many measures of physical symptoms have been found to be linked to state forgiveness and trait forgivingness, including the CHIPS checklist of physical symptoms, somatic symptoms, medication use, and sleep/fatigue, it is interesting to note that survey measures of physical health have not been found to be associated with forgivingness, including the physical health components of the SF-36 survey, a widely used instrument (Berry & Worthington, 2001; Green et al., 2013). As with the General Health Questionnaire discussed above, the SF-36 contains fewer items that directly assess physical symptoms. The physical components of the SF-36 are more focused on physical functioning and general health, though it does also assess pain (Ware, Snow, Kosinski, & Gandek, 1993). This pattern of association might suggest that state forgiveness and trait forgivingness are related to reports of physical symptoms more so than general self-rated health. However, much of the research linking trait forgivingness and state forgiveness to physical symptoms has been conducted by one research team. Findings should be replicated by others before conclusions are drawn.

In addition to state forgiveness and trait forgivingness generally, other aspects of forgiveness appear to be importantly associated with physical health. Research suggests that both the tendency to forgive others and the tendency to forgive the self are related to physical health as measured by single item self-ratings, self-ratings of symptoms, and somatic symptoms of illness. The tendency to forgive others may be related to health because it contributes to less stressful social relationships and promotes social support (McCullough, 2000). The tendency to forgive the self may be related to health because it reduces the stress of rumination, guilt, or shame (Thoresen, Harris, & Luskin, 2000). Both types of forgivingness could benefit from additional longitudinal study. The only study identified that assessed the associations of the tendency to forgive the self and the tendency to forgive of others to a cumulative health outcome did not find significant relationships between these types of forgivingness and mortality (Toussaint et al., 2012). This is in contrast to findings for unforgivingness and suggests that the health benefits of forgivingness may not be as lasting or as severe as the negative health consequences of unforgiveness. However, much more research is needed to explore these differential associations.

Two constructs related to unforgivingness also have been shown to be linked to poor physical health. Conditional forgiveness of others is characterized by requirements made of the transgressor by the victim before forgiveness is granted. By requiring such acts, it is likely that fewer instances of forgiveness occur in these peoples' lives, thus, it would be expected that a tendency to conditional forgivingness would be associated with poorer health (Toussaint et al., 2012). Conditional forgivingness has been related to both greater short-term symptoms and a cumulative health outcome, greater risk of mortality. Unforgivingness has also been related to poor health including poor self-rated heath and incidents of cardiovascular disease. Both findings that conditional forgivingness and unforgivingness are related to worse cumulative health outcomes support the hypothesis that unforgivingness is generative of stress that has negative long-term health consequences.

Future Directions for Forgiveness-Physical Health Research

Despite the variety of findings reviewed, extant research on associations of forgiveness and health is limited. The theoretical foundations of research on forgivingness, unforgivingness, and health must be strengthened in order to generate quality research. Conceptualizations of unforgiveness as a stressor must be clarified and tested. The function of forgiveness as a strategy to reduce the stress of unforgiveness must be explicitly tested along with the possibility that forgivingness has health benefits above and beyond the amelioration of the stress of unforgiveness. In order to do this, studies will have to assess both forgivingness and unforgivingness (Worthington & Scherer, 2004). The field of forgiveness and health research would be greatly improved by rigorous testing of theory-driven hypotheses.

Additionally, much of the extant research has been conducted with undergraduate populations (Toussaint et al., 2001). While this research is valuable, if it is expected that the health effects of forgivingness and unforgivingness are cumulative and may take years to develop, it is important to investigate associations in older populations for whom unforgiving or forgiving tendencies have had time to have an impact.

Furthermore, we know very little about moderators of the forgivingness-health link. Many moderators have been proposed, however. Theory might suggest that if forgivingness functions to reduce stress, being forgiving would be more health promoting among those experiencing greater stress or greater stress due to unforgivingness and hostility. Relatedly, as forgivingness may reduce social stress or promote social relationships, theory would suggest that forgivingness might be more important and more beneficial for physical health among individuals who greatly value social relationships. Furthermore, the impact of forgivingness may differ by type of relationship. If an individual is more forgiving of close others, that may be more beneficial than being more forgiving of others. Additionally, forgiving a person with whom one continues to have an active relationship may have different associations with health than forgiving a person with whom one does not have ongoing relationship. Lastly, for many, forgiveness is a religious or spiritual value or act. Forgivingness may have a differential association with physical health depending on its importance and the forgiver's overall religious or spiritual worldview. However, forgivingness is generally thought to be valued by and accessible to both secular and religious persons, so the associations may not differ. These and other possible moderating variables should be explored.

Much of the research on forgivingness and health hypothesizes that forgivingness is beneficial for health. However, it has also been suggested that costs of forgivingness should be explored. Forgivingness may open the door to further offense. Specifically, forgivingness may have costs to physical health if acts of forgiveness contribute to motivations to maintain relationships that are physically abusive. McNulty (2011) has conducted a number of studies on this topic. In a longitudinal study of newlywed couples, he found a positive association between spouses' reports of forgiveness of their partners and partners' reports of psychological and physical aggression (McNulty, 2011). However, other research suggests that acts of forgiveness do not increase the likelihood of future transgressions in general (Wallace, Exline, & Baumeister, 2008). More study is needed to explore the potential costs of forgivingness for physical health.

Extant research is also limited in its conceptualization of health. Studies have begun to move beyond single item measures of self-rated health, but research using physiological markers of health and disease outcomes is limited. As Worthington and colleagues advocated in 2007, more prospective studies documenting associations of forgivingness and incidence of disease must be conducted (Worthington, Witvliet, Pietrini, & Miller, 2007). As forgivingness and unforgivingness are expected to have effects through long-term stress processes, diseases of aging are prime candidates for research. Alternatively, studies that establish clear physiological response patterns associated with forgivingness and unforgivingness could be conducted to better understand how forgivingness might have cumulative effects on health. In Toussaint and colleagues', (2012) study on forgivingness and mortality, it was found that the association between conditional forgivingness and mortality was mediated by physical health. Thus, it may be that the effects of forgivingness on psychophysiology offer protection against disease and mortality.

Implications of the Forgivingness-Physical Health Connection

Forgiveness is of importance for health promotion. The evidence suggests that health could be promoted both by increasing forgivingness and decreasing unforgivingness. Forgivingness can be cultivated and taught. Forgivingness interventions have been shown to be effective in increasing forgivingness and decreasing unforgivingness in many populations. This research is reviewed in Chap. 18, in this volume. If forgiveness interventions increase forgivingness and decrease unforgivingness, they may also have an impact on physical health. However, given the hypothesized cumulative lifetime health effects of forgivingness, it is important that forgivingness skills be cultivated early. Forgivingness is often taught in the context of interventions with populations at risk for unforgivingness or for poor health or in psychotherapy with individuals who have similar risk profiles or who are actively experiencing extreme unforgivingness. Forgivingness must be promoted among the general population. Teaching forgivingness to children may be especially advantageous because the benefits will have a larger impact over the life course. Forgivingness interventions have been used among adolescents with mixed results; interventions and curricula likely need to be specially tailored to children and adolescents to be effective (Wade, Worthington, & Meyer, 2005).

While so many health promoting resources are available disproportionately to those with greater financial resources, forgivingness is available to all persons regardless of income status. There is substantial interest in identifying resources of this type among health psychologists and other researchers. Resources that can be cultivated by individuals regardless of status may play an important role in resilience. Conceptualizations vary, but resilience can be defined as the capacity, originating from individual traits and resources, to maintain health in the context of stress (Dunkel Schetter & Dolbier, 2011). If forgivingness is equally available to all persons, it may be an especially important resource for health among persons of low socioeconomic status for whom other health promoting resources are less accessible. Indeed, early research in this area is revealing intriguing findings in this regard (see Chap. 13; McFarland, Smith, Toussaint, & Thomas, 2012).

In addition to the importance of forgivingness in the lives of individuals, the study of forgivingness is important for psychologists. It provides a model for how to study the associations of physical and mental health and other virtues, positive behaviors, and religious values or practices. Forgivingness researchers have employed multiple methodologies to study forgivingness's associations with and impacts on physical health including laboratory studies of physiological effects, randomly controlled intervention trials, and cross-sectional and longitudinal correlation studies of self-report data. Such a pluralistic methodological approach can provide a model of programmatic research for other positive values gaining attention like gratitude, humility, and wisdom. In addition, evidence from multiple methods clarifies the picture of the mechanisms of the forgivingness-health link, giving rise to multiple theories of how forgivingness impacts health. These theories may be applicable to other positive values and practices as well as religious and spiritual beliefs and behaviors. Researchers of positive phenomena and religious and spiritual phenomena might look to the example of forgivingness research to further their programs of study.

Conclusions

Forgivingness is hypothesized to reduce stress and thereby improve health; in contrast, unforgivingness is hypothesized to increase stress and contribute to poor health. Many studies provide support for a link between forgivingness and aspects of physical health including self-rated health and reports of physical health symptoms. Limited research has illustrated links between unforgivingness and long-term health outcomes including cardiovascular disease and mortality.

Research suggests that forgivingness is an important resource for improving physical health in healthy populations. Further research on the forgivingness-health connection should clarify these implications and identify when and for whom forgivingness may be most beneficial to physical health.

References

Berry, J. W., & Worthington, E. L., Jr. (2001). Forgivingness, relationship quality, stress while imagining relationship events, and physical and mental health. *Journal of Counseling Psychology, 48*(4), 447–455. doi:10.1037//0022-0167.48.4.447.

Brosschot, J. F., Gerin, W., & Thayer, J. F. (2006). The perseverative cognition hypothesis: A review of worry, prolonged stress-related physiological activation, and health. *Journal of Psychosomatic Research, 60*(2), 113–124. doi:10.1016/j.jpsychores.2005.06.074.

Dunkel Schetter, C., & Dolbier, C. (2011). Resilience in the context of chronic stress and health in adults. *Social and Personality Psychology Compass, 5*(9), 634–652. doi:10.1111/j.1751-9004.2011.00379.x.

Enright, R. D., & Fitzgibbons, R. P. (2000). *Helping clients forgive*. Washington, DC: American Psychological Association.

Enright, R. D., Freedman, S., & Rique, J. (1998). The psychology of interpersonal forgiveness. In R. D. Enright & J. North (Eds.), *Exploring forgiveness* (pp. 46–62). Madison, WI: University of Wisconsin Press.

Fredrickson, B. (2001). The role of positive emotions in positive psychology: The broaden-and-build theory of positive emotions. *American Psychologist, 56*(3), 218–226.

Fredrickson, B. L., & Losada, M. F. (2005). Positive affect and the complex dynamics of human flourishing. *American Psychologist, 60*(7), 678–686. doi:10.1037/0003-066X.60.7.678.

Goldberg, D. P., & Hillier, V. F. (1979). A scaled version of the General Health Questionnaire. *Psychological Medicine, 9*(1), 139–145.

Green, M., Decourville, N., & Sadava, S. (2013). Positive affect, negative affect, stress, and social support as mediators of the forgiveness-health relationship. *Journal of Social Psychology, 152*(13), 288–307.

Hammen, C. (2006). Stress generation in expression: Reflections on origins, research, and future directions. *Journal of Clinical Psychology, 62*(9), 1065–1082. doi:10.1002/jclp.

Harris, A. H. S., & Thoresen, C. E. (2005). Forgiveness, unforgiveness, health, and disease. In E. L. Worthington (Ed.), *The handbook of forgiveness* (pp. 321–334). New York, NY: Routledge.

Hernandez, D. H., Larkin, K. T., & Whited, M. C. (2009). Cardiovascular response to interpersonal provocation and mental arithmetic among high and low hostile young adult males. *Applied Psychophysiology and Biofeedback, 34*(1), 27–35. doi:10.1007/s10484-009-9076-3.

Idler, E. (1992). Self-assessed health and mortality: A review of studies. In S. Maes, H. Leventhal, & M. Johnston (Eds.), *International review of health psychology* (pp. 33–54). New York, NY: Wiley.

Idler, E., & Benyamini, Y. (1997). Self-rated health and mortality: A review of twenty-seven community studies. *Journal of Health and Social Behavior, 38*, 21–37.

Krause, N., & Ellison, C. G. (2003). Forgiveness by god, forgiveness of others, and psychological well-being in late life. *Journal for the Scientific Study of Religion, 42*(1), 77–94.

Lawler, K. A., Younger, J. W., Piferi, R. L., Billington, E., Jobe, R., Edmondson, K., & Jones, W. H. (2003). A change of heart: cardiovascular correlates of forgiveness in response to interpersonal conflict. *Journal of Behavioral Medicine, 26*(5), 373–93.

Lawler, K. A., Younger, J. W., Piferi, R. L., Jobe, R. L., Edmondson, K. A., & Jones, W. H. (2005). The unique effects of forgiveness on health: An exploration of pathways. *Journal of Behavioral Medicine, 28*(2), 157–167.

Lawler-Row, K. A. (2010). Forgiveness as a mediator of the religiosity—Health relationship. *Psychology of Religion and Spirituality, 2*(1), 1–16. doi:10.1037/a0017584.

Lawler-Row, K. A., Karremans, J. C., Scott, C., Edlis-Matityahou, M., & Edwards, L. (2008). Forgiveness, physiological reactivity and health: The role of anger. *International Journal of Psychophysiology, 68*(1), 51–58. doi:10.1016/j.ijpsycho.2008.01.001.

Lyubomirsky, S., King, L., & Diener, E. (2005). The benefits of frequent positive affect: Does happiness lead to success? *Psychological Bulletin, 131*(6), 803–855. doi:10.1037/0033-2909.131.6.803.

Maltby, J., Macaskill, A., & Day, L. (2001). Failure to forgive self and others: A replication and extension of the relationship between forgiveness, personality, social desirability and general health. *Personality and Individual Differences, 30*(5), 881–885. doi:10.1016/S0191-8869(00)00080-5.

McCullough, M. E. (2000). Forgiveness as human strength: Theory, measurement, and links to well-being. *Journal of Social and Clinical Psychology, 19*(1), 43–55. doi:10.1521/jscp.2000.19.1.43.

McFarland, M., Smith, C., Toussaint, L., & Thomas, P. (2012). The relationship between forgiveness of others and health: Do race and neighborhood matter? *Journal of Gerontology: Social Sciences, 67B*, 66–75. doi:10.1093/geronb/gbr121.

McNulty, J. K. (2011). The dark side of forgiveness: The tendency to forgive predicts continued psychological and physical aggression in marriage. *Personality and Social Psychology Bulletin, 37*(6), 770–783. doi:10.1177/0146167211407077.

Merolla, A. J. (2008). Communicating forgiveness in friendships and dating relationships. *Communication Studies, 59*(2), 114–131. doi:10.1080/10510970802062428.

Miller, T. Q., Smith, T. W., Turner, C. W., Guijarro, M. L., & Hallet, A. J. (1996). A meta-analytic review of research on hostility and physical health. *Psychological Bulletin, 119*(2), 322–348.

Seligman, M. E. P., & Csikszentmihalyi, M. (2000). Positive psychology: An introduction. *American Psychologist, 55*(1), 5–14. doi:10.1037//0003-066X.55.1.5.

Strelan, P., & Covic, T. (2006). A review of forgiveness process models and a coping framework to guide future research. *Journal of Social and Clinical Psychology, 25*(10), 1059–1085.

Thoresen, C. E., Harris, A. H. S., & Luskin, F. (2000). Forgiveness and health: An unanswered question. In M. E. McCullough & K. I. Pargament (Eds.), *Forgiveness: Theory, research, and practice* (pp. 254–280). New York, NY: Guilford Press.

Toussaint, L., & Cheadle, A. C. D. (2009). Unforgiveness and the broken heart: Unforgiving tendencies, problems due to unforgiveness, and 12-month prevalence of cardiovascular health conditions. In M. T. Evans & E. D. Walker (Eds.), *Religion and psychology*. New York, NY: Nova Publishers.

Toussaint, L., & Cheadle, A. C. D. (2010, April). Forgiveness and physical health in elderly adults: A prospective study [Abstract]. *Annals of Behavioral Medicine, 39*, 2010 Supplement (p. s149).

Toussaint, L. L., Williams, D. R., Musick, M. A., & Everson, S. A. (2001). Forgiveness and health: Age differences in a U. S. probability sample. *Journal of Adult Development, 8*(4), 249–257.

Toussaint, L. L., Owen, A. D., & Cheadle, A. (2012). Forgive to live: Forgiveness, health, and longevity. *Journal of Behavioral Medicine, 35*(4), 375–386.

Uchino, B. N. (2009). Understanding the links between social support and physical health: A life-span perspective with emphasis on the separability of perceived and received support. *Perspectives on Psychological Science, 4*(3), 236–255. doi:10.1111/j.1745-6924.2009.01122.x.

Van Oyen Witvliet, C. (2001). Forgiveness and health: Review and reflections on a matter of faith, feelings, and physiology. *Journal of Psychology and Theology, 29*(3), 212–224.

Wade, N. G., Worthington, E. L., Jr., & Meyer, J. E. (2005). But do they really work? A meta-analysis of group interventions to promote forgiveness. In E. L. Worthington Jr. (Ed.), *Handbook of forgiveness* (pp. 423–439). New York, NY: Brunner-Routledge.

Wallace, H. M., Exline, J. J., & Baumeister, R. F. (2008). Interpersonal consequences of forgiveness: Does forgiveness deter or encourage repeat offenses? *Journal of Experimental Social Psychology, 44*(2), 453–460. doi:10.1016/j.jesp.2007.02.012.

Walrond-Skinner, S. (1998). The function and role of forgiveness in working with couples and families: Clearing the ground. *Journal of Family Therapy, 20*(1), 3–20. doi:10.1111/1467-6427.00065.

Ware, J. E., Snow, K. K., Kosinski, M., & Gandek, B. (1993). *SF-36 health survey: Manual and interpretation guide*. Lincoln, RI: QualityMetric Inc.

Webb, J. R., Toussaint, L., & Conway-Williams, E. (2012). Forgiveness and health: Psycho-spiritual integration and the promotion of better healthcare. *Journal of Health Care Chaplaincy, 18*(1–2), 57–73. doi:10.1080/08854726.2012.667317.

Wilson, T., Milosevic, A., Carroll, M., Hart, K., & Hibbard, S. (2008). Physical health status in relation to self-forgiveness and other-forgiveness in healthy college students. *Journal of Health Psychology, 13*(6), 798–803. doi:10.1177/1359105308093863.

Witvliet, C. V. O., Ludwig, T. E., & Vander Laan, K. L. (2001). Granting forgiveness or harboring grudges: Implications for emotion, physiology, and health. *Psychological Science, 12*(2), 117–123.

Worthington, E. L., Jr. (2001). Unforgiveness, forgiveness, and reconciliation in societies. In R. G. Helmick & R. L. Petersen (Eds.), *Forgiveness and reconciliation: Religion, public policy, and conflict transformation* (pp. 161–182). Philadelphia, PA: Templeton Foundation Press.

Worthington, E. L., Jr. (2006). *Forgiveness and reconciliation: Theory and application*. New York, NY: Routledge/Taylor & Francis Group.

Worthington, E. L., Jr. (2013). *Moving forward: Six steps to forgiving yourself and breaking free from the past*. Colorado Springs, CO: Waterbrook Press.

Worthington, E. L., Jr., & Langberg, D. (2012). Religious considerations and self-forgiveness in treating complex trauma and moral injury in present and former soldiers. *Journal of Psychology and Theology, 40*(4), 274–288.

Worthington, E. L., Jr., Sandage, S. J., & Berry, J. W. (2000). Group interventions to promote forgiveness: What researchers and clinicians out to know. In M. E. McCullough, K. I. Pargament, & C. E. Thoresen (Eds.), *Forgiveness: Theory, research and practice* (pp. 228–253). New York, NY: The Guilford Press.

Worthington, E. L., Jr., & Scherer, M. (2004). Forgiveness is an emotion-focused coping strategy that can reduce health risks and promote health resilience: Theory, review, and hypotheses. *Psychology & Health, 19*(3), 385–405. doi:10.1080/0887044042000196674.

Worthington, E. L., Jr., & Wade, N. G. (1999). The social psychology of unforgiveness and forgiveness and implications for clinical practice. *Journal of Social and Clinical Psychology, 18*, 385–418.

Worthington, E. L., Jr., Witvliet, C. V. O., Pietrini, P., & Miller, A. J. (2007). Forgiveness, health, and well-being: A review of evidence for emotional versus decisional forgiveness, dispositional forgivingness, and reduced unforgiveness. *Journal of Behavioral Medicine, 30*(4), 291–302. doi:10.1007/s10865-007-9105-8.

Chapter 8
Forgiveness and Health in Patient Populations

Jennifer P. Friedberg, Hillary Lewin Tuvia, and Rose Cha

There is a growing body of research on the potential benefits of forgiveness for patients in medical settings. This chapter will illustrate common patient populations for which the benefits of forgiveness have been empirically supported. The populations to be discussed include patients with terminal illness, cancer, fibromyalgia, HIV/AIDS, cardiovascular disease, chronic pain and traumatic brain injury. The role of forgiveness as an intervention in medical settings will be offered to help patients to better cope with illness.

The relationship between forgiveness and health has been explored in various disciplines including religion and spirituality, philosophy, medicine, ethics and public health. Only 110 scholarly works in any of these disciplines explored forgiveness from the fifth century through 1970 (Enright & North, 1998). In 1997, there were 58 empirical studies on forgiveness (McCullough, Exline, & Baumeister, 1998) and since then, the research has increased to well over 2,000 articles.

For thousands of years, religion and spirituality have promoted forgiveness as a pathway to improve emotional health, well-being, physical health and longevity (Luskin, 2002). From a philosophical perspective, there are many forms of forgiveness including self-forgiveness, forgiving wrongs done by others, forgiving the dead, God's forgiveness and forgiving God (Griswold, 2007). From a medical perspective, neuroimaging and psychophysiological studies have established potential biological mechanisms of forgiveness (Farrow & Woodruff, 2005; Friedberg, Suchday, &

J.P. Friedberg, Ph.D. (✉)
VA New York Harbor Healthcare System, New York, NY, USA

New York University School of Medicine, New York, NY, USA
e-mail: jennifer.friedberg@va.gov

H.L. Tuvia, Ph.D.
William Alanson White Institute, New York, NY, USA

R. Cha, MSW
Silver School of Social Work, New York, NY, USA

L.L. Toussaint et al. (eds.), *Forgiveness and Health*,
DOI 10.1007/978-94-017-9993-5_8

Shelov, 2007). From an ethical perspective, forgiveness is both a value and a weakness (Murphy, 2005). Research indicates forgiveness can promote resilience (Worthington, 2005) as well as physical and mental health (Thoresen, Harris, & Luskin, 2000) and, thus, forgiveness can be thought of as a beneficial public health intervention.

Definitions of Concepts

Dimensions of Health

In this chapter, we focus upon dimensions of the relationship of forgiveness and mental and physical health in patients with medical illnesses. Mental health and physical health are defined by both symptoms and diagnoses. Forgiveness can be viewed as a mediator between emotional stress and health. Most research on forgiveness emphasizes its relationship to emotions such as hostility, anxiety, anger, and depression (McCullough, 2000; Witvliet et al., 2001). Since those emotions have a negative impact on health, if forgiveness can reduce them, then it has an indirect effect on health (Williams & Williams, 1993).

Particularly Relevant Dimensions of Forgiveness

Forgiveness involves three entities: a hurt victim; a perceived transgression (or offense); and a transgressor (or offender). Forgiveness of others occurs because an individual has been wronged, and involves hostility, anger, and vengefulness. In contrast, forgiveness of self or by God occurs among individuals who have offended, and is generally related to guilt, shame, and self-recrimination. Individuals with physical illnesses are a unique category of victims. Medical conditions vary, but all can have multiple, devastating consequences on one's health and well-being, can permeate almost all aspects of one's life, and require one to change his or her life around an unpleasant reality. The illness itself becomes the transgression. Any medical condition could be considered a breach or violation of the boundaries of one's skin, one's personhood, and one's life. Identification of the offender, on the other hand, is vague. Research on attribution theory in patient populations has shown that different attribution targets for cause of disease (e.g., self-blame, other-blame, God-blame) can affect health variables (e.g., Lopez-Lopez, Montorio, Izal, & Velasco, 2008; Pargament & Hahn, 1986; Voth & Sirois, 2009). Thus, the target of the victim's blame becomes especially salient, as is the target of forgiveness.

Self-focused blame and forgiveness appear to trump other-focused blame and forgiveness in relation to health variables in individuals who are simultaneously rendered "victim" and "patient" (e.g., Martin, Vosvick, & Riggs, 2012; McCullough

& Witvliet, 2002; Svalina & Webb, 2012; Webb, Toussaint, Kalpakjian, & Tate, 2010). The need to forgive others, however, may become more salient in cases involving personal culpability such as traumatic brain injury, which may be related to the idea of forgiveness as a remedy for an "injustice gap" (Harris & Thoresen, 2006; Worthington & Scherer, 2004). Other-forgiveness is also associated with increased physical pain (Martin et al., 2012). Further investigation is required to explain such inconsistencies. Forgiveness could play a healing role in some diseases and not others. Self- and other-forgiveness could differentially affect health in different patient populations.

Theoretical/Conceptual Models of Forgiveness

Forgiveness is often defined as the inverse of blame, and self-forgiveness is frequently considered an antidote to self-blame (along with excessive guilt and self-hatred). Self-blame is associated with poor coping to chronic illness, and mediates the relationship between forgiveness and health in several studies (particularly in individuals with smoking-related diseases such as cancer and chronic obstructive pulmonary disease (COPD); Friedman et al., 2010; Plaufcan, Wamboldt, & Holm, 2012). Given this, self-forgiveness may be an important intervention in patient populations likely to self-blame, such as those in which the illness may be considered 'preventable' and in the patient's control. In some cases, however, self-forgiveness may be an inappropriate intervention, because self-blame could also lead to improved health (Hart, Hanks, Bogner, Millis, & Esselman, 2007). Self-blame could be the result of compensation for loss of control and can provide some relief from anxiety (Macleod, 1999). Regaining control through self-blame could motivate a patient to engage in healthy behaviors; sense of control over the disease is associated with better adjustment (Gulyn & Youssef, 2010).

Two types of self-blame are described in the literature: behavioral and characterological. Behavioral self-blame for the disease (what a person did or did not do) is typically associated with better adjustment to disease, whereas characterological self-blame (for being the kind of person they are) tends to predict poorer coping (Plaufcan et al., 2012; Roesch & Weiner, 2001). If self-forgiveness is an antidote to self-blame, then examining behavioral versus characterological self-forgiveness could expand our understanding of the benefits forgiveness may have on patients coping with illness. If behavioral versus characterological self-forgiveness can be considered synonyms for state versus trait forgiveness, researchers and clinicians can better understand how to incorporate these types of forgiveness into their work using existing state versus trait models.

Empirical Evidence of Forgiveness and Health

Several studies examined the associations between forgiveness and self-reported health, health behaviors, or health outcomes, but mainly in healthy samples. Fewer studies examined the link between forgiveness and health variables in patients. Most are cross-sectional and focus upon patients in rehabilitation settings or those with chronic pain, cardiovascular disease and cancer.

Cardiovascular Disease and Related Diseases It is not surprising that several researchers have investigated forgiveness in patients with cardiovascular disease, given the large body of work suggesting that hostility and anger, the antitheses of a forgiving attitude, are associated with the development of cardiovascular disease and hypertension (Miller, Smith, Turner, Guijarro, & Hallet, 1996; Siegman & Snow, 1997). Forgiveness has been associated with cardiovascular parameters in healthy samples, mostly in laboratory settings (e.g., Friedberg et al., 2007; Lawler et al., 2003; Lawler et al., 2005; Witvliet, Ludwig, & Vander Laan, 2001). Researchers have extended this work to patients with cardiovascular diseases. Work with hospitalized patients with coronary artery disease (CAD) suggested that individuals with higher levels of forgivingness had lower levels of anxiety, depression, and stress (Friedberg, Suchday, & Srinivas, 2009). Forgivingness was also negatively correlated with total cholesterol to HDL and LDL to HDL ratios after controlling for demographics. Some studies using healthy samples found that stress and negative affect mediated the relationship between forgiveness and physiological variables (Lawler et al., 2003; Lawler et al., 2005), but in our sample of CAD patients, this did not appear to be the case.

Park (2008) examined forgiveness in patients with congestive heart failure (CHF) at baseline and 6-month follow-up. Decreases in patients' estimates of their lifespan or uncertainty about longevity were related to increases in forgivingness. Essentially, CHF patients who shifted towards believing that they would pass away sooner or had more uncertainty about their longevity displayed greater increases in forgiveness. Toussaint and Cheadle (2009) examined the link between unforgiving, rather than forgiving, tendencies and cardiovascular diseases within the past 12 months using epidemiological data. Unforgivingness was associated with higher prevalence of cardiovascular conditions, particularly hypertension, angina, and tachycardia, in a survey of healthy people even after controlling for sociodemographic factors, depression, and anger. It was less consistently associated with myocardial infarction and arteriosclerosis.

DeWall and colleagues (2010) examined the relationship between self-control and both forgiveness and forgivingness in patients with diabetes, which is related to and often comorbid with cardiovascular disease. Diabetic symptoms were negatively associated with forgivingness, and positively correlated with unforgivingness of hypothetical and actual transgressions. The authors speculated this is because diabetic symptoms are a dimension of self-control as prior research has linked poor blood glucose control to aggression and lack of cooperative behavior.

Rehabilitation Patients There was no significant difference in forgivingness in patients with traumatic brain injury (TBI), cerebrovascular accident (CVA), and spinal cord injury (SCI) (Johnstone & Yoon, 2009). Forgivingness was associated with general health perceptions, but not general mental health, physical functioning, or bodily pain. In outpatients receiving physical therapy, forgivingness of self was associated with more healthy behavior, which was itself correlated with better overall health, physical health and current pain levels (thus forgivingness of self was only indirectly associated with these variables; Svalina & Webb, 2012). Self-forgivingness had a positive association with mental health status and a negative one with chronic pain, while feeling forgiven by God was associated with better health-related social functioning. Forgivingness of others was not related to health outcomes.

Other studies focused on specific rehabilitation populations. Forgivingness and anger were negatively associated in patients with mild to moderate TBI, though it should be noted that, with TBI, the anger could be organic and resulting from the injury itself, or could be a response to the debilitating injury (Gisi & D'Amato, 2000). If it is the latter, a forgiveness intervention might be beneficial for TBI patients. Webb and colleagues (2010) found that, in patients with traumatic SCI, after controlling for demographics, self-forgivingness was positively correlated with health behaviors and life satisfaction, while other-forgivingness was positively associated with health status. Johnstone and colleagues (2009) found that forgiveness was not associated with SF-36 variables in TBI patients. However, when conducting hierarchical regressions, the authors found that forgivingness and values/beliefs contributed to 16 % of the variance in SF-36 General Health Perception scores beyond that of demographic variables. Forgivingness may be more highly correlated with health factors in SCI patients than TBI patients because of the aforementioned organic changes that occurred as a result of TBI.

Chronic Pain In the aforementioned studies, forgivingness was not associated with bodily pain in a heterogeneous sample of rehabilitation patients (Johnstone & Yoon, 2009), while self-forgivingness was directly associated with chronic pain and indirectly associated with current pain levels through health behaviors in patients receiving outpatient physical therapy (Svalina & Webb, 2012). Forgiveness of a recent transgressor and forgiveness self-efficacy were both negatively associated with anger in, anger out, trait anger, state anger, distress, sensory pain, and affective pain in patients with chronic back pain (Carson et al., 2005). State anger mediated the relationship between forgiveness and distress, and partially mediated the relationship between forgiveness and pain. In patients with chronic musculoskeletal pain, forgiveness had a positive association with age (a finding also in non-patient populations, e.g., Toussaint, Williams, Musick, & Everson, 2001) and SF-36 mental component score (Rippentrop, Altmaier, Chen, Found, & Keffala, 2005). Forgiveness of the transgressor was also negatively associated with disability/compensation status, time in pain, pain level, and daily interference due to pain. This suggests that chronic pain patients who have difficulty forgiving may have more anger, mental health problems and disability due to pain than those who are higher in forgiveness. Thus, a forgiveness intervention may improve quality of life and functioning in patients with pain.

Cancer Two studies have examined the correlates of self-forgivingness in patients with breast cancer. Self-forgivingness was negatively associated with mood disturbance and positively associated with quality of life in patients at a breast cancer clinic (Romero et al., 2006). Similarly, women with stage 0-III breast cancer with higher levels of self-forgivingness had less mood disturbance and higher levels of quality of life than those with less self-forgivingness; forgivingness of self was also negatively associated with self-blame for cancer (Friedman et al., 2007). Self-blame partially mediated the relationship between self-forgivingness and quality of life. Van Laarhoven and colleagues (2012) found no difference in other-forgivingness between patients with advanced cancer and individuals with no disease. Self-forgivingness may be particularly salient when individuals face a potentially life-threatening illness such as cancer, while other-forgivingness may be less relevant for such patients.

Other Diseases A few researchers examined forgiveness in patients with other diseases. One study examined the relationship between bearing grudges and prevalence of a variety of health conditions (Messias, Saini, Sinato, & Welch, 2010). Bearing grudges, not surprisingly given the aforementioned research linking hostility and anger with a host of health issues especially cardiovascular disease, was significantly associated with history of heart attack, heart disease, high blood pressure, stomach ulcers, arthritis, back problems, headaches, and chronic pain, but not asthma, diabetes, epilepsy, allergies, stroke, or cancer.

Other studies examined specific unique patient populations. Patients with Parkinson's disease (PD) reported lower forgivingness levels than healthy age-matched controls (Butler, McNamara, Ghofrani, & Durso, 2011). A pilot sub-study was conducted to determine whether a common PD medication, levadopa, had an impact on religiosity and spirituality levels in PD patients; however, there was no difference in forgiveness when patients were off levadopa for a 12-h washout period as compared to when they were on the drug. The researchers used order randomization but did not provide information about masking in the paper. Forgivingness of self was positively correlated with quality of life in HIV patients (Martin et al., 2012). Interestingly, there was an interaction between forgiveness and attachment style such that, among individuals with greater attachment anxiety, forgiveness of others was associated with higher pain levels, while forgiveness of self was associated with greater perception of health. Anxiously attached individuals may receive fewer benefits from forgiving others, which is related to feelings of being a victim than from forgiving oneself, which is related to self-blame and guilt. The authors speculate that when trying to forgive the transgressions of others, they may constantly re-appraise interactions as negative. Thus, forgiveness interventions could have varying success rates among HIV patients depending on their attachment styles.

Interventions The aforementioned studies mainly examined the relationship between forgiveness and specific patient populations at one point in time or at two time points. The data suggest an association between tendency to forgive and various health outcomes in patient populations and point to the potential utility of forgiveness interventions in improving these health outcomes. Despite an expanding base of literature on the efficacy of forgiveness interventions in a variety of populations, few intervention studies utilized a patient population.

Hypertension patients randomized to an 8-week forgiveness intervention did not display a significant reduction in blood pressure after receiving the intervention, but they did show a decrease in anger expression, which was associated with lower mean arterial pressure post-intervention (Tibbits, Ellis, Piramelli, Luskin, & Lukman, 2006). Thus, a forgiveness intervention may reduce blood pressure not directly but indirectly through psychosocial variables such as anger. CAD patients receiving forgiveness therapy based on Enright's model had significant increases in forgiveness between pre-test and post-test and between pre-test and follow-up compared to the control group receiving sessions to cope with CAD (Waltman et al., 2009). There were no changes on anger-recall induced myocardial perfusion defects from pre-test to post-test in the intervention group, but there were differences from pre-test to 10-week follow-up. The authors suggest that forgiveness training may have a delayed impact on physiological parameters. A 4-week forgiveness therapy program for terminally ill cancer patients significantly improved forgiveness, hope, and quality of life and reduced anger compared to wait-list control (Hansen, Enright, Baskin, & Klatt, 2009).

While the above studies specifically tested the effectiveness of forgiveness therapy, two additional studies examined the effectiveness of therapies that had several components including forgiveness. Breast cancer patients receiving a group body-mind-spirit treatment including forgiveness displayed greater reductions in anxiety than the control group receiving standard of care, but patients in both groups had similar decreases in depression and increases in body-mind-spirit well-being (Liu et al., 2008). Patients who had less than 6 months to live who received a three-session treatment focusing on issues related to life completion and preparation (compared to relaxation meditation or no intervention) displayed improvements in functional status, anxiety, depression, and preparation for end of life, but the sample size was too small to detect significant differences (Steinhauser et al., 2008). Participants only discussed issues related to self- and other-forgiveness in the second session. Qualitative interviews with a subset of participants (Steinhauser, Alexander, Byock, George, & Tulsky, 2009) revealed that about two-thirds did not have forgiveness to ask for, half recalled asking for forgiveness in an ongoing basis and about half recalled giving forgiveness throughout their lives (not at end of life); thus, this forgiveness intervention may not be effective for palliative care patients. The prior cross-sectional studies with patients with cancer suggest that an intervention focusing on self-forgivingness may be more beneficial for patients facing end of life issues.

Limitations of Existing Work

Although there has been an increase in studies examining forgiveness in patients with physical illnesses, they are still few and far between. Many of the studies are cross sectional and rely on the Brief Multidimensional Measure of Religiousness/Spirituality (BMMRS) to assess trait forgiveness levels. The forgiveness factor is made up of three questions taking into account forgivingness of others, of self, and by God (Johnstone, Yoon, Franklin, Schopp, & Hinkebein, 2009). Forgiveness is a complex process that cannot simply be measured with only three items that separately assess forgiveness of self, of others, and by God, which are separate constructs that are quite different. Forgiveness of others is a process in which negative emotions, cognitions, and behaviors associated with anger, resentment, and hostility are reduced with a simultaneous increase in those associated with empathy, compassion, and affection for the transgressor (Worthington & Wade, 1999), while feeling forgiven by God and forgiving oneself involves a different process that results in freedom from guilt and self-blame. Similarly, the few longitudinal investigations of forgiveness in individuals with physical illness have been limited by the use of poor forgiveness measures. Park's (2008) examination of forgiveness in CHF patients over time used the BMMRS. While the studies by Toussaint and Cheadle (2009) and Messias and colleagues (2010) are notable for their use of large, nationally representative datasets, Toussaint and Cheadle's study assessed tendency to be unforgiving using two items, while Messias and colleagues' study used one question about bearing grudges.

Nearly all of the aforementioned studies, both cross-sectional and longitudinal, assessed health status and symptoms via self-report rather than with objective physiological measures. Studies examining the link between forgiveness and health in general adult populations have found forgiveness is associated with outcomes like blood pressure, cardiovascular reactivity, and heart rate (Larkin, Goulet, & Cavanagh, 2015), suggesting that forgiveness can buffer against future development of health problems. The relationship between physiological parameters and forgiveness has not been established in patient populations, and thus it is unclear if forgiveness can protect against worsening symptoms in patients who have already developed conditions such as CAD, cancer, CVA, TBI, SCI, or chronic pain. Furthermore, the data do not yet make a case for using forgiveness interventions to improve symptoms or functioning in such patients.

The only known intervention studies were RCTs with sample sizes that are likely too small to detect significant intervention effects. Two of the studies assessed the effect of specific forgiveness interventions on physiological variables (Tibbits et al., 2006; Waltman et al., 2009). A third RCT only examined the impact upon psychosocial variables (Hansen et al., 2009). The other two known RCTs were of interventions in which forgiveness therapy was only one component of several, and had psychosocial outcomes (Liu et al., 2008; Steinhauser et al., 2008).

Future Research Agenda

More research is needed to further establish the link between forgiveness and health in patients with medical illnesses. It would be beneficial to examine how forgiveness impacts physiological parameters that are measured objectively (e.g., from medical records or objective methods like measuring blood pressure) rather than only by self-report. It would be helpful for forgiveness to be measured using valid and reliable assessment tools with multiple items (e.g., Heartland Forgiveness Scale, Trait Forgiveness Scale). Most of the work has been done in patients with cardiovascular disease or a related condition and rehabilitation patients, and even in those conditions, only a few studies have been conducted to date. Future research should expand the work in these areas as well as in less studied disease conditions.

Future research in forgiveness may benefit from incorporating specific concepts and findings from attribution theory, such as the behavioral versus characterological distinction in self-blame, the "responsibility" (adaptive) versus "blame" (maladaptive) distinction, as well as the potential role of self-blame (for the illness) as a compensatory strategy in response to loss of control (by the illness). Researchers could also examine the relationships among blame target, forgiveness target, and self- versus other "just-world beliefs" (Lucas, Young, Zhdanova, & Alexander, 2010; (Mullet, 2007; Strelan & Sutton, 2011). Healthcare providers are urged to assess the presence, as well as the target of, patients' blame for their illness, along with their just-world beliefs, on a case-by-case basis.

More longitudinal work must be done to establish whether forgiveness impacts health in patient populations over time. Furthermore, it is essential to examine whether forgiveness intervention programs (such as those by Enright, Worthington or Luskin described below) can improve mental and physical health in patients with physical illnesses via rigorous RCTs.

Implications for Health Enhancement, Medicine, Integrative Treatment

Forgiveness can enhance health in the general population and can be beneficial for patients receiving medical treatment. Forgiveness interventions are beneficial for both mind and body, but are seldom used in medical settings (Harris & Thoresen, 2006). Research suggests clinical and psycho-educational forgiveness interventions generate health benefits (see Baskin & Enright, 2004; Burchard et al., 2003; Lampton, Oliver, Worthington, & Berry, 2005; Ripley & Worthington, 2002;

Wade & Worthington, 2003). Literature on the effects of forgiveness training on health is emerging and encouraging results are being documented (Toussaint et al., 2010). For example, forgiveness training helps individuals with chronic physical conditions decrease their anger and resentment toward others (Carson et al., 2005), which reduces physical and psychological symptoms leading to improvement in overall well-being (Kautz, 2008). It is evident the ability to forgive is a teachable skill gaining some acceptance in health care settings as a feasible treatment goal (Harris & Thoresen, 2006). Following are examples of forgiveness programs implemented in patient populations that yielded positive results for patient's physical and emotional health.

Intervention Research

Enright Process Model The first training program, developed by Enright and The Human Development Study Group (1996) utilizes a 20—step model of forgiveness. The model consists of four phases: "uncovering," "deciding," "working," and "deepening." Enright and Fitzgibbons (2000) *Helping Clients Forgive* is a book written for clinicians from different theoretical orientations to offer forgiveness-focused counseling to patients. This training program was only empirically tested once in CAD patients to our knowledge (Waltman et al., 2009), and, as mentioned above, resulted in immediate increases in forgiveness post-intervention and delayed effects on anger-recall induced myocardial perfusion defects. The other forgiveness training programs described below have not been used in any RCTs in medical patient samples.

Worthington's REACH Forgiveness Model Worthington's (2001) Five Steps to Forgiveness is a training program also known as REACH Forgiveness (leader and participant manuals are available at www.people.vcu.edu/~eworth), which promotes forgiveness for a specific wrongdoing and seeks to promote changes in forgivingness as well. The model involves psycho-educational group work focused on Recalling the hurt, building Empathy, giving an Altruistic gift of forgiveness, Committing to forgiveness, and Holding onto the forgiveness achieved.

Luskin's Forgive-for-Good Model Luskin's (2002) book *Forgive for Good* is an adaptation of the treatment used in the Stanford Forgiveness Project; ongoing workshops and research projects examine the effectiveness of his forgiveness methods on various populations (Harris & Thoresen, 2006). The Forgiveness Project consists of nine steps to forgiveness aimed at reducing anger, depression and stress and increasing feelings of hope, compassion and self-confidence (Luskin, 2002).

Assessment of the Models In a meta-analysis (Wade, Hoyt, & Worthington, 2014) of interventions to promote forgiveness, it was found that Enright's model had been tested in 23 RCTs, the REACH Forgiveness model in 22 RCTs and all others put together in 22 combined RCTs. The meta-analysis showed forgiveness was strongly related to time of intervention and the correlated severity of the problem. Once those two factors were removed, the Enright, Worthington, and other interventions were equal in outcomes—both forgiveness (of a specific offense) and mental health outcomes.

Conclusion

Despite limited research on the impact of forgiveness on physical and mental health in patient populations, it is evident there is legitimacy to the relationship between these variables in those with medical illnesses. Several types of forgiveness (e.g. self-forgiveness, forgiveness of others) should be considered when assessing the impact of forgiveness upon health. Patients with medical conditions have unique responses to the dimensions of forgiveness as described throughout this chapter. It would be useful to implement forgiveness training in medical settings as needed. It is worthwhile to invest in more research and implement forgiveness training programs to further understand and benefit from the relationship of forgiveness and health.

References

Baskin, T. W., & Enright, R. D. (2004). Intervention studies on forgiveness: A meta-analysis. *Journal of Counseling and Development, 82*, 79–90.

Burchard, G. A., Yarhouse, M. A., Kilian, M. K., Worthington, E. L., Jr., Berry, J. W., & Canter, D. E. (2003). A study of two marital enrichment programs and couples' quality of life. *Journal of Psychology and Theology, 31*, 240–252.

Butler, P., McNamara, P., Ghofrani, J., & Durso, R. (2011). Disease-associated differences in religious cognition in patients with Parkinson's disease. *Journal of Clinical and Experimental Neuropsychology, 33*(8), 917–928. doi:10.1080/13803395.2011.575768.

Carson, J. W., Keefe, F. J., Goli, V., Fras, A. M., Lynch, T. R., Thorp, S. R., & Buechler, J. L. (2005). Forgiveness and chronic low back pain: A preliminary study examining the relationship of forgiveness to pain, anger, and psychological distress. *Journal of Pain, 6*(2), 84–91. doi:10.1016/j.jpain.2004.10.012

DeWall, C. N., Pond, R. S., Jr., & Bushman, B. J. (2010). Sweet revenge: Diabetic symptoms predict less forgiveness. *Personality and Individual Differences, 49*(7), 823–826. doi:10.1016/j.paid.2010.06.030.

Enright, R. D., & Fitzgibbons, R. P. (2000). *Helping clients forgive: An empirical guide for resolving anger and restoring hope*. Washington, DC: American Psychological Association.

Enright, R. D., & North, J. (1998). Introducing forgiveness. In R. D. Enright & J. North (Eds.), *Exploring forgiveness* (pp. 3–8). Madison, WI: University of Wisconsin Press.

Enright, R. D., & The Human Development Study Group. (1996). Counseling within the forgiveness triad: On forgiving, receiving forgiveness, and self-forgiveness. *Counseling and Values, 40*, 107–126.

Farrow, T. F., & Woodruff, P. W. (2005). Neuroimaging of forgivability. In E. L. Worthington Jr. (Ed.), *Handbook of forgiveness* (pp. 259–272). New York, NY: Brunner-Routledge.

Friedberg, J. P., Suchday, S., & Shelov, D. V. (2007). The impact of forgiveness on cardiovascular reactivity and recovery. *International Journal of Psychophysiology, 65*(2), 87–94. doi:10.1016/j.ijpsycho.2007.03.006.

Friedberg, J. P., Suchday, S., & Srinivas, V. S. (2009). Relationship between forgiveness and psychological indices in cardiac patients. *International Journal of Behavioral Medicine, 16*(3), 205–211. doi:10.1007/s12529-008-9016-2.

Friedman, L. C., Barber, C. R., Chang, J., Tham, Y. L., Kalidas, M., Rimawi, M. F., ... Elledge, R. (2010). Self-blame, self-forgiveness, and spirituality in breast cancer survivors in a public sector setting. *Journal of Cancer Education, 25*(3), 343–348. doi:10.1007/s13187-010-0048-3

Friedman, L. C., Romero, C., Elledge, R., Chang, J., Kalidas, M., Dulay, M. F., ... Osborne, C. K. (2007). Attribution of blame, self-forgiving attitude and psychological adjustment in women with breast cancer. *Journal of Behavioral Medicine, 30*(4), 351–357. doi:10.1007/s10865-007-9108-5

Gisi, T. M., & D'Amato, R. C. (2000). What factors should be considered in rehabilitation: Are anger, social desirability, and forgiveness related in adults with traumatic brain injuries? *International Journal of Neuroscience, 105*(1–4), 121–133. doi:10.3109/00207450009003271.

Griswold, C. L. (2007). *Forgiveness: A philosophical exploration Cambridge*. Cambridge, UK: Cambridge University Press.

Gulyn, L. M., & Youssef, F. (2010). Attribution of blame for breast and lung cancers in women. *Journal of Psychosocial Oncology, 28*(3), 291–301. doi:10.1080/07347331003689052.

Hansen, M. J., Enright, R. D., Baskin, T. W., & Klatt, J. (2009). A palliative care intervention in forgiveness therapy for elderly terminally ill cancer patients. *Journal of Palliative Care, 25*(1), 51–60.

Harris, A. H. S., & Thoresen, C. E. (2006). Extending the influence of positive psychology interventions into health care settings: Lessons from self-efficacy and forgiveness. *Journal of Positive Psychology, 1*, 27–36.

Hart, T., Hanks, R., Bogner, J. A., Millis, S., & Esselman, P. (2007). Blame attribution in intentional and unintentional traumatic brain injury: Longitudinal changes and impact on subjective well-being. *Rehabilitation Psychology, 52*(2), 152–161. doi:10.1037/0090-5550.52.2.152.

Johnstone, B., & Yoon, D. P. (2009). Relationships between the Brief Multidimensional Measure of Religiousness/Spirituality and health outcomes for a heterogeneous rehabilitation population. *Rehabilitation Psychology, 54*(4), 422–431. doi:10.1037/a0017758.

Johnstone, B., Yoon, D. P., Franklin, K. L., Schopp, L., & Hinkebein, J. (2009). Re-conceptualizing the factor structure of the Brief Multidimensional Measure of Religiousness/Spirituality. *Journal of Religion and Health, 48*(2), 146–163. doi:10.1007/s10943-008-9179-9.

Johnstone, B., Yoon, D. P., Rupright, J., & Reid-Arndt, S. (2009). Relationships among spiritual beliefs, religious practises, congregational support and health for individuals with traumatic brain injury. *Brain Injury, 23*(5), 411–419. doi:10.1080/02699050902788501.

Kautz, D. (2008). Inspiring hope in our rehabilitation patients, their families, and ourselves. *Rehabilitation Nursing, 33*, 148–153, 177.

Lampton, C., Oliver, C. J., Worthington, E. L., & Berry, J. W. (2005). Helping college students become more forgiving: An intervention study to promote forgiveness as part of a program to shape Christian character. *Journal of Psychology and Theology, 33*(4), 278–281.

Larkin, K. T., Goulet, C., & Cavanagh, C. (2015). Forgiveness and physiological concomitants and outcomes. In L. L. Toussaint, E. L. Worthington, Jr., & D. Williams (Eds.), *Forgiveness and health: Scientific evidence and theories relating forgiveness to better health*. Dordrecht, Netherlands: Springer.

Lawler, K. A., Younger, J. W., Piferi, R. L., Billington, E., Jobe, R., Edmondson, K., & Jones, W. H. (2003). A change of heart: Cardiovascular correlates of forgiveness in response to interpersonal conflict. *Journal of Behavioral Medicine, 26*(5), 373–393. doi:10.1023/A:1025771716686

Lawler, K. A., Younger, J. W., Piferi, R. L., Jobe, R. L., Edmondson, K. A., & Jones, W. H. (2005). The unique effects of forgiveness on health: An exploration of pathways. *Journal of Behavioral Medicine, 28*(2), 157–167. doi:10.1007/s10865-005-3665-2.

Liu, C. V., Hsiung, P. C., Liu, Y. F., Wang, K. C., Hsiao, F. H., Ng, S. M., et al. (2008). A study on the efficacy of body-mind-spirit group therapy for patients with breast cancer. *Journal of Clinical Nursing, 17*(19), 2539–2549.

Lopez-Lopez, A., Montorio, I., Izal, M., & Velasco, L. (2008). The role of psychological variables in explaining depression in older people with chronic pain. *Aging Mental Health, 12*(6), 735–745.

Lucas, T., Young, J. D., Zhdanova, L., & Alexander, S. (2010). Self and other justice beliefs, impulsivity, rumination, and forgiveness: Justice beliefs can both prevent and promote forgiveness. *Personality and Individual Differences, 49*(8), 851–856. doi:10.1016/j.paid.2010.07.014.

Luskin, F. (2002). *Forgive for good: A proven prescription for health and happiness*. San Francisco, CA: HarperSanFrancisco.

Macleod, M. (1999). Why did it happen to me? Social cognition processes in adjustment and recovery from criminal victimisation and illness. *Current Psychology, 18*(1), 18–31. doi:10.1007/s12144-999-1014-2.

Martin, L. A., Vosvick, M., & Riggs, S. A. (2012). Attachment, forgiveness, and physical health quality of life in HIV+ adults. *AIDS Care, 24*(11), 1333–1340. doi:10.1080/09540121.2011.648598.

McCullough, M. E. (2000). Forgiveness as human strength: Theory, measurement, and links to well being. *Journal of Social and Clinical Psychology, 19*(1), 43–55.

McCullough, M. E., Exline, J. J., & Baumeister, R. F. (1998). An annotated bibliography of research on forgiveness and related concepts. In E. L. Worthington Jr. (Ed.), *Dimensions of forgiveness: Psychological research and theological perspectives* (pp. 193–317). Philadelphia, PA: Templeton Foundation Press.

McCullough, M. E., & Witvliet, C. V. (2002). The psychology of forgiveness. In *Handbook of positive psychology* (pp. 446–455). Oxford, UK: Oxford University Press.

Messias, E., Saini, A., Sinato, P., & Welch, S. (2010). Bearing grudges and physical health: Relationship to smoking, cardiovascular health and ulcers. *Social Psychiatry and Psychiatric Epidemiology, 45*(2), 183–187. doi:10.1007/s00127-009-0054-0.

Miller, T. Q., Smith, T. W., Turner, C. W., Guijarro, M. L., & Hallet, A. J. (1996). A meta-analytic review of research on hostility and physical health. *Psychological Bulletin, 119*(2), 322–348.

Mullet, E. (2007). Cognitive processes involved in blame and blame-like judgments and in forgiveness and forgiveness-like judgments. *American Journal of Psychology, 120*(1), 25–46.

Murphy, G. (2005). Forgiveness, self-respect, and the value of resentment. In E. L. Worthington Jr. (Ed.), *Handbook of forgiveness* (pp. 33–40). New York, NY: Brunner-Routledge.

Pargament, K., & Hahn, J. (1986). God and the just world: Causal and coping attributions to God in health situations. *Journal for the Scientific Study of Religion, 25*, 193–207.

Park, C. L. (2008). Estimated longevity and changes in spirituality in the context of advanced congestive heart failure. *Palliative & Supportive Care, 6*(1), 3–11.

Plaufcan, M. R., Wamboldt, F. S., & Holm, K. E. (2012). Behavioral and characterological self-blame in chronic obstructive pulmonary disease. *Journal of Psychosomatic Research, 72*(1), 78–83. doi:10.1016/j.jpsychores.2011.10.004.

Ripley, J. S., & Worthington, E. L., Jr. (2002). Hope-focused and forgiveness-based group interventions to promote marital enrichment. *Journal of Counseling and Development, 80*, 452–463.

Rippentrop, A. E., Altmaier, E. M., Chen, J. J., Found, E. M., & Keffala, V. J. (2005). The relationship between religion/spirituality and physical health, mental health, and pain in a chronic pain population. *Pain, 116*(3), 311–321. doi:10.1016/j.pain.2005.05.008.

Roesch, S. C., & Weiner, B. (2001). A meta-analytic review of coping with illness: Do causal attributions matter? *Journal of Psychosomatic Research, 50*(4), 205–219. doi:http://dx.doi.org/10.1016/S0022-3999(01)00188-X

Romero, C., Kalidas, M., Elledge, R., Chang, J., Liscum, K. R., & Friedman, L. C. (2006). Self-forgiveness, spirituality, and psychological adjustment in women with breast cancer. *Journal of Behavioral Medicine, 29*(1), 29–36. doi:10.1007/s10865-005-9038-z.

Siegman, A. W., & Snow, S. C. (1997). The outward expression of anger, the inward experience of anger and CVR: The role of vocal expression. *Journal of Behavioral Medicine, 20*(1), 29–45.

Steinhauser, K. E., Alexander, S. C., Byock, I. R., George, L. K., Olsen, M. K., & Tulsky, J. A. (2008). Do preparation and life completion discussions improve functioning and quality of life in seriously ill patients? Pilot randomized control trial. *Journal of Palliative Medicine, 11*(9), 1234–1240. doi:10.1089/jpm.2008.0078.

Steinhauser, K. E., Alexander, S. C., Byock, I. R., George, L. K., & Tulsky, J. (2009). Seriously ill patients' discussions with preparation and life completion: An intervention to assist with the transition at the end of life. *Palliative & Supportive Care, 7*(4), 393–404. doi:10.1017/S147895150999040X.

Strelan, P., & Sutton, R. M. (2011). When just-world beliefs promote and when they inhibit forgiveness. *Personality and Individual Differences, 50*(2), 163–168. doi:http://dx.doi.org/10.1016/j.paid.2010.09.019

Svalina, S. S., & Webb, J. R. (2012). Forgiveness and health among people in outpatient physical therapy. *Disability and Rehabilitation: An International, Multidisciplinary Journal, 34*(5), 383–392. doi:10.3109/09638288.2011.607216.

Thoresen, C. E., Harris, A. H. S., & Luskin, F. (2000). Forgiveness and health: An unanswered question. In M. E. McCullough, K. I. Pargament, & C. E. Thoresen (Eds.), *Forgiveness: Theory, research, and practice* (pp. 254–280). New York, NY: Guilford Press.

Tibbits, D., Ellis, G., Piramelli, C., Luskin, F., & Lukman, R. (2006). Hypertension reduction through forgiveness training. *Journal of Pastoral Care & Counseling, 60*(1–2), 27–34.

Toussaint, L., & Cheadle, A. C. D. (2009). Unforgiveness and the broken heart: Unforgiving tendencies, problems due to unforgiveness, and 12-month prevalence of cardiovascular health conditions. In M. T. Evans & E. D. Walker (Eds.), *Religion and psychology* (pp. 135–170). New York, NY: Nova Publishers.

Toussaint, L., Overvold-Ronningen, M., Vincent, A., Luedtke, C., Whipple, M., Schriever, T., & Luskin, F. (2010). Implications of forgiveness enhancement in patients with fibromyalgia and chronic fatigue syndrome. *Journal of Health Care Chaplaincy, 16*(3–4), 123–139. doi:10.1080/08854726.2010.492713

Toussaint, L. L., Williams, D. R., Musick, M. A., & Everson, S. A. (2001). Forgiveness and health: Age differences in a U.S. probability sample. *Journal of Adult Development, 8*, 249–257.

van Laarhoven, H. W., Schilderman, J., Verhagen, C. A., & Prins, J. B. (2012). Comparison of attitudes of guilt and forgiveness in cancer patients without evidence of disease and advanced cancer patients in a palliative care setting. *Cancer Nursing, 35*(6), 483–492. doi:10.1097/NCC.0b013e318243fb30.

Voth, J., & Sirois, F. M. (2009). The role of self-blame and responsibility in adjustment to inflammatory bowel disease. *Rehabilitation Psychology, 54*(1), 99–108. doi:10.1037/a0014739.

Wade, N. G., Hoyt, W. T., Kidwell, J. E. M., & Worthington, E. L. (2014). Efficacy of psychotherapeutic interventions to promote forgiveness: A meta-analysis. *Journal of Consulting and Clinical Psychology, 82*, 154–170.

Wade, N. G., & Worthington, E. L., Jr. (2003). Overcoming interpersonal offenses: Is forgiveness the only way to deal with unforgiveness? *Journal of Counseling and Development, 81*, 343–353.

Waltman, M. A., Russell, D. C., Coyle, C. T., Enright, R. D., Holter, A. C., & Swoboda, C. M. (2009). The effects of a forgiveness intervention on patients with coronary artery disease. *Psychology & Health, 24*(1), 11–27. doi:10.1080/08870440801975127.

Webb, J. R., Toussaint, L., Kalpakjian, C. Z., & Tate, D. G. (2010). Forgiveness and health-related outcomes among people with spinal cord injury. *Disability and Rehabilitation: An International, Multidisciplinary Journal, 32*(5), 360–366. doi:10.3109/09638280903166360.

Williams, R., & Williams, V. (1993). *Anger kills: Seventeen strategies for controlling the hostility that can harm your health*. New York, NY: Harper Perennial.

Witvliet, C. V., Ludwig, T. E., & Vander Laan, K. L. (2001). Granting forgiveness or harboring grudges: Implications for emotion, physiology, and health. *Psychological Science, 12*, 117–123.

Worthington, E. L., Jr. (2001). *Five steps to forgiveness: The art and science of forgiving: Bridges to wholeness and hope*. New York, NY: Crown Publishers.
Worthington, E. L., Jr., & Scherer, M. (2004). Forgiveness is an emotion-focused coping strategy that can reduce health risks and promote health resilience: Theory, review, and hypotheses. *Psychology & Health, 19*(3), 385–405. doi:10.1080/0887044042000196674.
Worthington, E. L., Jr. (Ed.). (2005). *Handbook of forgiveness*. New York, NY: Brunner-Routledge.
Worthington, E. L., Jr., & Wade, N. G. (1999). The social psychology of unforgiveness and forgiveness and implications for clinical practice. *Journal of Social and Clinical Psychology, 18*, 385–418.

Chapter 9
The Role of Forgiveness in Chronic Pain and Fibromyalgia

Martin Offenbächer, Jessie Dezutter, Miguel A. Vallejo, and Loren L. Toussaint

A commonly overlooked connection between forgiveness and holistic health is its connection with pain. Although pain takes many forms, this chapter will review research and build a conceptual argument for forgiveness' relevance to two specific types of pain conditions: (a) chronic widespread pain (CWP) and fibromyalgia syndrome (FMS). It is in reviewing these two pain disorders that a picture emerges from a biopsychosocial model of health that suggests an important connection between social stress, coping, and forgiveness.

In brief, we argue that many of the intrapersonal and interpersonal sources of stress that are confronted by patients with CWP and FMS can be effectively and appropriately addressed through forgiveness of oneself or others. Our logic is built upon the conceptual model depicted in Fig. 9.1, originally developed by Toussaint et al. (2010), and adapted here for the present purposes. The model depicts common sources of stress for patients with CWP and FMS and reflects the known effects of this stress on health. Also depicted in the model is the influence of stress on central and autonomic function (a hallmark physiological marker of FMS) and impaired functioning of the hypothalamic-pituitary adrenal cortical axis (HPA) commonly associated with FMS. Forgiveness is conceptualized as a coping mechanism that helps to relieve common sources of stress but also has direct and indirect (through stress) effects on health and nervous and endocrine function (see Chap. 4). Because

M. Offenbächer (✉)
University of Munich, 80336 Munich, Germany
e-mail: martin.offenbaecher@med.uni-muenchen.de

J. Dezutter
Katholieke Universiteit Leuven, Tiensestraat 102, 3000 Leuven, Belgium

M.A. Vallejo
Universidad Nacional de Educación a Distancia, Juan del Rosal 10, 28040 Madrid, Spain

L.L. Toussaint
Department of Psychology, Luther College, Decorah, IA, USA

L.L. Toussaint et al. (eds.), *Forgiveness and Health*,
DOI 10.1007/978-94-017-9993-5_9

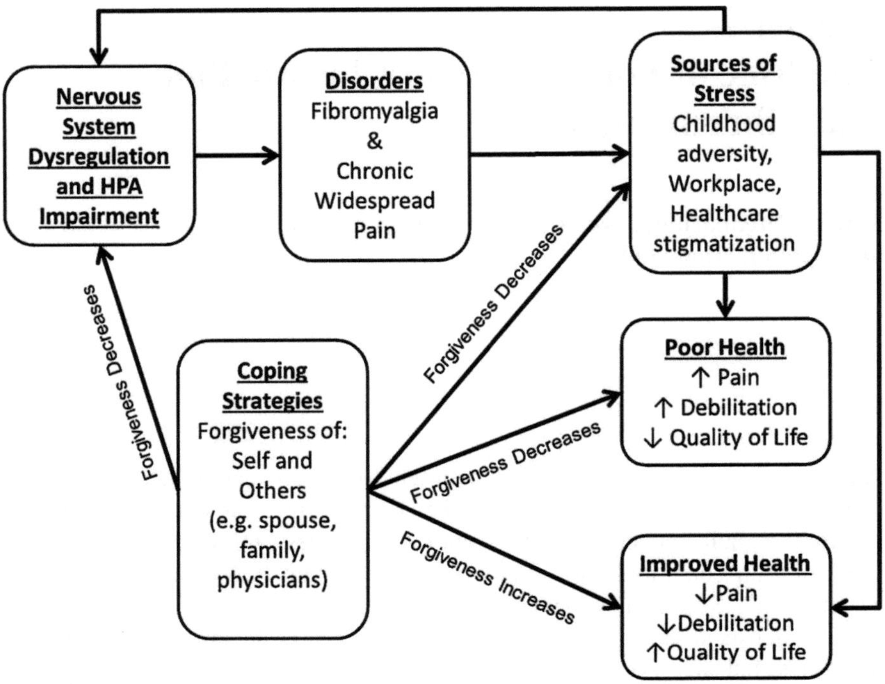

Fig. 9.1 Conceptual model of the stressful consequences of fibromyalgia and chronic widespread pain and the role of forgiveness as a coping mechanism that positively impacts health

this argument is relatively new in the literature on forgiveness and health, we first develop the conceptual classification and structure of the sources of stress that are relevant to forgiveness. The second focus is then on how these forms of stress are effectively coped with, and we suggest that an especially healthy means of coping is through forgiveness.

Chronic Wide Spread Pain and Fibromyalgia Syndrome (FMS)

Chronic wide spread pain (CWP) is a prevalent disease. Population-based studies of CWP have suggested that approximately 10–11 % of the population has this symptom at any given time (Bergman et al., 2001; Buskila, Abramov, Biton, & Neumann, 2000). CWP, defined as pain on both sides of the body above and below the waist and in the axial skeleton present for at least 3 months, is the cardinal feature of fibromyalgia syndrome (FMS) (Wolfe et al., 1990). The population-based prevalence of FMS has been reported in the industrialized world to be 3 % (White, Speechley, Harth, & Ostbye, 1999), indicating that this is an important subgroup of CWP. Both CWP and FMS are health conditions of unknown etiology that predominantly affect middle-aged adults, women somewhat more than men.

FMS is associated with debilitating widespread pain, fatigue, non-restorative sleep (Wolfe, Ross, Anderson, & Russell, 1995), and other symptoms (Bennett, 1996; Bou-Holaigah et al., 1997; Landro, Stiles, & Sletvold, 1997). Depression is a common comorbidity in patients with FMS (Uguz et al., 2010). Both conditions, as well as, anxiety have independent, as well as, additive adverse effects on pain severity, pain interference, functional limitations and quality of life (Bair, Wu, Damush, Sutherland, & Kroenke, 2008). Patients with FMS report reduced physical functioning and exhibit a lower health-related quality of life (Neumann, Berzak, & Buskila, 2000). Furthermore, patients with CWP or FMS may develop so-called "pain behaviors", such as expression or suppression of emotional distress, avoidance of activities believed to cause pain, distressed interpersonal communication, and maladaptive coping strategies (Burckhardt, Clark, O'Reilly, & Bennett, 1997). It has been suggested that the costs of health care for patients with chronic pain may exceed the combined costs of treating patients with coronary artery disease, cancer, and AIDS (Cousins, 1995).

Stress and FMS

Stress results when environmental demands exceed an individual's perceived ability to cope producing a response composed of negative cognitive and emotional states (Lazarus & Folkman, 1984). This includes chronic stressors such as caring for a spouse with dementia (Roepke et al., 2011) or brief events, such as sexual assault, that continue to be experienced as stressful long after they have ended (Baum, Cohen, & Hall, 1993).

Stressors activate the hypothalamic-pituitary-adrenal (HPA) axis and/or the sympathetic nervous system (SNS) to help the organism adapt physiologically with the threat (Black, 2003). The HPA axis and the SNS regulate via their central effectors (i.e., hypothalamic hormones and norepinephrine) and peripheral effectors (i.e., glucocorticoids, norepinephrine and epinephrine) the physiological stress response thereby influencing wake-sleep cycles, growth, thyroid axis response, and reproductive, gastrointestinal, cardiorespiratory, metabolic, and immune systems (Chrousos, 2009). HPA and SNS mediated effects of stress on disease are supported by animal and human studies (Cohen, Janicki-Deverts, & Miller, 2007).

There is growing evidence that FMS is a stress related syndrome. Studies in FMS have generally demonstrated altered functioning of the HPA axis and SNS (Martinez-Lavin, 2012; Williams & Clauw, 2009). However, studies have demonstrated both hypo- and hyper-activity of the HPA axis and the SNS in FMS, and often the degree of abnormality is small or occurs in a subgroup of patients with substantial overlap between patients and controls. Some researchers have proposed that FMS can be viewed as a failed attempt of our complex adaptive system to accommodate to a hostile external environment. FMS is, in this view, a disease in which distress is transformed into pain through sympathetic system rigidity (Martinez-Lavin, 2012).

Sources of Stress in CWP and FMS

Given the relevance of stress to pain, a number of sources of stress that are particularly important, unique, and impactful for CWP and particularly for FMS are reviewed below. The following review focuses especially on those sources of stress that are of an interpersonally stressful nature or involve stress that results from the wrongdoing of others. In short, we review stressors that are prevalent in individuals with CWP or FMS and for which forgiveness would seem to be an effective and healing coping response. Table 9.1 summarizes this discussion including sources of stress and the best-fitting forgiveness coping response(s).

Childhood Adversity Childhood adversities including sexual abuse, abuse and neglect, are extremely common in western societies (Kessler et al., 2010). Multiple converging lines of evidence point to the role of childhood adversities in pain

Table 9.1 Sources of stress for chronic wide-spread pain and fibromyalgia patients and relevant dimensions of forgiveness coping

	Relevant forgiveness coping dimensions	
Source of stress	Forgiveness of self	Forgiveness of others
Childhood adversity: Emotional, physical, sexual trauma		✓
Workplace: Bullying, harassment, discrimination		✓
Spouse, family, friends: Lack of affection and support from others; difficulties with parenting and marital strife	✓	✓
Healthcare stigmatization: Scepticism from healthcare staff, difficulties with insurance providers, misdiagnosis		✓
Overcommitment: Levels of dissatisfaction with oneself, insecurity, and a lack of social recognition	✓	✓
Perfectionism: Dealing with exceedingly high and unreachable expectations for oneself and others	✓	✓
Anger: Anger at: (a) the person responsible for the injury/illness, (b) the health care provider, (c) the mental health professional, (d) the legal system, (e) insurance and third party payers, (f) employers, (g) significant others, (h) God, (i) self, and (j) the whole world	✓	✓
Shame: Shame and self-blame over interference with activities of daily living resulting from pain; struggles with self-esteem and dignity	✓	
Social exclusion: Feeling alienated by physicians, health authorities, significant others and friends. Feeling unappreciated.		✓

disorders such as FMS. Cross sectional studies have shown that FMS patients have histories of higher rates of emotional and physical maltreatment and sexual abuse compared to controls (Boisset-Pioro, Esdaile, & Fitzcharles, 1995; Hauser, Kosseva, Uceyler, Klose, & Sommer, 2011). In addition to sexual and physical maltreatment, FMS patients more frequently report a poor emotional relationship with both parents, a lack of physical affection, experiencing parents' physical quarrels, as well as, alcohol or other problems of addiction in the mother, separation, and a poor financial situation before the age of 7 (Imbierowicz & Egle, 2003). Not surprisingly, abused FMS patients show significantly higher pain, fatigue, functional disability, and stress compared to the non-abused FMS patients.

Qualitative research offers additional insight into the connection between adversity and pain disorders. Sigurdardottir and Halldorsdottir (2013) interviewed seven women with a history of childhood sexual abuse. All suffered CWP and five had FMS. All the women described repressed and silent suffering in all aspects of life, and felt the abuse was still seriously affecting them and their loved ones at the time of the interview. As children, they reported having learning problems, experiencing bullying, and suffering unexplained physical symptoms. As adults, all had trouble trusting others. According to their accounts, time does not heal all wounds.

The weight of the evidence suggests a pivotal role for childhood adversity in FMS and this may have important therapeutic implications. Sexual, physical, and emotional trauma, potentially mediated by shame and self-blame, appear to be important factors in the development and maintenance of FMS and its associated disability. This is exemplified in the following case:

Case Description The 54 year old female patient grew up in a very tough family environment. Her father was an aggressive alcoholic who beat and sexually abused her mother. Very early in her childhood the patient was a silent witness of the brutal incidents. At the age of 7 her mother left her father. She then grew up at her grandmother's house, where she was able to start anew. She was very active in the religious community in her town. Her mother married again and her father insisted, enforced by law, that she had to visit him every 2 weeks. At these visits he was often drunk and beat her. She silently endured her martyrdom. At the age of 12 she lost her 3-year old brother in a motorcycle accident. She lost her faith and left her religious community. She was mad at God, because of the death of her brother. At the age of 14 she was sexually abused by her father. Again she kept silent. Her emotional pain, trauma, anger and grief were still very present when she decided to start therapy in 2006. The main focus of the holistic and spiritual therapeutic process was a shift from being victimised to developing a more reflective and gentle perspective of the self in order to foster forgiveness towards her father. In this process she started to realize that to stop her suffering it would be necessary to forgive her father and herself. She intensively reflected about her father and took responsibility for her life. She began to understand that her hate and anger towards him and her pain kept her in limbo. This realization helped her find harmony and inner peace. Her chronic pain gradually improved. In the next step she effectively worked to reduce feelings of guilt about her brother's death. Later on she acknowledged that repressed anger and feelings of powerlessness were being expressed as chronic pain.

Though childhood adversities may be an impactful stressor with long-term consequences, other sources of chronic stress that are concomitant with adult pain disorders also exist. Though not an exhaustive review, we provide some of the key sources of chronic stress for individuals living with pain disorders in the following.

Workplace It is well known that CWP and FMS affect working ability (Reisine, Fifield, Walsh, & Forrest, 2008). In one study (Henriksson, 1994) 75 % of the FMS patients reported symptoms that had influenced the work situation and 69 % found their work stressful. Fifty two percent worked shorter hours than prior to the FMS symptoms, 34 % worked at a slower pace, and 38 % needed frequent rest periods. Forty-five percent reported that specific work tasks were difficult to perform (e.g. sitting or standing for long periods, operating machines, typing, etc.). Despite numerous challenges, women with FMS indicate that work roles are very important for their identity and self-esteem (Liedberg & Henriksson, 2002). Non-working patients lose social contacts and become isolated resulting in feelings of diminished dignity and meaning in life. FMS patients mention often the importance of the interpersonal environment at work referring to understanding, help, and support from colleagues (Bossema et al., 2012). To the contrary, FMS patients often encounter disapproval of their peers due to their reduced working capacity and frequent sick days. It is not uncommon that this results in bullying, harassment, offending behavior, and social exclusion that ultimately affects work and productivity (Einarsen, Hoel, Zapf, & Cooper, 2003). Eventual stigmatisation and repeated victimization are not uncommon.

Spouse, Family, and Friends Couples dealing with chronic pain have more psychological and relationship distress than healthy couples (Cano, Johansen, Leonard, & Hanawalt, 2005). Chronic pain appears to affect family functioning in multiple ways: (a) cohesiveness (e.g., lower family commitment and support provision for affected partner), (b) couples' affection/sexual relations (e.g., decrease in marital and sexual satisfaction in both partners), (c) family finances (e.g., lower income due to inability to work), (d) friends (e.g., less and infrequent contacts due to illness), (e) household tasks (e.g., inability to manage household chores), and (f) recreation (e.g. inability to engage in joint activities). Each of these factors holds potential for increased interpersonal distress leading to more pain symptoms.

Other studies point to an important connection between spousal and family discord and difficulties with pain. Spousal anger, contempt, and sadness have been shown to have a negative effect on depressive symptoms and pain in the partner suffering from pain (Johansen & Cano, 2007). However, when both partners reported chronic pain the effect of negative emotional expression on symptoms was less pronounced indicating that it may instead promote emotion regulation because the affect is experienced with a spouse who may be more empathic (and perhaps more able to forgive). In another study, FMS patients that self-reported family stressors, strains, and distress showed increased health problems and functional disability (Preece & Sandberg, 2005). Studies such as these suggest that hostile marriage and family environments have negative consequences in patients with FMS.

Stigmatization in the Health Care System Medical conditions vary dramatically in the extent to which they are socially accepted. For instance, patients with incontinence or schizophrenia are often stigmatized, whereas, those with hypertension or bone fractures are accepted. This may seem trivial medically, but consider that if all stigmatised conditions were taken together and all outcomes examined, stigma would be shown to have a major impact on peoples' lives (Link & Phelan, 2006).

FMS is commonly stigmatized because no identifiable organic pathology can be found. This causes uncertainty among doctors (Perrot, Choy, Petersel, Ginovker, & Kramer, 2012) and patients, enhancing stigmatization. Lengthy debates have developed in the medical literature (Hadler, 2003; Winfield, 2001) often with the result that FMS is considered a psychogenic disorder that is "all in the head" of the patients. This results in undermining the personal legitimacy of FMS patients (Cohen, Quintner, Buchanan, Nielsen, & Guy, 2011). As a result of stigmatization, FMS patients withdraw from several areas of social life (Asbring & Narvanen, 2002) further enhancing the feeling of rejection and worthless.

Focus group research shows that apart from the pain, the attitude of others regarding FMS was the most important theme (Hieblinger, Coenen, Stucki, Winkelmann, & Cieza, 2009). Patients describe often feeling left alone with their illness, due to a lack of understanding and acceptance from others. Several patients reported feeling as if FMS is not accepted as a legitimate illness by many doctors and health care professionals and is often trivialised by friends, relatives and colleagues. Women with FMS have also emphasized the impact of a physician's negative attitude and disbelief of FMS resulting in a feeling of being doomed and not being able to move on with one's life (Sylvain & Talbot, 2002).

Over-committment Female FMS patients often have a history of chronic psychosocial burden consisting of caring for their families, going to work, and looking after needy relatives (e.g. one's own or spouse's parents or grandparents) prior to the onset of FMS related symptoms. FMS patients describe themselves as "very action-oriented" (Van Houdenhove, Neerinckx, Onghena, Lysens, & Vertommen, 2001). This self-image can lead to self-blame and feelings of guilt and anger when faced with functional limitations due to pain and fatigue. This notion is corroborated by a small study of FMS and chronic fatigue patients showing high reported levels of dissatisfaction with oneself, insecurity, and a lack of social recognition (Van Houdenhove et al., 2002).

Perfectionism Perfectionism is the tendency to impose extremely high standards on performance and to interpret perceived shortcomings as failures (Hart, Gilner, Handal, & Gfeller, 1998). Perfectionism has been further differentiated into three types: (a) self-oriented perfectionism which is critical self-scrutiny and unrealistic self-imposed personal standards, (b) other-oriented perfectionism which is the expectation that others should achieve unrealistic standards and a tendency toward dominance and authoritarianism, and (c) socially prescribed perfectionism which is the need to achieve standards and goals given by others (Hewitt & Flett, 1991). Research with patients suffering from chronic insomnia, a key symptom of FMS, supports the connection between perfectionism and negative health outcomes (Vincent & Walker, 2000). Chronic insomniac patients were more likely to report doubts about action, frequent parental criticism, and concern over mistakes. Our own clinical observations suggest that especially high demands towards oneself and overestimation of one's own capabilities often result in a self-induced failure. We illustrate this in the following case example:

Case Description Mrs. Smith's only source of self-esteem and -approval is her work. She puts all her resources into her work without realizing that her high standards are a source of conflict with peers and superiors. These conflicts trigger anxiety and she has to increase her efforts to live up to her high standards. This results in increased fatigue, pain, exhaustion, and withdrawal. She also has high expectations toward her friends, but they are not prepared to live up to her high expectations. This leads to frustrations and challenges but she avoids talking about things with her friends. Her friends sense her suppressed anger and bring this to her attention. She feels like no one understands her and she withdraws even more: "Nobody can see how bad I feel."

Anger Anger is an emotion that can be defined as a strong, uncomfortable emotional response to a provocation that is unwanted and incongruent with one's values, beliefs, or rights (Thomas, 1995). One study identified 10 potential targets of anger in patients with chronic pain: (a) the person responsible for the injury/illness, (b) the health care provider, (c) the mental health professional, (d) the legal system, (e) insurance and third party payers, (f) employers, (g) significant others, (h) God, (i) self, and (j) the whole world (Fernandez & Turk, 1995). A high proportion of chronic pain patients experience angry feelings. In a cross-sectional study with 96 patients, 74 % reported anger at oneself and 62 % were angry with a health care professional (Okifuji, Turk, & Curran, 1999). These kinds of anger were shown to be related to perceived disability, and anger towards oneself was significantly associated with pain and depression.

Styles of anger expression have been shown to have unique connections to pain. In a recent 28-day study of 333 women with FMS, only trait anger inhibition was significantly related to more pain (van Middendorp et al., 2010). Another smaller study showed that anger-in (i.e. suppressed and unexpressed anger style) was consistently higher in fibromyalgia patients as compared to patients with rheumatoid arthritis (Sayar, Gulec, & Topbas, 2004). These findings are further supported by a small qualitative study where chronic pain patients presented themselves as conscientious, compliant, passive, and rule-bound, viewing life and emotional expression as dangerous, avoiding conflict and risk, and denying their own emotional needs (Corbishley, Hendrickson, Beutler, & Engle, 1990). These studies suggest that the presence, intensity, and expression of anger may be important to better understand psychological adaptation to chronic pain.

Shame Shame and guilt are negative emotions and as such, both can cause intrapsychic pain (Tangney, Stuewig, & Mashek, 2007). Shame is considered the more painful emotion because one's core self is at stake. Feelings of shame are typically accompanied by a sense of shrinking or of "being small" and by a sense of worthlessness and powerlessness.

Patients with chronic pain and FMS often experience feelings of shame and self-blame for different reasons, some of which we have already alluded to. They feel shame because of their sickness, or they doubt their feelings of pain and think of themselves as hypochondriacs, or they feel questioned from healthcare professionals and misunderstood by family and friends, and they struggle for self-esteem and dignity as patients and women (Gustafsson, Ekholm, & Ohman, 2004; Werner & Malterud, 2003).

Social Exclusion Social exclusion, sometimes dubbed social pain, is common in FMS patients whose suffering is not recognized by physicians, health authorities, significant others and friends. Often people who are not feeling pain or fatigue underestimate the pain of the patient (Kappesser, Williams, & Prkachin, 2006), and this is valid in relation to social exclusion and pain (Nordgren, Banas, & MacDonald, 2011). Further, it is not infrequent that FMS patients perceive this stigma (Asbring & Narvanen, 2002; Looper & Kirmayer, 2004). In short, humans are social animals and exclusion, as a social threat, is as important as biological threats (Williams, 1997). Neural overlap in processing physical and social sources of pain has been described in several studies (Eisenberger & Lieberman, 2004) suggesting that social exclusion has a strong potential for exacerbating or contributing independently to increased pain intensity. For pain patients, experiencing social exclusion is likely associated with negative emotions such as anger, shame, and guilt, the adverse effects of which have already been described.

Coping Mechanisms in CWP and FMS

CWP and FMS patients are not only confronted with enduring pain, but also with the detrimental and stressful conditions and environments that were reviewed above. Consequently, it is critical to study coping as it can reduce *or* amplify the effects of these stressors on pain and adjustment (Skinner, Edge, Altman, & Sherwood, 2003).

Emotion Regulation Researchers largely agree that problem-focused coping can be useful for changeable situations, whereas emotion-focused coping might be most useful for situations not amenable to change (Strelan & Covic, 2006). Therefore, emotion regulation is an important and often studied process in coping with chronic pain (Keefe et al., 2001). Emotion regulation can be both maladaptive and adaptive in nature (Stanton, Danoff-Burg, Cameron, & Ellis, 1994). With this in mind, we examine anger as a maladaptive or failed attempt at emotion regulation and contrast it with forgiveness as a complementary positive coping process.

Anger Anger is one of the most salient properties of pain (Fernandez & Turk, 1995), and can exacerbate pain (Greenwood, Thurston, Rumble, Waters, & Keefe, 2003). A positive correlation between anger and pain intensity has been shown in patients with chronic back pain (Kerns, Rosenberg, & Jacob, 1994), spinal cord injury (Conant, 1998), and cancer (Glover, Dibble, Dodd, & Miaskowski, 1995). Anger-in (i.e., suppressing feelings of anger) and anger-out (i.e., displaying anger in an overtly aggressive manner) have both shown detrimental effects on cardiovascular health (Gallacher, Yarnell, Sweetnam, Elwood, & Stansfeld, 1999), hypertension (Gentry, Chesney, Gary, Hall, & Harburg, 1982) and somatic complaints (Martin et al., 1999). Recent research suggests that anger coping is a multidimensional construct and other dimensions of anger coping should be studied as well (Miers, Rieffe, Meerum Terwogt, Cowan, & Linden, 2007).

One aspect of anger coping that is receiving increasing attention, especially in relation to chronic pain, is angry rumination. Rumination can be defined as a passive and repetitive focus on the negative and damaging aspects of a situation (McCullough, Orsulak, Brandon, & Akers, 2007). Angry rumination is associated with increased physical complaints in both children (Miers et al., 2007) and adults (Hogan & Linden, 2004). Biological (e.g., increased muscle reactivity), behavioral (e.g. anger disrupting important social relationships), and affective pathways (e.g. anger leading to depression) may connect angry rumination to chronic pain disorders.

Forgiveness Forgiveness is currently receiving growing interest as a valuable coping mechanism in chronic pain. A unique method of coping, forgiveness involves affective, behavioral, motivational and cognitive components (Strelan & Covic, 2006). Growing evidence suggests health benefits of forgiveness in a variety of groups such as the general population (Toussaint, Williams, Musick, & Everson, 2001; Toussaint, Owen, & Cheadle, 2012), elderly blacks (McFarland, Smith, Toussaint, & Thomas, 2012), and patients with spinal cord injury (Webb, Toussaint, Kalpakjian, & Tate, 2010). Furthermore, forgiveness has been shown to be inversely related to pain in physical therapy outpatients (Svalina & Webb, 2012), chronic pain patients (Parenteau, Hamilton, Twillman, & Khan, 2008), and low-back pain patients (Carson et al., 2005).

Though often thought of as a personality characteristic, forgiveness can be conceptualized as an emotion-focused coping mechanism for dealing with interpersonal and social stress (Worthington & Scherer, 2004). There are at least six ways in which the forgiveness process is analogous to the coping process, namely forgiveness: (a) is a reaction to a stressor, (b) involves appraisals, (c) is emotion regulation, (d) is future-oriented, (e) can be both intra- and inter-personal, and (f) is dynamic and unfolds over time (Strelan & Covic, 2006). Given the broad spectrum of interpersonal and social stressors that are unique and powerful contributors to

CWP and FMS, forgiveness as an emotion-focused coping process would seem an ideal and productive response.

Conclusions and Implications

Because it may not be immediately apparent why forgiveness would be relevant to pain disorders, we have offered a review of several unique sources of stress that pain patients confront that have a high relevance to forgiveness. In addition, we briefly reviewed anger and forgiveness as ways of responding to these stressors. Though CWP and FMS patients often report adversity in childhood, personality characteristics that exacerbate pain, and family, social, and stigmatization experiences that could easily elicit chronic anger and angry rumination, forgiveness might potentially offer a more productive approach to handling these adversities and chronic stressors. We provided a couple of case examples to illustrate the relevance to forgiveness in pain disorders and hope that healthcare professionals will consider the importance of appropriate emotion regulation through forgiveness to help patients cope with life situations that undoubtedly take a significant toll on their health and well-being. To that end, we offer a couple of additional ways in which common stressors might be coped with through forgiveness in pain patients: (a) Interference due to symptoms of pain, fatigue, depression, muscle stiffness, and disability could be coped with through self-forgiveness. (b) Not being able to fulfil demands of a spouse (e.g., sports, leisure time activities) because of symptoms could be coped with through self-forgiveness. (c) Spousal negativity, showing displeasure, criticism, anger, could be dealt with through forgiveness of others. (d) Stigmatization and discrimination faced by patients from friends, family, and healthcare providers could be coped with through forgiveness of others. Certainly other examples exist of how the unique social stressors and circumstances surrounding CWP and FMS could provide opportunities for coping through forgiveness. We hope that our review of the most common sources of social stress and suggestion for the positive outcomes of coping with it through forgiveness instead of anger will inspire both patients and providers to consider the potential healing of coping through forgiveness.

References

Asbring, P., & Narvanen, A. L. (2002). Women's experiences of stigma in relation to chronic fatigue syndrome and fibromyalgia. *Qualitative Health Research, 12*(2), 148–160.

Bair, M. J., Wu, J., Damush, T. M., Sutherland, J. M., & Kroenke, K. (2008). Association of depression and anxiety alone and in combination with chronic musculoskeletal pain in primary care patients. *Psychosomatic Medicine, 70*(8), 890–897.

Baum, A., Cohen, L., & Hall, M. (1993). Control and intrusive memories as possible determinants of chronic stress. *Psychosomatic Medicine, 55*(3), 274–286.

Bennett, R. M. (1996). The contribution of muscle to the generation of fibromyalgia symptomatology. *Journal of Musculoskeletal Pain, 4*, 35–59.

Bergman, S., Herrstrom, P., Hogstrom, K., Petersson, I. F., Svensson, B., & Jacobsson, L. T. (2001). Chronic musculoskeletal pain, prevalence rates, and sociodemographic associations in a Swedish population study. *Journal of Rheumatology, 28*(6), 1369–1377.

Black, P. H. (2003). The inflammatory response is an integral part of the stress response: Implications for atherosclerosis, insulin resistance, type II diabetes and metabolic syndrome X. *Brain, Behavior, and Immunity, 17*(5), 350–364.

Boisset-Pioro, M. H., Esdaile, J. M., & Fitzcharles, M. A. (1995). Sexual and physical abuse in women with fibromyalgia syndrome. *Arthritis and Rheumatism, 38*(2), 235–241.

Bossema, E. R., Kool, M. B., Cornet, D., Vermaas, P., de Jong, M., van Middendorp, H., & Geenen, R. (2012). Characteristics of suitable work from the perspective of patients with fibromyalgia. *Rheumatology (Oxford), 51*(2), 311–318.

Bou-Holaigah, I., Calkins, H., Flynn, J. A., Tunin, C., Chang, H. C., Kan, J. S., & Rowe, P. C. (1997). Provocation of hypotension and pain during upright tilt table testing in adults with fibromyalgia. *Clinical and Experimental Rheumatology, 15*(3), 239–246.

Burckhardt, C. S., Clark, S. R., O'Reilly, C. A., & Bennett, R. M. (1997). Pain-coping strategies of women with fibromyalgia: Relationship to pain, fatigue, and quality of life. *Journal of Musculoskeletal Pain, 5*(3), 5–21.

Buskila, D., Abramov, G., Biton, A., & Neumann, L. (2000). The prevalence of pain complaints in a general population in Israel and its implications for utilization of health services. *Journal of Rheumatology, 27*(6), 1521–1525.

Cano, A., Johansen, A. B., Leonard, M. T., & Hanawalt, J. D. (2005). What are the marital problems of patients with chronic pain? *Current Pain and Headache Reports, 9*(2), 96–100.

Carson, J. W., Keefe, F. J., Goli, V., Fras, A. M., Lynch, T. R., Thorp, S. R., & Buechler, J. L. (2005). Forgiveness and chronic low back pain: a preliminary study examining the relationship of forgiveness to pain, anger, and psychological distress. *The Journal of Pain, 6*(2), 84–91.

Chrousos, G. P. (2009). Stress and disorders of the stress system. *Nature Reviews Endocrinology, 5*(7), 374–381.

Cohen, M., Quintner, J., Buchanan, D., Nielsen, M., & Guy, L. (2011). Stigmatization of patients with chronic pain: The extinction of empathy. *Pain Medicine, 12*(11), 1637–1643.

Cohen, S., Janicki-Deverts, D., & Miller, G. E. (2007). Psychological stress and disease. *JAMA, 298*(14), 1685–1687.

Conant, L. (1998). Psychological variables associated with pain perceptions among individuals with chronic spinal cord injury pain. *Journal of Clinical Psychology in Medical Settings, 5*, 71–90.

Corbishley, M. A., Hendrickson, R., Beutler, L. E., & Engle, D. (1990). Behavior, affect, and cognition among psychogenic pain patients in group expressive psychotherapy. *Journal of Pain and Symptom Management, 5*(4), 241–248.

Cousins, M. J. (1995). Foreword. In W. E. Fordyce (Ed.), *Back pain in the workplace management of disability in nonspecific conditions task force report* (Vol. IX). Seattle, WA: IASP Press.

Einarsen, S., Hoel, H., Zapf, D., & Cooper, C. L. (Eds.). (2003). *The concept of bullying at work. The European tradition*. London, UK: Taylor & Francis.

Eisenberger, N. L., & Lieberman, M. D. (2004). Why rejection hurts: A common neural alarm system for physical and social pain. *Trends in Cognitive Sciences, 8*, 294–300.

Fernandez, E., & Turk, D. C. (1995). The scope and significance of anger in the experience of chronic pain. *Pain, 61*(2), 165–175.

Gallacher, J. E., Yarnell, J. W., Sweetnam, P. M., Elwood, P. C., & Stansfeld, S. A. (1999). Anger and incident heart disease in the caerphilly study. *Psychosomatic Medicine, 61*(4), 446–453.

Gentry, W. D., Chesney, A. P., Gary, H. E., Jr., Hall, R. P., & Harburg, E. (1982). Habitual anger-coping styles: I. Effect on mean blood pressure and risk for essential hypertension. *Psychosomatic Medicine, 44*(2), 195–202.

Glover, J., Dibble, S. L., Dodd, M. J., & Miaskowski, C. (1995). Mood states of oncology outpatients: Does pain make a difference? *Journal of Pain and Symptom Management, 10*(2), 120–128.

Greenwood, K. A., Thurston, R., Rumble, M., Waters, S. J., & Keefe, F. J. (2003). Anger and persistent pain: Current status and future directions. *Pain, 103*(1–2), 1–5.

Gustafsson, M., Ekholm, J., & Ohman, A. (2004). From shame to respect: Musculoskeletal pain patients' experience of a rehabilitation programme, a qualitative study. *Journal of Rehabilitation Medicine, 36*(3), 97–103.

Hadler, N. M. (2003). "Fibromyalgia" and the medicalization of misery. *Journal of Rheumatology, 30*(8), 1668–1670.

Hart, B. A., Gilner, F. H., Handal, P. J., & Gfeller, J. D. (1998). The relationship between perfectionism and self-efficacy. *Personality and Individual Differences, 24*, 109–113.

Hauser, W., Kosseva, M., Uceyler, N., Klose, P., & Sommer, C. (2011). Emotional, physical, and sexual abuse in fibromyalgia syndrome: A systematic review with meta-analysis. *Arthritis Care & Research (Hoboken), 63*(6), 808–820.

Henriksson, C. M. (1994). Longterm effects of fibromyalgia on everyday life. A study of 56 patients. *Scandinavian Journal of Rheumatology, 23*(1), 36–41.

Hewitt, P. L., & Flett, G. L. (1991). Perfectionism in the self and social contexts: Conceptualization, assessment, and association with psychopathology. *Journal of Personal and Social Psychology, 60*(3), 456–470.

Hieblinger, R., Coenen, M., Stucki, G., Winkelmann, A., & Cieza, A. (2009). Validation of the international classification of functioning, disability and health core Set for chronic widespread pain from the perspective of fibromyalgia patients. *Arthritis Research & Therapy, 11*(3), R67.

Hogan, B. E., & Linden, W. (2004). Anger response styles and blood pressure: At least don't ruminate about it! *Annals of Behavioral Medicine, 27*(1), 38–49.

Imbierowicz, K., & Egle, U. T. (2003). Childhood adversities in patients with fibromyalgia and somatoform pain disorder. *European Journal of Pain, 7*(2), 113–119.

Johansen, A. B., & Cano, A. (2007). A preliminary investigation of affective interaction in chronic pain couples. *Pain, 132*(Suppl 1), S86–S95.

Kappesser, J., Williams, A. C., & Prkachin, K. M. (2006). Testing two accounts of pain underestimation. *Pain, 124*(1–2), 109–116.

Keefe, F. J., Lumley, M., Anderson, T., Lynch, T., Studts, J. L., & Carson, K. L. (2001). Pain and emotion: New research directions. *Journal of Clinical Psychology, 57*(4), 587–607.

Kerns, R. D., Rosenberg, R., & Jacob, M. C. (1994). Anger expression and chronic pain. *Journal of Behavioral Medicine, 17*(1), 57–67.

Kessler, R. C., McLaughlin, K. A., Green, J. G., Gruber, M. J., Sampson, N. A., Zaslavsky, A. M., & Williams, D. R. (2010). Childhood adversities and adult psychopathology in the WHO World Mental Health Surveys. *British Journal of Psychiatry, 197*(5), 378–385.

Landro, N. I., Stiles, T. C., & Sletvold, H. (1997). Memory functioning in patients with primary fibromyalgia and major depression and healthy controls. *Journal of Psychosomatic Research, 42*(3), 297–306.

Lazarus, R. S., & Folkman, S. (1984). *Stress, appraisal and coping*. New York, NY: Springer.

Liedberg, G. M., & Henriksson, C. M. (2002). Factors of importance for work disability in women with fibromyalgia: An interview study. *Arthritis and Rheumatism, 47*(3), 266–274.

Link, B. G., & Phelan, J. C. (2006). Stigma and its public health implications. *Lancet, 367*(9509), 528–529.

Looper, K. J., & Kirmayer, L. J. (2004). Perceived stigma in functional somatic syndromes and comparable medical conditions. *Journal of Psychosomatic Research, 57*(4), 373–378.

Martin, R., Wan, C., David, J., Wegner, E., Olson, B., & Watson, D. (1999). Style of anger expression: Relation to expressivity, personality, and health. *Personality and Social Psychology Bulletin, 25*, 1196–1207.

Martinez-Lavin, M. (2012). Fibromyalgia: When distress becomes (un)sympathetic pain. *Pain Research and Treatment, 2012*, 981565.

McCullough, M. E., Orsulak, P., Brandon, A., & Akers, L. (2007). Rumination, fear, and cortisol: An in vivo study of interpersonal transgressions. *Health Psychology, 26*(1), 126–132.

McFarland, M. J., Smith, C. A., Toussaint, L., & Thomas, P. A. (2012). Forgiveness of others and health: Do race and neighborhood matter? *Journals of Gerontology. Series B, Psychological Sciences and Social Sciences, 67*(1), 66–75.

Miers, A. C., Rieffe, C., Meerum Terwogt, M., Cowan, R., & Linden, W. (2007). The relation between anger coping strategies, anger mood and somatic complaints in children and adolescents. *Journal of Abnormal Child Psychology, 35*(4), 653–664.

Neumann, L., Berzak, A., & Buskila, D. (2000). Measuring health status in Israeli patients with fibromyalgia syndrome and widespread pain and healthy individuals: Utility of the short form 36-item health survey (SF-36). *Seminars in Arthritis and Rheumatism, 29*(6), 400–408.

Nordgren, L. F., Banas, K., & MacDonald, G. (2011). Empathy gaps for social pain: Why people underestimate the pain of social suffering. *Journal of Personal and Social Psychology, 100*(1), 120–128.

Okifuji, A., Turk, D. C., & Curran, S. L. (1999). Anger in chronic pain: Investigations of anger targets and intensity. *Journal of Psychosomatic Research, 47*(1), 1–12.

Parenteau, S., Hamilton, N., Twillman, R., & Khan, T. (2008). To forgive is divine, but does it help patients adjust to chronic pain?: The role of forgiveness and offense-taking in chronic pain. *Annals of Behavioral Medicine, 35*, S155.

Perrot, S., Choy, E., Petersel, D., Ginovker, A., & Kramer, E. (2012). Survey of physician experiences and perceptions about the diagnosis and treatment of fibromyalgia. *BMC Health Services Research, 12*, 356.

Preece, J. C., & Sandberg, J. G. (2005). Family resilience and teh management of fibromyalgia: Implications for family therapists. *Contemporary Family Therapy, 27*, 559–576.

Reisine, S., Fifield, J., Walsh, S., & Forrest, D. D. (2008). Employment and health status changes among women with fibromyalgia: A five-year study. *Arthritis and Rheumatism, 59*(12), 1735–1741.

Roepke, S. K., Chattillion, E. A., von Kanel, R., Allison, M., Ziegler, M. G., Dimsdale, J. E., & Grant, I. (2011). Carotid plaque in Alzheimer caregivers and the role of sympathoadrenal arousal. *Psychosomatic Medicine, 73*(2), 206–213.

Sayar, K., Gulec, H., & Topbas, M. (2004). Alexithymia and anger in patients with fibromyalgia. *Clinical Rheumatology, 23*(5), 441–448.

Sigurdardottir, S., & Halldorsdottir, S. (2013). Repressed and silent suffering: Consequences of childhood sexual abuse for women's health and well-being. *Scandinavian Journal of Caring Sciences, 27*(2), 422–432.

Skinner, E. A., Edge, K., Altman, J., & Sherwood, H. (2003). Searching for the structure of coping: A review and critique of category systems for classifying ways of coping. *Psychological Bulletin, 129*(2), 216–269.

Stanton, A. L., Danoff-Burg, S., Cameron, C. L., & Ellis, A. P. (1994). Coping through emotional approach: Problems of conceptualization and confounding. *Journal of Personal and Social Psychology, 66*(2), 350–362.

Strelan, P., & Covic, T. (2006). A review of forgiveness process models and a coping framework to guide future research. *Journal of Social and Clinical Psychology, 25*, 1059–1085.

Svalina, S. S., & Webb, J. R. (2012). Forgiveness and health among people in outpatient physical therapy. *Disability and Rehabilitation, 34*(5), 383–392.

Sylvain, H., & Talbot, L. R. (2002). Synergy towards health: A nursing intervention model for women living with fibromyalgia, and their spouses. *Journal of Advanced Nursing, 38*(3), 264–273.

Tangney, J. P., Stuewig, J., & Mashek, D. J. (2007). Moral emotions and moral behavior. *Annual Review of Psychology, 58*, 345–372.

Thomas, S. P. (1995). Women's anger: Causes, manifestations and correlates. In C. D. Spielberger & I. Sarason (Eds.), *Stress and emotions* (Vol. 15, pp. 53–74). Washington, DC: Taylor and Francis.

Toussaint, L. L., Owen, A. D., & Cheadle, A. (2012). Forgive to live: Forgiveness, health, and longevity. *Journal of Behavioral Medicine, 35*(4), 375–386.

Toussaint, L., Overvold-Ronningen, M., Vincent, A., Luedtke, C., Whipple, M., Schriever, T., & Luskin, F. (2010). Implications of forgiveness enhancement in patients with fibromyalgia and chronic fatigue syndrome. *Journal of Health Care Chaplaincy, 16*(3–4), 123–139.

Toussaint, L., Williams, D., Musick, M., & Everson, S. (2001). Forgiveness and health: Age differences in a U.S. probability sample. *Journal of Adult Development, 8*, 249–257.

Uguz, F., Cicek, E., Salli, A., Karahan, A. Y., Albayrak, I., Kaya, N., & Ugurlu, H. (2010). Axis I and Axis II psychiatric disorders in patients with fibromyalgia. *General Hospital Psychiatry, 32*(1), 105–107.

Van Houdenhove, B., Neerinckx, E., Onghena, P., Lysens, R., & Vertommen, H. (2001). Premorbid "overactive" lifestyle in chronic fatigue syndrome and fibromyalgia. An etiological factor or proof of good citizenship? *Journal of Psychosomatic Research, 51*(4), 571–576.

Van Houdenhove, B., Neerinckx, E., Onghena, P., Vingerhoets, A., Lysens, R., & Vertommen, H. (2002). Daily hassles reported by chronic fatigue syndrome and fibromyalgia patients in tertiary care: A controlled quantitative and qualitative study. *Psychotherapy and Psychosomatics, 71*, 207–213.

van Middendorp, H., Lumley, M. A., Moerbeek, M., Jacobs, J. W., Bijlsma, J. W., & Geenen, R. (2010). Effects of anger and anger regulation styles on pain in daily life of women with fibromyalgia: A diary study. *European Journal of Pain, 14*(2), 176–182.

Vincent, N. K., & Walker, J. R. (2000). Perfectionism and chronic insomnia. *Journal of Psychosomatic Research, 49*(5), 349–354.

Webb, J. R., Toussaint, L., Kalpakjian, C. Z., & Tate, D. G. (2010). Forgiveness and health-related outcomes among people with spinal cord injury. *Disability and Rehabilitation, 32*(5), 360–366.

Werner, A., & Malterud, K. (2003). It is hard work behaving as a credible patient: Encounters between women with chronic pain and their doctors. *Social Science and Medicine, 57*(8), 1409–1419.

White, K. P., Speechley, M., Harth, M., & Ostbye, T. (1999). The London fibromyalgia epidemiology study: The prevalence of fibromyalgia syndrome in London, Ontario. *Journal of Rheumatology, 26*(7), 1570–1576.

Williams, D. A., & Clauw, D. J. (2009). Understanding fibromyalgia: Lessons from the broader pain research community. *The Journal of Pain, 10*(8), 777–791.

Williams, K. D. (Ed.). (1997). *Social ostracism*. New York, NY: Plenum Press.

Winfield, J. B. (2001). Does pain in fibromyalgia reflect somatization? *Arthritis and Rheumatism, 44*(4), 751–753.

Wolfe, F., Ross, K., Anderson, J., & Russell, I. J. (1995). Aspects of fibromyalgia in the general population: Sex, pain threshold, and fibromyalgia symptoms. *Journal of Rheumatology, 22*(1), 151–156.

Wolfe, F., Smythe, H. A., Yunus, M. B., Bennett, R. M., Bombardier, C., Goldenberg, D. L., et al. (1990). The American college of rheumatology 1990 criteria for the classification of fibromyalgia. Report of the multicenter criteria committee. *Arthritis and Rheumatism, 33*(2), 160–172.

Worthington, E., & Scherer, M. (2004). Forgiveness as an emotion focused coping strategy that can reduce health risks and promote health resilience: Theory, review, and hypotheses. *Psychology and Health, 19*, 385–405.

Chapter 10
Forgiveness and Problematic Substance Use

Jon R. Webb and Bridget R. Jeter

> ... we saw that we were not only in conflict with *ourselves*, but also with *people* and *situations* in the world in which we lived. We had to begin to make our peace ... – *Twelve Steps & Twelve Traditions* (Alcoholics Anonymous, 1981, p. 108; emphasis added).

Since the 1930s, the Twelve-Step Model of addiction and recovery, originating and most notably associated with Alcoholics Anonymous (AA), has *anecdotally* included resentment and forgiveness as key components in the course of addiction and recovery (AA, 1981, 1998, 2001). The Twelve-Step Model also has been adapted for use in the context of many other substances, including various narcotics, marijuana, and nicotine, as well as other compulsive behaviors, such as gambling, overeating, and sexual activity. Over 15 years ago, Worthington (1998) included substance abuse problems as one of many areas of psychological research in health and well-being to which forgiveness would be applicable. In 2007, the then Deputy Director of the National Institute on Alcohol Abuse and Alcoholism argued for the prioritization of research on forgiveness (Calhoun, 2007). More recently, scholars have explicitly identified the construct and process of forgiveness in standardized, evidence-based, federally funded treatments for alcohol use disorders (Webb & Trautman, 2010). Although the lay mutual-help community, scholars, and policymakers have agreed that forgiveness is likely a critical factor in problematic substance use, only a small number of *empirical* examinations of such have been conducted. Of that which has been conducted (for a review, see Webb, Hirsch, & Toussaint, 2011), the long-held assumption of the salutary role of forgiveness in recovery has found preliminary support. In this chapter, we provide an overview of the psychology of forgiveness as it pertains to problematic substance use, including: (a) relevant dimensions of each in their relationship to one another, (b) theoretical

J.R. Webb (✉) • B.R. Jeter
Department of Psychology, East Tennessee State University, Johnson City, TN, USA
e-mail: webbjr@etsu.edu

L.L. Toussaint et al. (eds.), *Forgiveness and Health*,
DOI 10.1007/978-94-017-9993-5_10

modeling, (c) empirical evidence, (d) a research agenda, and (e) implications for health and well-being.

Dimensions of Problematic Substance Use

Recently updated diagnostic guidelines (American Psychiatric Association, 2013), while keeping the relevant conceptual criteria, no longer make a categorical distinction between Substance *Abuse* (maladaptive use and negative consequences) and Substance *Dependence* (continued abuse, often including tolerance, withdrawal, *and/or* compulsive behavior). Rather, the severity of a Substance *Use* Disorder is determined by the number of overall criteria present. More importantly, perhaps, many dimensional aspects of substance use are relevant when seeking a comprehensive understanding of problematic use and the implications and consequences thereof. As such, in addition to the *basic* diagnostic criteria for substance use disorders, the health-related outcome of problematic substance use necessarily includes more *complex* dimensional qualities, such as quantity, frequency, and/or intensity of use, problems associated with use (e.g., health, driving under the influence, unwanted sexual activity, financial strain), prevention, recovery (i.e., natural or treatment-based), relapse, and the impact of problematic substance use on others (e.g., partners, family, friends, individuals raised by parents with substance use problems). Given its fundamental role in the Twelve-Step Model and its consistency with evidence-based treatments, we maintain that forgiveness is critically relevant to each of the aforementioned aspects of problematic substance use. That is, whether in the context of: (a) resentments and the *lack* of forgiveness leading to problematic use itself or (b) working to resolve resentments and the *presence* of forgiveness leading to recovery from problematic use.

Dimensions of Forgiveness

There are *many* distinct dimensions of forgiveness, including state, trait, target (e.g., self, others, uncontrollable situations, and deity), and method (e.g., offering, seeking, feeling; see Toussaint & Webb, 2005). Referring back to the opening quote of this chapter, it is clear that multiple dimensions of forgiveness are likely to be relevant in the context of problematic substance use. Furthermore, when warning against and addressing the pitfalls of "hostility, grudges, [and] resentments" (AA, 1998, p. 38), thereby attaining and maintaining sobriety and recovery, the Twelve-Step Model stresses the importance of explicitly identifying the offending "people, institutions, [and] principles" (AA, 2001, p. 64). However, underlying this approach, the reader/consumer of *The Big Book* is reminded that, "First, we searched out the flaws in our make-up which caused our failure. Being convinced that *self*, manifested in various ways, was what had defeated us, we considered its common manifestations" (AA, 2001, p. 64; emphasis added). Importantly, individuals are encouraged also to balance their recovery with responsible self-compassion (AA, 1998), which can include self-forgiveness (Neff, 2003). As such, according to the Twelve-Step Model, it appears that while many dimensions of forgiveness are likely relevant, forgiveness of self may be the most important dimension when addressing problematic substance use.

Models of the Association Between Forgiveness and Problematic Substance Use

Basic models regarding the relationship between forgiveness and health, in general, as well as the process of forgiveness itself have been developed. Respectively, these models have been: (a) expanded to include the specific relationship with problematic substance use and (b) identified as inherent to and/or consistent with evidenced-based treatments for problematic substance use. Addressed extensively elsewhere in this volume, we will briefly mention relevant aspects of said models here, in order to provide important context for our ensuing discussion of their expansion to problematic substance use and consistency with evidence-based treatments.

General Health Worthington and colleagues have proposed a model that claims that trait forgiveness, or forgivingness, as a component of the larger relationship between religion and health, is associated with a variety of aspects of physical health, mental health, and well-being through both direct and indirect mechanisms (e.g., Worthington, 1998; Worthington, Berry, & Parrott, 2001). The direct effect is thought to be a function of its inextricable association with rumination and stress (see Toussaint & Webb, 2005) arising in response to the process of *un*forgiveness, which encompasses a variety of negative emotional responses to offense, including *resentment*, anger, bitterness, hostility, fear, and hatred (emphasis added). The indirect effect is thought to be a function of mediating relationships with other distinct variables, such as health behavior, social support, and interpersonal functioning. For example, it is thought that higher levels of forgiveness are likely to be associated with higher levels of social support, which in turn is likely to be associated with better health-related outcomes. Evidence in support of the salutary association of forgiveness with health is burgeoning and while less work focused on the particular context of Worthington's model has been done, it is accumulating (see Webb, Hirsch, Visser, & Brewer, 2013; Webb, Toussaint, & Conway-Williams, 2012).

Problematic Substance Use We have proposed that the association between forgiveness and problematic substance use also is likely to operate through direct and indirect mechanisms (Fig. 10.1; Webb et al., 2011). Consistent with Worthington's model regarding the role of rumination, stress, and resentment in the otherwise direct effect of forgiveness on health, our model of the direct effect is focused on the fundamental interplay between resentments and forgiveness in the Twelve-

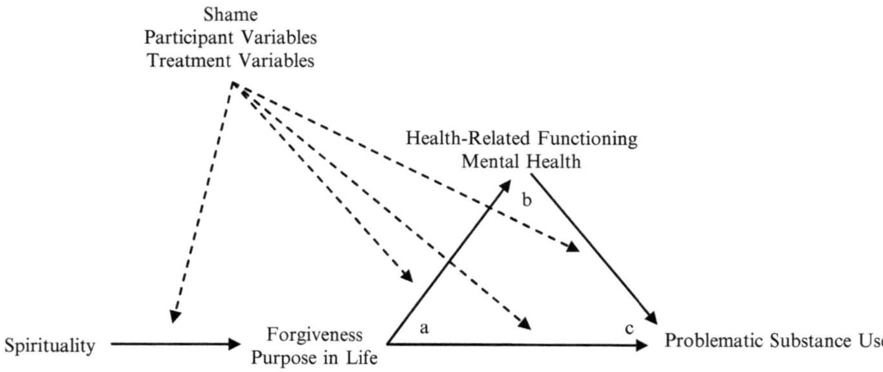

Fig. 10.1 A model of the forgiveness–problematic substance use association. a→c = Direct Effect of Forgiveness on Dependent Variable(s). a→b = Direct Effect of Forgiveness on Mediator Variable(s). b→c = Direct Effect of Mediator Variable(s) on Dependent Variable(s). a→b→c = Indirect Effect of Forgiveness on Dependent Variable(s) through Mediator Variable(s). Dotted → = Moderation Effect (Note. This figure is a conceptual representation of the relationship between forgiveness and problematic substance use. For statistical modeling and analyses relevant to various manifestations of this model, see Hayes (2013). Adapted from Worthington et al. (2001), Webb et al. (2011), and Lyons et al. (2010))

Step Model. That is, "*resentment* is the 'number one' offender. It destroys more alcoholics than anything else" (AA, 2001, p. 64; emphasis added). Arguably *the* core component of the Twelve-Step Model designed to address the problem of resentments is the development and resolution of a "grudge list" (AA, 2001, p. 65). One is carefully, honestly, and thoroughly to identify all resentments based in anger, hurt, and perception of threat, including all targets of such resentments. Of note, this grudge list is meant to be a *living* document, such that in order to attain and maintain recovery, one must include and address *all* resentments; past, present, and future. As such, within the Twelve-Step Model, the process and practice of forgiveness is thought to be embedded in recovery from problematic substance use. We argue that the direct effect of forgiveness is likely to result from its relationship to several, if not all, of the steps in the Twelve-Step Model (Webb et al., 2011; Webb & Trautman, 2010). Importantly, Lyons, Deane, and Kelly (2010) also have proposed a model wherein forgiveness, along with purpose in life, plays a role in the relationship between spirituality and recovery (Fig. 10.1).

Our model of the indirect effect involves two categories of distinct mediators (Fig. 10.1; Webb et al., 2011). Consistent with Worthington's general model, Health-Related Functioning includes health behavior, social support, and interpersonal functioning as mediators. Expanding upon Worthington's model, Mental Health includes psychological distress (i.e., symptoms of depression and anxiety) and suicidal behavior as mediators. In developing this model of the indirect effect, we have *begun* to identify a variety of potential mediators based upon said variables being associated, theoretically and/or empirically, with both forgiveness and a variety of the dimensions of problematic substance use. This identification process, whether in the context of Worthington's general model or any additional mediators, involves identifying variables individually associated with forgiveness and problematic substance use. For example, given that depressive symptoms are: (a) negatively associated with forgiveness (see Webb et al., 2012) and (b) positively associated with problematic substance use (see Webb et al., 2011), it may be that depression plays a role in the relationship *between* forgiveness and substance use.

Such variables may be considered proximal players in the forgiveness–problematic substance use association. Variables otherwise known to be associated with proximal mediators, but not necessarily associated with forgiveness and/or problematic substance use may also play a role. For example, psychache [intense, unrelenting, and unremitting psychological pain (e.g., an aching soul; Holden, Mehta, Cunningham, & McLeod, 2001)] is related to depression and suicidal behavior (DeLisle & Holden, 2009). While forgiveness is associated with depression and suicidal behavior (see Webb et al., 2012), its association with psychache is unknown, given a lack of published research. Nonetheless, given its close association with otherwise proximal mediators and its intuitive, but again, unknown association with problematic substance use, it seems likely that psychache may also be a mediator. Using these methods to identify potential indirect mechanisms, it is feasible that there may be many mediators *and* moderators (see McFarland, Smith, Toussaint, & Thomas, 2012) of the association between forgiveness and problematic substance use.

Process of Forgiveness Extensive models of the practice of forgiveness have been developed. For example, Enright, Freedman, and Rique (1998) culled and summarized 20 units of forgiveness from the literature and divided them into four broad phases, herein denoted by the first letter of each phase: $UDWD_2$. *Uncovering* refers to an awareness of the problem and emotional pain following an offense, including anger and insight; *Decision* includes realizing the need for an alternate resolution; *Work* includes processes such as, reframing, empathy, and acceptance of pain; and *Deepening* includes finding meaning and universality. Similarly, Worthington's (2006) REACH Forgiveness model involves *Recall*ing an offense, developing *Empathy*, choosing forgiveness as an *Altruistic* gift, making a public, formal *Commitment* to forgive, and *Holding on* to progress.

Evidence-Based Treatment Twelve-Step Facilitation Therapy, Motivational Enhancement Therapy, and Cognitive-Behavioral Coping Skills Therapy, individually (e.g., Project MATCH; Longabaugh & Wirtz, 2001) and collectively (e.g., COMBINE; Miller, 2004), have received ample scientific evaluation as standardized treatment(s) for problematic substance use. Webb and Trautman (2010) argue that the process of forgiveness is inherent to *each* of these empirically-supported psychosocial treatments (see Table 10.1).

Concentrating on the first three steps of the Twelve-Step Model (AA, 1981, 1998, 2001), Twelve-Step Facilitation Therapy (Nowinski, Baker, & Carroll, 1994) is focused on the underlying principles of acceptance and surrender. However,

Table 10.1 The process of forgiveness among evidence-based treatments for problematic substance use

Forgiveness phase		Corresponding aspects of empirically-based treatments		
Enright ($UDWD_2$)	Worthington (REACH)	TSF	MET/SoC[a]	CBCST
Uncovering	Recall	Step 1[b]	Contemplation	Introduction;
				Cravings and urges;
				Emergencies and relapse
Decision	Empathy;	Steps 2 & 3	Determination;	Managing thoughts;
	Altruism;		development of discrepancy	Irrelevant decisions;
	Commitment			Refusal skills
Work	Commitment	Steps 4, 5, 6, 7, 8, & 9	Action; empathy	Cravings and urges;
				Managing thoughts;
				Irrelevant decisions;
				Problem solving;
				Refusal skills;
				Reframing; role-playing
D_2eepening	Hold On	Steps 10, 11, & 12	Maintenance	Managing thoughts;
				Irrelevant decisions;
				Universality

TSF Twelve-step facilitation therapy, *MET/SoC* motivational enhancement therapy/stages of change, *CBCST* cognitive-behavioral coping skills therapy

[a]Precontemplation and Relapse are consistent with the ebb and flow of forgiveness

[b]While Uncovering and Recall are overwhelmingly associated with Step 1, they also are likely associated with Steps 2–12, albeit to a lesser degree

Adapted from Webb and Trautman (2010)

it also can incorporate a variety of elective components, thereby potentially including each of the Twelve Steps. Admitting powerlessness over substances, Step 1 addresses developing accurate and appropriate self-regulation, including understanding the interplay of defenses, anger, and shame [Forgiveness: Enright's *U* and Worthington's *R* phases (see Table 10.1)]. Believing in a higher power (Step 2) and making the decision to submit to one's conceptualization thereof (Step 3) involves recognizing and considering the personal need for both change and help, and making a commitment thereto (Enright's *D* and Worthington's *E*, *A*, and *C*). Developing a personal moral inventory (i.e., a grudge list; Step 4) identifies resentments and striving for forgiveness, which can be directed toward a variety of targets (e.g., self, others, and God). Appropriate self disclosure of one's grudge list (Step 5) and active submission to one's higher power (Steps 6 & 7) involve continued and focused efforts to reframe, accept, and find resolution to issues heretofore uncovered. Becoming willing to make amends (Step 8) and making amends when possible and appropriate (Step 9) have been explicitly described as the *forgiveness steps* of AA (Hart, 1999). Considering Steps 4 through 9 together, much time and arduous effort is necessarily invested in Enright's *W* and Worthington's *C* phases of the process of forgiveness. Proactive continuation of the processes involved in Steps 4 and 5 (Step 10), consistent pursuit of one's higher power (Step 11), and assisting peers with recovery and the broad personal application of the entire Twelve-Step Model to *everyday living* (Step 12) foster vigilance and serve to strengthen recovery (Enright's D_2 and Worthington's *H*).

Designed to catalyze change through internal motivation (Miller, Zweben, DiClemente, & Rychtarik, 1994), Motivational Enhancement Therapy incorporates Prochaska and DiClemente's (1986) model of the Stages of Change (SoC). Consistent with SoC *Contemplation*, both Enright's *U* and Worthington's *R* phases involve an individual developing an awareness of their problematic circumstances (see Table 10.1). Consistent with SoC *Determination*, Enright's *D* and Worthington's *E*, *A*, and *C* each involve a deliberate cognitive resolution to pursue a different course of action. Consistent with SoC *Action*, both Enright's *W* and Worthington's *C* expand the previous task to include purposeful activities and behavior to address the problem at hand. Likewise, consistent with SoC *Maintenance*, Enright's D_2 and Worthington's *H* are designed to preserve, strengthen, and develop the progress heretofore achieved. Additionally, SOC *Precontemplation* and *Relapse* are consistent with the ebb and flow of forgiveness (see Enright et al., 1998; Toussaint & Webb, 2005; Webb & Trautman, 2010) in that individuals may fluctuate back and forth between a lack of consideration of forgiveness, the process of forgiveness, and a return to problematic behavior.

The expression of empathy and the development of discrepancy also are important components in the clinical practice of Motivational Enhancement Therapy (Miller & Rollnick, 1991). While the function of empathy may differ between forgiveness and Motivational Enhancement Therapy, each approach similarly requires a level of understanding to proceed; whether given or received. The development of discrepancy in Motivational Enhancement Therapy is similar to Enright's *D* and Worthington's *E*, *A*, and *C* wherein the task is to recognize and choose an alternative option(s) more likely to lead to growth.

Consisting of eight core sessions followed by up to four electives, Cognitive-Behavioral Coping Skills Therapy (CBCST) is designed to entail up to 12 sessions (Kadden et al., 1994). Building rapport and understanding of rationale (CBCST *Introduction*) facilitates many components of Enright's *U* and Worthington's *R* phases through identifying one's patterns, motivations, and defenses and recognizing the various harms of substance use (see Table 10.1). Addressing triggers for relapse (CBCST *Craving and Urges*) facilitates both Enright's *U* and Worthington's *R* through continued recognition of cathexis and Enright's *W* and Worthington's

C through consistent acceptance and reframing of urges and thoughts. *Managing Thoughts* and *Irrelevant Decisions* (CBCST) involves each of the phases of forgiveness, except Enright's *U* and Worthington's *R*, such that it is important to *maintain* a firm commitment to recovery and continued vigilance in identifying, recognizing, and countering relapse-provoking thought processes. *Problem Solving* and *Refusal Skills* (CBCST) include the management of interpersonal tension wherein reframing social situations (Enright's *W* and Worthington's *C*) will likely relieve pressure for relapse. *Refusal Skills* also mirrors Enright's *D* and Worthington's *E*, *A*, and *C*, given the need to avoid high-risk situations and to be quick to refuse immediate demands. Dealing with the effects of guilt and shame following relapse (CBCST *Emergencies and Relapse*) will necessitate a return to Enright's *U* and Worthington's *R* as one struggles to prevent sustained relapse. Also, the general CBCST themes of universality, reframing thoughts, and role-playing newly acquired skills are central to Enright's *W* and D_2 and Worthington's *C* and *H* phases of the process of forgiveness.

In sum, Webb and Trautman (2010) have conceptually linked the process of forgiveness to Twelve-Step Facilitation Therapy, each step in the Twelve-Step Model, and many of the principles of Motivational Enhancement Therapy and Cognitive-Behavioral Coping Skills Therapy. Lyons et al. (2010) also described the extensive conceptual tie between forgiveness and the Twelve-Step Model. Forgiveness, from a psychosocial point of view, may very well be the primary antidote to problematic substance use, in particular, and addiction, in general.

Empirical Evidence

Webb et al. (2011) reviewed the scientific literature available through early 2011 and found 59 relevant references; 13 were published studies explicitly focused on the *empirical* relationship of forgiveness with problematic *alcohol* use. In early 2013, using the same search tools and phrase [PsycINFO and PUBMED; "(alcohol OR substance OR drug) AND forgiv*"], we found 10 additional references; 8 were empirical studies focused in a similar fashion.

Literature Through Early 2011 Webb et al. (2011) reviewed empirical literature pertaining to each of the associations portrayed in the aforementioned model (see Fig. 10.1). Across and within most of these studies multiple dimensions of forgiveness were examined; mostly trait forgivingness of self, of others, and/or by God.

In summarizing the aforementioned literature, Webb et al. (2011) observed that "forgiveness, primarily forgiveness of self operating through mental health, may have a robust and salutary relationship with alcohol-related outcomes, whether it is in the context of use, problems, or recovery" (p. 261). It was also noted that: (a) religious culture may influence whether other dimensions of forgiveness (i.e., of others and by God) are associated, (b) for negative consequences of use, such relationships may be present longitudinally at 6-month follow-up, (c) social undermining, rather than general social support, may be a mediator, (d) shame may be a moderator, and (e) forgiveness *itself* may be an indirect mechanism of the association of numerous psychosocial issues with alcohol-related outcomes.

Updated Literature Review In the context of our model (see Fig. 10.1), 7 of the new empirical studies were focused on health and well-being related outcomes ($a \rightarrow b$) and 1 was focused on problematic use outcomes ($a \rightarrow c$). Again, across and within most of these studies multiple dimensions of forgiveness were examined, including forgivingness of self, of others, of uncontrollable situations, by others, and by God and/or state forgiveness of self and of others.

Half of the studies were conducted among individuals in alcohol and/or drug related treatment programs. Deane, Wootton, Hsu, and Kelly (2012) examined predictors of treatment dropout at 3 months, including forgivingness of self and of others. Of self was observed to be associated with higher odds of dropout, whereas of others was not associated therewith. Langman and Chung (2013) examined cross-sectional predictors of PTSD symptoms and psychological co-morbidity, including forgivingness of self, of others, and of situations and found no forgiveness-based associations. Lyons, Deane, Caputi, and Kelly (2011) cross-sectionally examined forgivingness of self, of others, by others, and by God as: (a) predictors of resentment and (b) mediators of the association between spirituality and purpose in life. Each dimension of forgivingness was associated with less resentment. Likewise, each dimension, except of others, was observed to be a partial mediator of the association between daily spiritual experiences and purpose in life. However, the association between Twelve-Step spiritual beliefs and purpose in life appeared to be indirect only – operating through feeling forgiven by God. Scherer, Worthington, Hook, and Campana (2011) compared the effect of a forgiveness of self intervention against treatment as usual on state forgiveness of self (re: alcohol problems), drinking refusal self-efficacy, guilt, and shame. Those receiving the forgiveness intervention showed greater improvements on each of the outcome measures.

Two studies individually examined forgiveness in the context of drinking and smoking. Krentzman, Cranford, and Robinson (2013) included forgivingness of self and of others in a longitudinal study of the effect of AA on frequency and intensity of drinking, as mediated by spirituality, among individuals diagnosed with alcohol dependence. AA involvement at 6 months was found to predict of others, but not of self, at 12 months. However, 12-month of others was not observed to be a mediator of the relationship between 6-month AA involvement and the drinking indicators at 18 months. Wohl and Thompson (2011) cross-sectionally examined state forgiveness of self (re: smoking) in association with Prochaska and

DiClemente's (1986) model of the Stages of Change. In support of their general hypothesis, forgiveness of self was observed to be negatively associated with stages of smoking behavior change.

Two studies examined forgiveness among people impacted by the problematic substance use of others. Osterndorf, Enright, Holter, and Klatt (2011) examined the effect of a forgiveness of others intervention on a variety of psychological variables among adult children of alcoholics, including state forgiveness of others, anxiety, depression, anger, self-esteem, and positive relationships with others. The forgiveness intervention was observed to have a salutary effect on each of the outcome measures, except anxiety, for adult children of alcoholics. Scherer et al. (2012) cross-sectionally examined relationships among state and trait forgiveness of others, trust, family cohesion, and perception of another's drinking refusal self-efficacy among participants who had an alcohol misuser in their family. In one study, trust and state forgiveness of others were lower in regard to a misusing drinker in the family versus a non-misusing drinker in the family. In a second SEM-based study, salutary associations were observed; forgivingness of others and family cohesion were associated with state forgiveness of others, which was associated with trust, which in turn was associated with participants' perception of the drinking refusal self-efficacy of a misusing drinker in the family.

Empirical examination of the relationship between forgiveness and problematic substance use continues to suggest a consistent, broad, and salutary association. Of the various dimensions of forgiveness measured, of self continues to play a prominent role. Yet, it was *also* observed to play a *deleterious* role in the context of treatment dropout and smoking behavior change. Lastly, the impact of one's problematic use on others (e.g., family) appears amenable to forgiveness.

Limitations

Although the benefit of forgiveness for recovery from addiction has been known from an anecdotal mutual-help perspective for *at least* 75 years (AA, 2001), scientific examination and verification has only recently begun. We are aware of but 21 empirical studies explicitly focused thereon. There are, of course, limitations local to each particular study. However, there are consistent concerns across studies as well and, in this regard, more important *global* limitations in need of attention. Of the research published to date, it is largely cross-sectional, naturalistic, and, when used, consists of short follow-up intervals. As such, conclusions cannot be drawn regarding a cause and effect relationship between forgiveness and problematic substance use. Furthermore, most of the studies are only in the context of alcohol, including all of the studies that measure actual use (i.e., quantity, frequency, and/or intensity of use). Last, although AA and related groups are well-established international organizations (see www.aa.org; www.na.org), much of the aforementioned research is also limited by Western cultural and religious bias.

Conclusions

While relevant empirical work is limited in terms of availability and research design, the existing scientific data appear to confirm what the Twelve-Step Model has tirelessly advocated since the 1930s. That is, the process of (un)forgiveness appears likely to be a critical factor in addiction and recovery. Together, 19 of 21 studies (90 %) suggest that multiple dimensions of forgiveness are meaningful and perhaps essential in addressing problematic substance use. Moreover, of the dimensions measured, forgivingness of self may be the most important thereto.

Future Research Agenda

In addition to the aforementioned limitations and as outlined in our model (Fig. 10.1), there are many aspects of the relationship between forgiveness and problematic substance use remaining to be identified and examined. When considering the limited availability of and design limitations to the existing studies, it is safe to say that all aspects of our model are in need of rigorous and continued empirical examination.

Elsewhere (Webb et al., 2011), we have called for a prioritized focus on intervention-based research, including the use of both clinical and non-clinical samples, multiple dimensions of forgiveness, and sophisticated design and analysis of indirect effects, including forgiveness itself examined as an indirect mechanism. Of critical importance for such research, we urged the use of sufficient follow-up intervals in order to prevent a variety of threats regarding Type I and Type II error. Early in treatment and recovery, individuals are less likely to use substances making analysis of relapse and relapse prevention more difficult. Likewise, limited statistical variation in substance use/problem related data prevents the utilization of more sophisticated analytical procedures and the ebb and flow of forgiveness may preclude confidence in short term results, whether salutary or deleterious. Lastly, we encouraged the use of Worthington's REACH Forgiveness intervention, given its explicit adaptation to problematic substance use *and* forgiveness of self in the context thereof (e.g., Scherer et al., 2011; Worthington, 2006).

Here, we will focus our recommendations for future directions on additional areas in need of attention. First and foremost, going forward it is imperative that we incorporate a wide range of substances in this program of research. While there is considerable overlap, it is critical to remember that there are salient differences in the process of addiction and recovery across substances of abuse. Second, in addition to potential differences among clinical versus non-clinical samples, a variety of other treatment-related (e.g., natural recovery, differing treatment modalities, etc.) and/or participant-related (e.g., gender, age, ethnicity, education, SES, spirituality, college environment, social environment (i.e., victim of others' problematic substance use), etc.) variables may come into play. Similarly, we must examine the full scope of forgiveness dimensions in this program of study. For example, the core component of the Twelve-Step Model regarding the development (Step 4) and resolution (Steps 8 and 9) of one's grudge list necessarily involves the identification and elimination of resentments (AA, 2001). While forgiveness *of* others is conceptually and anecdotally part of this process (and has received some empirical support), *seeking* forgiveness *from* others and *feeling* forgiveness *from* others are as well, and this process (seeking *and* feeling) may well be as important as forgiveness of self. Nevertheless, very little empirical attention has been paid to the separate constructs of seeking and feeling forgiveness from others (e.g., Lyons et al., 2011). Moderated differences may arise in one or more of the relationships proposed in our model (see Fig. 10.1). For example, ethnicity may moderate the association of forgiveness with problematic substance use (a → c; see McFarland et al., 2012), forgiveness with depression (a → b), the association of depression with problematic substance use (b → c), and/or the indirect association of forgiveness with problematic substance use, operating through depression (a → b → c). In terms of statistical analyses of indirect effects, Hayes (2013) describes myriad possibilities applicable to a model such as ours.

Third, we, and Lyons et al. (2010) also, have described the many links between forgiveness and specific evidence-based treatments for problematic substance use. Aside from Krentzman et al. (2013) said associations have not been empirically investigated. Lastly, consistent with the aforementioned models regarding forgiveness playing a role in the relationship between religion/spirituality and both health and problematic substance use (Lyons et al., 2010; Worthington et al., 2001), ritualistic, theistic, and/or existential spirituality (Webb, Toussaint, & Dula, 2014) may impact the associations portrayed in Fig. 10.1. That is, the association between spirituality, forgiveness, purpose in life, and problematic substance use may vary based on the particular aspects or dimensions thereof under consideration. For example, ritualistic spirituality (i.e., a structured connection with deity) may be associated with feeling forgiven by God and less problematic use, whereas existential spirituality (i.e., a non-theistic search for meaning and purpose) may be associated with forgiveness of self and fewer negative consequences of substance use.

Implications for Health and Well-Being

Understanding the influence of forgiveness in the process of addiction and recovery holds great potential not only for individuals struggling therewith (re: treatment), but public health (re: prevention) and society (re: education), at large. In previous reviews of the literature (Toussaint & Webb, 2005; Webb et al., 2011, 2012), we have stressed that the construct of forgiveness, while common to all mainstream world religions (Eastern, Western, monotheistic, polytheistic), is also central to psychology and philosophy, and thus, while not a panacea, is applicable to all people, regardless of culture, historical context, or geography. Forgiveness is an internally based process, largely independent of subsequent interaction with the offender and can be tailored to fit individual needs based on its multidimensional nature (e.g., state, trait, target, and method). Indeed, "given the universal, independent, and individual nature of forgiveness as a construct and intervention it is potentially very flexible in its application to [problematic substance use] and the effective and efficient treatment thereof" (Webb et al., 2011, p. 265).

Verification of the hypothesized effects of forgiveness in recovery likely will have a significant impact on current treatments for problematic substance use. For Twelve-Step Facilitation Therapy, an otherwise explicit and overt spirituality-based treatment, it will provide clarity and focus on a particular aspect of spirituality, rather than the general application thereof. For Motivational Enhancement Therapy, Cognitive-Behavioral Coping Skills Therapy, and other treatment modalities, the shift may be more profound, given a deliberate infusion of the explicit principles and practices of forgiveness, rather than simply sharing the otherwise underlying processes. In addition to the aforementioned scenario of forgiveness being an "Add-On" to well-established treatments, it may be that the science warrants the development of forgiveness as a "Stand-Alone" treatment for problematic substance use. Again, we encourage the continued expansion and application of Worthington's REACH Forgiveness model and intervention as it seems ready made for this purpose (see Scherer et al., 2011; Worthington, 2006).

More broadly, verification of the role of forgiveness in the process of addiction and recovery can be employed to the betterment of humanity through public health related efforts. In this regard, there can be efforts aimed at individuals at risk for developing problematic substance use, including substance use disorders. For example, outreach and prevention programs could be established on college campuses in an effort to combat the so-called substance abuse culture common thereto. Likewise, the reality is that most people engaging in problematic substance use, including those with substance use disorders, do not seek treatment and many people ultimately attain *natural* recovery through mutual-help programs, spiritual communities, or other means. As such, Public Service campaigns and other efforts (e.g., social networking) of local and national governments, as well as international leaders (i.e., individuals) and organizations (e.g., World Health Organization) may be effective in disseminating the relevant science and reducing the overwhelming biopsychosocial public burden of problematic substance use. Lastly, we advocate that society at large should *recognize* the science and engage in educating each other (individually and more generally through formal forgiveness education programs) regarding the merits of the construct and practice of forgiveness as a means of preventing the seeds of resentment from being planted in the first place.

Finally, the empirical examination of the direct and indirect effects of forgiveness in the context of addiction and recovery should carry wide appeal to a variety of funding agencies, both public and private. In the USA alone, a number of agencies under the umbrella of the National Institutes of Health (www.nih.gov) are charged with addressing issues core to our model. For example, the National Institute (NI) on Alcohol Abuse and Alcoholism, the NI on Drug Abuse, the NI of Mental Health, and the National Center for Complementary and Alternative Medicine. Likewise, the Substance Abuse and Mental Health Services Administration (www.samhsa.

gov) of the Department of Health & Human Services (www.hhs.gov) shares similar purposes. Relevant private agencies include the John Templeton Foundation (www.templeton.org) and the Fetzer Institute (www.fetzer.org). We call on such agencies to prioritize research in this area. The scientific field of forgiveness and problematic substance use is in a unique position to catalyze research. Not only to serve its own purposes, but more broadly in that once society fully recognizes the value of forgiveness from a scientific perspective, meaningful increases in funding, and the potential force for good thereof, may spread to other principles and practices common to positive psychology and/or spirituality and likely to promote health and well-being.

References[1]

Alcoholics Anonymous. (1981). *Twelve steps and twelve traditions*. New York, NY: Author.

Alcoholics Anonymous. (1998). *Living sober*. New York, NY: Author.

Alcoholics Anonymous. (2001). *Alcoholics Anonymous: The story of how many thousands of men and women have recovered from alcoholism* (4th ed.). New York, NY: Author.

American Psychiatric Association. (2013). *Diagnostic and statistical manual of mental disorders* (5th ed.). Washington, DC: Author.

Calhoun, F. J. (2007). Developmental research on alcohol and spirituality: What we know and what we don't know. *Southern Medical Journal, 100*(4), 427–429. doi:10.1097/SMJ.0b013e3180315de4.

*Deane, F. P., Wootton, D. J., Hsu, C.-I., & Kelly, P. J. (2012). Predicting dropout in the first 3 months of 12-step residential drug and alcohol treatment in an Australian sample. *Journal of Studies on Alcohol and Drugs, 73*(2), 216–225.

DeLisle, M. M., & Holden, R. R. (2009). Differentiating between depression, hopelessness, and psychache in university undergraduates. *Measurement and Evaluation in Counseling and Development, 42*(1), 46–63. doi:10.1177/0748175609333562.

Enright, R. D., Freedman, S., & Rique, J. (1998). The psychology of interpersonal forgiveness. In R. D. Enright & J. North (Eds.), *Exploring forgiveness* (pp. 46–62). Madison, WI: University of Wisconsin Press.

Hart, K. E. (1999). A spiritual interpretation of the 12-steps of alcoholics anonymous: From resentment to forgiveness to love. *Journal of Ministry in Addiction and Recovery, 6*, 25–39.

Hayes, A. F. (2013). *Introduction to mediation, moderation, and conditional process analysis: A regression-based approach*. New York, NY: Guilford Press.

Holden, R. R., Mehta, K., Cunningham, E. J., & McLeod, L. D. (2001). Development and preliminary validation of a scale of psychache. *Canadian Journal of Behavioural Science/Revue Canadienne des Sciences du Comportement, 33*(4), 224–232. doi:10.1037/h0087144.

Kadden, R., Carroll, K. M., Donovan, D., Cooney, N., Monti, P., Abrams, D., et al. (1994). *Cognitive-behavioral coping skills therapy manual: A clinical research guide for therapists treating individuals with alcohol abuse and dependence*. Rockville, MD: National Institute on Alcohol Abuse and Alcoholism.

*Krentzman, A. R., Cranford, J. A., & Robinson, E. A. R. (2013). Multiple dimensions of spirituality in recovery: A lagged mediational analysis of Alcoholics Anonymous'

[1] *Studies included in the updated literature review.

principal theoretical mechanism of behavioral change. *Substance Abuse, 34*(1), 20–32. doi:10.1080/08897077.2012.691449.
* Langman, L., & Chung, M. (2013). The relationship between forgiveness, spirituality, traumatic guilt and Posttraumatic Stress Disorder (PTSD) among people with addiction. *Psychiatric Quarterly, 84*(1), 11–26. doi:10.1007/s11126-012-9223-5.
Longabaugh, R., & Wirtz, P. W. (Eds.). (2001). *Project MATCH: Hypotheses, results, and causal chain analyses*. Rockville, MD: National Institute on Alcohol Abuse and Alcoholism.
* Lyons, G. C. B., Deane, F. P., Caputi, P., & Kelly, P. J. (2011). Spirituality and the treatment of substance use disorders: An exploration of forgiveness, resentment and purpose in life. *Addiction Research & Theory, 19*(5), 459–469. doi:10.3109/16066359.2011.555022.
Lyons, G. C. B., Deane, F. P., & Kelly, P. J. (2010). Forgiveness and purpose in life as spiritual mechanisms of recovery from substance use disorders. *Addiction Research & Theory, 18*(5), 528–543. doi:10.3109/16066351003660619.
McFarland, M. J., Smith, C. A., Toussaint, L., & Thomas, P. A. (2012). Forgiveness of others and health: Do race and neighborhood matter? *Journals of Gerontology. Series B, Psychological Sciences and Social Sciences, 67B*(1), 66–75. doi:10.1093/geronb/gbr121.
Miller, W. R. (Ed.). (2004). *COMBINE monograph series, volume 1. Combined behavioral intervention manual: A clinical research guide for therapists treating people with alcohol abuse and dependence* (DHHS publication no. (NIH) 04-5288). Bethesda, MD: National Institute on Alcohol Abuse and Alcoholism.
Miller, W. R., & Rollnick, S. (1991). *Motivational interviewing: Preparing people for change*. New York, NY: Guilford Press.
Miller, W. R., Zweben, A., DiClemente, C. C., & Rychtarik, R. G. (1994). *Motivational enhancement therapy manual: A clinical research guide for therapists treating individuals with alcohol abuse and dependence*. Rockville, MD: National Institute on Alcohol Abuse and Alcoholism.
Neff, K. D. (2003). Self-compassion: An alternative conceptualization of a healthy attitude toward oneself. *Self and Identity, 2*(2), 85–101. doi:10.1080/15298860309032.
Nowinski, J., Baker, S., & Carroll, K. M. (1994). *Twelve step facilitation therapy manual: A clinical research guide for therapists treating individuals with alcohol abuse and dependence*. Rockville, MD: National Institute on Alcohol Abuse and Alcoholism.
*Osterndorf, C., Enright, R., Holter, A., & Klatt, J. (2011). Treating adult children of alcoholics through forgiveness therapy. *Alcoholism Treatment Quarterly, 29*(3), 274–292. doi:10.1080/07347324.2011.586285.
Prochaska, J. O., & DiClemente, C. C. (1986). Toward a comprehensive model of change. In W. R. Miller & N. Heather (Eds.), *Treating addictive behaviors: Processes of change* (pp. 3–27). New York, NY: Plenum Press.
* Scherer, M., Worthington, E. L., Jr., Hook, J. N., Campana, K. L., West, S. L., & Gartner, A. L. (2012). Forgiveness and cohesion in familial perceptions of alcohol misuse. *Journal of Counseling & Development, 90*(2), 160–168. doi:10.1111/j.1556-6676.2012.00021.x.
* Scherer, M., Worthington, E. L., Jr., Hook, J. N., & Campana, K. L. (2011). Forgiveness and the bottle: Promoting self-forgiveness in individuals who abuse alcohol. *Journal of Addictive Diseases, 30*(4), 382–395. doi:10.1080/10550887.2011.609804.
Toussaint, L., & Webb, J. R. (2005). Theoretical and empirical connections between forgiveness, mental health, and well-being. In E. L. Worthington Jr. (Ed.), *Handbook of forgiveness* (pp. 349–362). New York, NY: Brunner-Routledge.
Webb, J. R., Hirsch, J. K., Visser, P. L., & Brewer, K. G. (2013). Forgiveness and health: Assessing the mediating effect of health behavior, social support, and interpersonal functioning. *Journal of Psychology: Interdisciplinary and Applied, 147*(5), 391–414. doi:10.1080/00223980.2012.700964.
Webb, J. R., Hirsch, J. K., & Toussaint, L. (2011). Forgiveness and alcohol problems: A review of the literature and a call for intervention-based research. *Alcoholism Treatment Quarterly, 29*(3), 245–273. doi:10.1080/07347324.2011.585922.

Webb, J. R., Toussaint, L., & Conway-Williams, E. (2012). Forgiveness and health: Psycho-spiritual integration and the promotion of better healthcare. *Journal of Health Care Chaplaincy, 18*, 57–73. doi:10.1080/08854726.2012.667317.

Webb, J. R., Toussaint, L., & Dula, C. S. (2014). Ritualistic, theistic, and existential spirituality: Initial psychometric qualities of the RiTE measure of spirituality. Journal of Religion & Health, 53(4), 972–985. doi:10.1007/s10943-013-9697-y.

Webb, J. R., & Trautman, R. P. (2010). Forgiveness and alcohol use: Applying a specific spiritual principle to substance abuse problems. *Addictive Disorders & Their Treatment, 9*(1), 8–17. doi:10.1097/ADT.0b013e318195000d.

* Wohl, M. J. A., & Thompson, A. (2011). A dark side to self-forgiveness: Forgiving the self and its association with chronic unhealthy behaviour. *British Journal of Social Psychology, 50*(2), 354–364. doi:10.1111/j.2044-8309.2010.02010.x.

Worthington, E. L., Jr. (1998). Empirical research in forgiveness: Looking backward, looking forward. In E. L. Worthington Jr. (Ed.), *Dimensions of forgiveness: Psychological research and theological perspectives* (pp. 321–339). Philadelphia, PA: Templeton Foundation Press.

Worthington, E. L., Jr. (2006). *Forgiveness and reconciliation: Theory and application*. New York, NY: Brunner-Routledge.

Worthington, E. L., Jr., Berry, J. W., & Parrott, L., III. (2001). Unforgiveness, forgiveness, religion, and health. In T. G. Plante & A. C. Sherman (Eds.), *Faith and health: Psychological perspectives* (pp. 107–138). New York, NY: Guilford Press.

Chapter 11
Forgiveness and Subjective Well-Being: Discussing Mechanisms, Contexts, and Rationales

Patrick L. Hill, Marie E. Heffernan, and Mathias Allemand

Forgiveness has been described as a virtue (e.g., Downie, 1965; Kurzynski, 1998; McGary, 1989), a strength (McCullough, 2000), and a benchmark of moral development (e.g., Enright et al., 1992; Enright, 1994). These conceptualizations often point to either the act of forgiveness, or being dispositionally forgiving as an indicator of a "prosocial" individual or one of high character. However, in addition to helping others and promoting social well-being, forgiveness also appears to benefit the forgiver insofar that it appears to promote personal well-being across multiple domains (see e.g., Hill, Allemand, & Heffernan, in press; Worthington, Witvliet, Pietrini, & Miller, 2007 for reviews).

The current chapter will discuss the role of forgiveness on personal well-being, focusing on whether and why forgiving individuals tend to report greater satisfaction and happiness across different domains. First, we begin by briefly defining forgiveness as a state and as a trait, the latter typically referred to as forgivingness (e.g., Roberts, 1995), as well as the concept of self-forgiveness. Second, we provide a theoretical model to explain the potential for forgiveness to promote life satisfaction, happiness, and domain-specific satisfaction across different relationship contexts. Third, we review the extant literature demonstrating a link between forgiveness or forgivingness and subjective well-being. Fourth, we conclude by discussing the need for future research that examines (a) state and trait forgiveness together in order to better understand their benefits, and (b) whether benefits may differ in kind or extent across the lifespan.

P.L. Hill (✉)
Department of Psychology, Carleton University, Ottawa, ON, Canada
e-mail: Patrick.Hill@carleton.ca

M.E. Heffernan
Department of Psychology, University of Illinois at Urbana-Champaign, Champaign, IL, USA

M. Allemand
Department of Psychology, University of Zurich, Zurich, Switzerland

L.L. Toussaint et al. (eds.), *Forgiveness and Health*,
DOI 10.1007/978-94-017-9993-5_11

Defining Forgiveness and Forgivingness

The act of forgiveness has received significant attention from psychological researchers over the years (e.g., Worthington, 2005). For our purposes, we borrow from McCullough and Witvliet (2002) in suggesting that forgiveness "may be understood as a prosocial change in a victim's thoughts, emotions, and/or behaviors toward a blameworthy transgression" (p. 447). Others too have noted how forgiveness portends an adaptive change from negative emotions toward the transgressor, to more prosocial or other-focused ones (e.g., Worthington & Wade, 1999). Three points are worth emphasizing regarding this definition. First, forgiveness need not require reconciliation, or a reestablishment of relations between the transgressor and victim, although in several cases both forgiveness and reconciliation may occur. Second, while the definition clearly establishes the prosocial benefits, it fails to suggest why it would lead to positive self-focused outcomes as well, a point that serves as the central catalyst for the current chapter. Third, forgiveness refers to a single act and a single transgressor. In other words, whether one forgives a given hurt need not suggest that the individual will forgive in a different future scenario.

To address this point, researchers have begun examining forgivingness, defined as a dispositional tendency to forgive others across different transgressions and transgressors (Roberts, 1995). In other words, forgivingness should predict an increased likelihood to forgive any specific transgression, and as such has been described as an attribute of a moral individual (Hill et al., in press). It therefore is important to note that forgivingness has been linked to state-level forgiveness (Allemand, Amberg, Zimprich, & Fincham, 2007), and meta-analytic work confirms that the disposition is a significant predictor of whether one forgives in a single scenario (Fehr, Gelfand, & Nag, 2010). However, these effect sizes tend to be moderate in nature, in line with the notion that a personality trait reflects a generally enduring, but not perfect tendency to act in a certain fashion (Roberts, 2009).

Another variable that merits consideration is self-forgiveness. Self-forgiveness refers to the ability to forgive the self either for personal failures or for transgressions against others (Hall & Fincham, 2005; Mauger et al., 1992; Tangney, Boone, & Dearing, 2005). Self-forgiveness has been assessed both in a given scenario (Wohl, DeShea, & Wahkinney, 2008), and as a greater dispositional tendency (Mauger et al., 1992; Thompson et al., 2005). Though trait self-forgiveness appears related to forgivingness (Thompson et al., 2005), research has demonstrated how self-forgiveness is empirically distinct from other forms of forgiveness (see e.g., Wohl et al., 2008). Indeed, work consistently has demonstrated that self- and other-forgiveness are distinct constructs with different correlates (e.g., Macaskill, 2012b; Ross, Kendall, Matters, Rye, & Wrobel, 2004).

Given this definitional multiplicity, describing the literature can quickly prove very complicated, particularly given that all three have been referred to under the umbrella term of "forgiveness." In order to avoid unnecessary complexity, we too will occasionally employ this universal term, as several points below will pertain to all forms of forgiveness. However, when describing specific findings, or predictions that may differ by form, we will employ terms such as "state forgiveness" as a contrast from trait "forgivingness," as well as state and trait "self-forgiveness" to differentiate the types discussed above. For instance, when describing why forgiveness can lead to subjective well-being, distinctive rationales and mechanisms can be posited for self-forgiveness compared to the other forms. Several of these distinctions reflect how the effects of forgiveness may change depending on the offender (e.g., yourself or someone else), given the vastly different subjective experiences involved.

The Scaffolding Self and Social Systems Model of Forgiveness and Subjective Well-Being

Researchers often focus on how forgiveness benefits the forgiver by virtue of releasing him or her from rumination, vengefulness, or other ill-thoughts. Indeed, it has been suggested that the primary goal of forgiveness is to "attenuate the bad" (e.g., Allemand, Hill, Ghaemmaghami, & Martin, 2012; Allemand, Job, Christen, & Keller, 2008; Worthington & Scherer, 2004), despite the fact that lay perceptions of forgiveness tend to focus more on its positive features (Kearns & Fincham, 2004). A conceptual corollary can be found in the emotion regulation literature, which notes the potential for down-regulating negative and up-regulating positive emotions (e.g., Parrott, 1993), although the focus tends to be on down-regulation (see e.g., Gross, Richards, & John, 2006). As such, several mediators previously discussed in the literature may fail to describe why forgiveness promotes well-being, rather than just reducing ill-being. Accordingly, Fig. 11.1 provides an organizing framework for future research to consider how forgiveness can lead to greater satisfaction and happiness. Such work could prove particularly valuable given that, as we discuss later, linking forgiveness to subjective well-being may be one pathway that motivates individuals toward a forgiving disposition. For now, we discuss the Scaffolding Self and Social Systems (4S) Model without this potential feedback loop, in order to simplify the introduction of potential mediators and mechanisms.

Increasing Relationship Harmony

Clearly, one of the larger roadblocks to having a satisfying relationship in any context is whether one experiences a large number of conflicts and strife. Such discord reduces relationship harmony. For instance, whether couples have conflicts, how they resolve them, and whether they restore relationship harmony are strong predictors of relationship satisfaction (e.g., Cramer, 2000; Fincham, Beach, & Davila, 2007; Schneewind & Gerhard, 2002). In this respect, one mechanism by

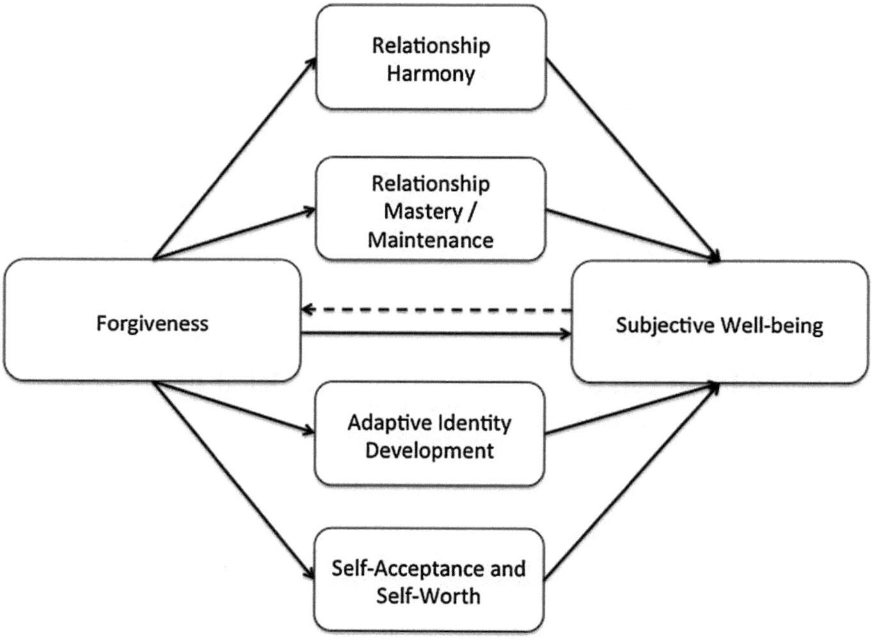

Fig. 11.1 The Scaffolding Self and Social Systems (4S) model of forgiveness and subjective well-being

which forgiveness could promote subjective well-being is through promoting more positive conflict resolution strategies when they do occur. Whether with respect to workplace, friend, romantic, or family relationships, one would predict that forgiving a relationship partner should lessen the likelihood for strife in that relationship. Additionally, self-forgiveness can lead to better relationships through making amends and repairing social damage (Worthington, 2013). Therefore, this pathway may better reflect the potential positives of state forgiveness or forgivingness than it does for self-forgiveness.

Promoting Relationship Mastery and Maintenance

Similarly, our second pathway also may represent the benefits of state forgiveness or forgivingness than self-forgiveness, as it again focuses on how forgiveness can promote subjective well-being through influencing one's social life. Specifically, in addition to reducing relationship strife, forgiveness may help to contour or promote relationship mastery and maintenance. By this, we mean to suggest that forgiving others can help people maintain close contacts, and have greater control over a given relationship. Put differently, an unforgiving person is likely to experience greater variability in their day-to-day relations with a given social partner, and as such will perceive less control over the social situation. As such, it is unsurprising that forgiveness has been described as a "core social construct" (Fincham, 2000), and possibly an evolutionary adaptation focused on promoting social cohesion and success (McCullough, 2008).

Fostering Adaptive Identity Development

Turning our focus to the self, forgiveness could play an important role in whether and how one explores and commits to an identity. Identity development has been demonstrated as a prominent influence on well-being and adaptation, particularly during the adolescent and emerging adult years (e.g., Berzonsky, 2003; Marcia, 1980; Meeus, Iedema, Helsen, & Vollebergh, 1999). Forgiveness could play one of two potential roles in promoting adaptive identity development. First, being able to forgive oneself for past transgressions, rather than linger and ruminate about whether these reflect self-failures, is likely to "free" an individual to more fully self-reflect and determine his or her identity. Second, as exploring the self often entails gaining information from significant others, being a dispositionally forgiving person should facilitate the process, insofar that it allows one to more freely navigate his or her social relationships. Put differently, if one is generally unforgiving of others, that individual may have few social resources from which to gain insight about his or her identity.

Increasing Self-Acceptance and Self-Worth

As noted above, people often view forgiveness as a moral virtue, and as such being a forgiving person could bolster one's self-perception. However, the potential exists for the alternative directionality as well: transgressions can come as an affront to one's sense of self (e.g., Scobie & Scobie, 1998), and in turn diminish the likelihood that one forgives the transgressor (Eaton, Struthers, & Santelli, 2006). As such, predictions on how state forgiveness and forgivingness may influence self-worth can prove complicated. A clearer prediction, though, can be made for self-forgiveness. By definition, forgiving the self means coming to terms with one's faults from the past, and thus should entail greater self-acceptance (see also Worthington, 2013). Similarly, relieving oneself from guilt over past affairs should increase self-worth as well, which then could increase subjective well-being (see Hall & Fincham, 2005).

Additional Model Notes

In addition to positing these pathways, we would like to point out three notes regarding the model. First, and most importantly, the model should be viewed both as a diagram for how forgiveness may promote satisfaction and happiness *in general* as well as how it may operate within a given context. For instance, these pathways can provide some rationale behind both why dispositionally forgiving people report better life satisfaction, and why forgiving your spouse can lead to better romantic relationship satisfaction. It remains an important question for future empirical work then to test whether these pathways are equally relevant for different contexts. Second, the value of these pathways also should differ by age group. For instance, the benefits linked to identity development are likely more valuable during adolescence and emerging adulthood, while relationship maintenance and quality appears a more important goal later in life (e.g., Lang & Carstensen, 2002), and as such this pathway could become a stronger mediator with age. Third, the model is left intentionally broad with respect to the specific indicators of each mediator and outcome. We do not intend to circumscribe the model by suggesting that it pertains only to life satisfaction, or happiness, or relationship satisfaction. Instead, we leave it to researchers to consider how different indicators may influence model results, and thus have tried to construct a relatively broad literature review below.

Forgiveness and Subjective Well-Being: A Review of the Extant Literature

Throughout our empirical review, we will describe studies that (a) link forgiveness with subjective well-being as well as (b) link forgiveness to the potential mediators in a causal pathway leading to greater well-being. Given our central focus on forgiveness, we refrain from providing a full description of how the mediators themselves link to subjective well-being, leaving the reader to consult the relevant literature in each specific domain (e.g., identity development, relationships, and well-being) for more on the linkages between the proposed mediators and well-being. However, as will become evident, much more research is needed that examines all three variables (predictor, mediator, and outcome) simultaneously.

Prior to the review, it is worth acknowledging the different roles that state and trait forgiveness may play when looking at broader or domain-specific well-being. For instance, forgiving a relatively minor transgression has the potential to influence one's well-being within that specific relationship, but may only have an effect on broader life satisfaction if that domain is especially valued or salient. Instead, forgivingness, reflecting a tendency to forgive across different relationship domains, is more susceptible to influencing overall life satisfaction. One can make similar claims regarding the potential benefits of state versus trait self-forgiveness. Accordingly, as will be shown below, the relationship between state forgiveness and well-being is more frequently examined within a specific domain, while broader measures of well-being are more commonly linked to trait measures. We will return to this point in the discussion section though, when considering whether well-being can motivate forgiveness.

Forgiveness and Global Well-Being

Life Satisfaction First, a number of studies have linked forgiveness positively to overall life satisfaction. Most frequently, researchers have examined this link with respect to the trait form of forgiveness. Indeed, the relationship between forgivingness and life satisfaction has been frequently substantiated, across different forgivingness measures (e.g., Brown & Phillips, 2005; Lawler-Row & Piferi, 2006; Thompson et al., 2005). Some work has suggested that the effect may be stronger, or even only occur, for older individuals (Sastre, Vinsonneau, Neto, Girard, & Mullet, 2003; Toussaint, Williams, Musick, & Everson, 2001), but one study found that no significant interaction effects with age, sex, or marital status (Hill & Allemand, 2011). A possible explanation for the occasional age interaction effects is that the benefits (and perceived benefits) of forgivingness may build up with time, leading to a stronger effect on overall life satisfaction for older than younger individuals. Alternatively, forgiveness may serve different functions across the life span, given that social goals tend to fluctuate during adulthood (e.g., Lang & Carstensen, 2002), as discussed further below.

Although it is more difficult to examine state forgiveness as a predictor of life satisfaction, given that it requires looking at single acts, some work does suggest that adaptive fluctuations in forgiveness-related motivations on a daily basis does predict increased later well-being, a composite measure that included life satisfaction (Bono, McCullough, & Root, 2008). For instance, increases in benevolence toward a transgressor coincided with increases in well-being.

Moreover, given that self-forgiveness is linked to greater psychological health (e.g., Mauger et al., 1992), it is unsurprising that research has demonstrated a link between the construct and life satisfaction. Indeed, some research even suggests that this relationship may be stronger than that evidenced for forgivingness (Macaskill, 2012b; Thompson et al., 2005), though they likely work on entirely different emotions and motivations. While our review focuses on self-forgiveness as a disposition, it is worth noting that some work on state self-forgiveness has failed to find a relationship with life satisfaction (Wohl, DeShea, & Wahkinney, 2008). Accordingly, again, when discussing overall satisfaction across multiple life domains, dispositional characteristics may prove better predictors than measures of forgiveness in a specific setting.

Happiness While infrequent, studies also have examined the role of forgiveness on dispositional happiness. For instance, one study demonstrated that both negative and positive aspects of state forgiveness are predictive (negatively and positively, respectively) of happiness across multiple measures (Maltby, Day, & Barber, 2005). In addition, some work suggests a link between forgivingness and happiness or general well-being (e.g., Toussaint & Friedman, 2009), as well as being forgiving and general positive affect (Hill & Allemand, 2011). Finally, one study found that self-forgiveness was related to more adaptive scores on a depression-to-happiness scale, suggesting that either they were happier, less susceptible to depression, or both (Macaskill, 2012a).

Mediator Analyses Very few studies have provided formal mediational tests of the link between forgiveness and global well-being, but some possible mechanisms have been suggested. For instance, one study has suggested potential roles for health behaviors, social support, religious well-being, and existential well-being in linking forgivingness to life satisfaction (Lawler-Row & Piferi, 2006). While this work failed to differentiate which variables played a stronger explanatory role than others, the potential role for social support underscores the promise for the social systems pathways in our 4S Model. In addition, work with psychotherapy outpatients found that the well-being benefits of forgivingness and self-forgiveness were mediated by whether individuals (a) reported greater positive than negative affect and (b) held more positive self-beliefs (Toussaint & Friedman, 2009). Here, one can find initial support for the possible role of scaffolding one's self as an explanatory mechanism. Though preliminary and with a circumscribed sample, these results suggest that forgiveness may promote well-being through increasing self-worth and self-esteem.

Forgiveness and Romantic Relationship Well-Being

Given the prosocial nature of forgiveness, it is unsurprising that it consistently correlates with or predicts greater relationship success. Indeed, state forgiveness of one's partner consistently correlates with greater romantic relationship satisfaction (e.g., Gordon, Hughes, Tomcik, Dixon, & Litzinger, 2009; Pansera & La Guardia, 2012; Schumann, 2012; Wieselquist, 2009). Given the importance of forgiveness for marital success, researchers have recently developed a scale focused on forgiveness of marital-specific transgressions, which points to the importance of increased benevolence and decreased resentment from both partners for marital quality and life satisfaction (Paleari, Regalia, & Fincham, 2009). It is interesting to note, then, that the effects do appear to differ by partner when looking at longitudinal effects. For instance, one study found that state forgiveness longitudinally predicted higher levels of later marital quality, but only when looking at the wives' forgiveness (Fincham & Beach, 2007). A potential reason for this sex difference may be that while wives' motives for forgiveness help predict their husbands' later conflict resolution, this effect does not appear to hold when examining the reverse (Fincham, Beach, & Davila, 2007). In other words, wives' state forgiveness and their motives for forgiving may mean more for later resolution of the transgression and ultimately marital satisfaction.

While most studies have looked at state forgiveness, its other forms also may play a role. Indeed, forgivingness has been shown to be positively associated with relationship satisfaction both in cross-sectional (Allemand, Amberg, Zimprich, & Fincham, 2007; Kachadourian, Fincham, & Davila, 2004) and longitudinal

(Braithwaite, Selby, & Fincham, 2011) data. Though these effects often are modest, such magnitudes may be expected given that these findings reflect evidence that forgiveness construed as a broad disposition can influence context-specific outcomes. Finally, with respect to self-forgiveness, researchers have discussed the potential for marriages to be negatively influenced when one partner is unforgiving of himself or herself (Fincham, Hall, & Beach, 2006; Hall & Fincham, 2005), but relatively little work has empirically tested this prediction.

Mediator Analyses Again, research is needed that formally tests the mediational mechanisms linking forgiveness to relationship satisfaction, but some studies have been conducted along this front. For instance, forgivingness appears to influence relationship satisfaction, because forgiving individuals put greater effort into a relationship and employ fewer negative conflict tactics (Braithwaite et al., 2011). In addition, forgiveness may promote dyadic trust, which in turn predicts greater satisfaction (Gordon et al., 2009). As such, this work provides initial support that forgiveness should decrease relationship strife (and increase relationship harmony), through promoting positive resolution tactics, as well as promote relationship maintenance and success, which should be concomitant with dyadic trust. Moreover, given that forgivingness does predict state forgiveness in a relationship (Allemand et al., 2007), it is likely that the trait predicts relationship satisfaction by promoting forgiveness of any specific incident, a point we elaborate upon below when discussing the importance of including both state and trait models in future research.

Forgiveness and Family Well-Being

Another relationship domain of interest is whether and how forgiveness may promote well-being within the family domain. Though few studies have assessed its role in family contexts, the results thus far are promising. For instance, adolescents' willingness to forgive their parents appears to coincide with greater child-parent relationship quality (Paleari, Regalia, & Fincham, 2003). In addition, when parents have a greater tendency to forgive their children, it longitudinally predicts greater relationship quality (Maio, Thomas, Fincham, & Carnelley, 2008). While quality is not synonymous with subjective satisfaction, these results do point for the potential role of forgiveness in promoting family-specific well-being. However, additional research is particularly needed in this domain, given the relative lack of studies both providing initial links to family well-being, as well as those describing and testing possible explanatory mechanisms. Of particular interest may be the pathway through identity development, given the prominent role that families play in influencing adaptive or maladaptive individuation (e.g., Allison & Sabatelli, 1988; Rice, Cole, & Lapsley, 1990).

Returning to the Model and Future Directions

While this model-specific review is by no means intended to be exhaustive, it points to the potential for the 4S Model to help direct future research in the field. Moreover, the model allows for clear predictions regarding which pathways may prove more important for the well-being outcome of interest. For instance, when predicting relationship or family well-being from forgiveness, it likely will be of greater interest to test the pathways involving relationship harmony and mastery/maintenance. Alternatively, when looking at global well-being, or potential explanations for the benefits of self-forgiveness, the self-scaffolding pathways (identity development and self-acceptance/self-worth) are potentially more valuable. In addition, three further predictions of the model warrant further discussion and testing in future research.

A Feedback Loop

A common finding is that forgiveness across most forms tends to increase with age (Allemand, 2008; Bono & McCullough, 2004; Girard & Mullet, 1997; Steiner, Allemand, & McCullough, 2011, 2012; see Allemand & Steiner, 2010, 2012 for reviews), although the age trends for self-forgiveness are less clear (e.g., Toussaint et al., 2001). A potential explanation is that older individuals have greater experience dealing with transgressions and transgressors, and as such have built a more positive repertoire of techniques and skills to deal with such scenarios (Allemand & Steiner, 2012). Similarly, one could suggest that these individuals have greater experience with forgiveness, and know of its potential for bolstering well-being. In turn, with a greater accumulation of the benefits conferred by forgiveness, one should be more inclined to deepen his or her forgiving tendencies. In other words, subjective well-being may provide feedback in the form of promoting positive development on constructs like forgivingness and trait self-forgiveness.

Such a prediction has received recent empirical support in the personality development literature. For instance, adults who increase in social well-being with time also tend to show correlated increases on positive personality traits (Hill, Turiano, Mroczek, & Roberts, 2012), including those known to predict forgivingness, such as emotional stability, agreeableness, and conscientiousness. In addition, adults higher on initial life satisfaction are more prone to gain on these traits over time (Specht, Egloff, & Schmukle, 2011). Accordingly, we would make a similar prediction regarding the potential for subjective well-being to in turn promote forgiveness, and the 4S Model thus provides a novel and potentially useful explanation for the well-replicated age effects in the field.

This process also speaks to the need for including measures of both state forgiveness and forgivingness into a single longitudinal study when testing the model, to examine the interplay between whether one has forgiven recent transgressions and his or her later dispositional tendency to forgive. State forgiveness may lead to greater well-being in the moment, which then should encourage forgiveness in a future state. Over time, these effects will accrue, "building" a disposition toward forgiveness. In this respect, we can discuss the interplay between states and traits as influencing personality development, a point discussed frequently in that literature (e.g., Fleeson, 2001; Roberts, 2009). As such, we encourage researchers to include measures that assess multiple forms of forgiveness in future work, not only to address this point, but also to understand whether the efficacy of the 4S Model may differ across forgiveness subtypes.

Lack of Additional Feedback Loops

Perhaps a more intriguing question is whether the mediators could themselves provide feedback to forgiveness, without having an influence on subjective well-being. As an example, one could think of mechanisms by which committing to an identity could promote forgiveness outside of subjective well-being (e.g., identity commitment leads to a stronger sense of who one is, which leads to a decreased likelihood that one feels that any single transgression is an attack on the self). We certainly agree that such alternative pathways are possible and in fact, quite likely. Indeed, after testing the feedback loop posited above, a particularly valuable contribution would be to investigate whether subjective well-being serves as the catalyst for forgiveness change, or if it proves a proxy for the "true" mechanism involved. For instance, the study cited above (Specht et al., 2011) suggested that life satisfaction may serve to approximate how closely one fits one's roles for life, and thus this role commitment piece may serve as the true driving mechanism of personality development (see also, Roberts, Wood, & Caspi, 2008). Similarly, it would be valuable to see whether it is subjective well-being itself that drives forgiveness development, or if this posited feedback loop dissipates when including alternatives.

Accentuate the Positive?

Finally, it will prove valuable to formally test how forgiveness "promotes the good" uniquely from how it "attenuates the bad." In most cases, the subjective well-being outcomes examined have clear correlates on the other end of the spectrum (e.g., positive versus negative affect; relationship satisfaction versus dissatisfaction). For instance, negative affect can be employed as a reverse indicator of subjective well-being (e.g., Diener, 2000), given its clear empirical connection to variables like happiness and life satisfaction, but we have refrained from discussing it here to maintain our focus on how forgiveness may lead to positive outcomes. However, a central goal for future researchers is to examine whether the effects of forgiveness on positive well-being can be empirically distinguished from those on the reduction of negative ill-being. Testing these claims will provide a better understanding of whether the 4S Model serves to uniquely describe the role of forgiveness on subjective well-being, or alternatively, if the suggested pathways may play similar explanatory roles for positive and negative outcomes.

Conclusion

In the current chapter, we sought to present a potential model for understanding the role of forgiveness in promoting happiness and subjective well-being. In so doing, it becomes clear that while the field has progressed greatly over the past decade, several important questions remain for future inquiry into the benefits of forgiveness. We hope that the 4S Model can help direct researchers toward generating better hypotheses regarding the potential subjective well-being benefits conferred by forgiveness. While the model presents four potential pathways linking forgiveness to satisfaction, we are certain that several others may present over the decade to come.

References

Allemand, M. (2008). Age differences in forgivingness: The role of future time perspective. *Journal of Research in Personality, 42*, 1137–1147.

Allemand, M., Amberg, I., Zimprich, D., & Fincham, F. D. (2007). The role of trait forgiveness and relationship satisfaction in episodic forgiveness. *Journal of Social and Clinical Psychology, 26*, 199–217.

Allemand, M., Hill, P. L., Ghaemmaghami, P., & Martin, M. (2012). Forgivingness and subjective well-being in adulthood: The moderating role of future time perspective. *Journal of Research in Personality, 46*, 32–39.

Allemand, M., Job, V., Christen, S., & Keller, M. (2008). Forgivingness and action orientation. *Personality and Individual Differences, 45*, 762–766.

Allemand, M., & Steiner, M. (2010). Verzeihen und Selbstverzeihen über die Lebensspanne: Gegenwärtiger Forschungsstand und Forschungsperspektiven. [Forgiveness and self-forgiveness across the lifespan: Present state of research and research perspectives]. *Zeitschrift für Entwicklungspsychologie und Pädagogische Psychologie, 42*, 63–78.

Allemand, M., & Steiner, M. (2012). Situation-specific forgiveness and dispositional forgiveness: A lifespan perspective. In E. Kahls & J. Maes (Eds.), *Justice psychology ad conflicts: Theoretical and empirical contributions* (pp. 361–375). New York, NY: Springer.

Allison, M. D., & Sabatelli, R. M. (1988). Differentiation and individuation as mediators of identity and intimacy in adolescence. *Journal of Adolescent Research, 3*, 1–16.

Berzonsky, M. D. (2003). Identity style and well-being: Does commitment matter? *Identity: An International Journal of Theory and Research, 3*, 131–142.

Bono, G., & McCullough, M. E. (2004). Religion, forgiveness, and adjustment in older adults. In K. W. Schaie, N. Krause, & A. Booth (Eds.), *Religious influences on health and well-being in the elderly* (pp. 163–186). New York, NY: Springer.

Bono, G., McCullough, M. E., & Root, L. M. (2008). Forgiveness, feeling connected to others, and well-being: Two longitudinal studies. *Personality and Social Psychology Bulletin, 34*, 182–195.

Braithwaite, S. R., Selby, E. A., & Fincham, F. D. (2011). Forgiveness and relationship satisfaction: Mediating mechanisms. *Journal of Family Psychology, 25*, 551–559.
Brown, R. P., & Phillips, A. (2005). Letting bygones be bygones: Further evidence for the validity of the tendency to forgive scale. *Personality and Individual Differences, 38*, 627–638.
Cramer, D. (2000). Relationship satisfaction and conflict style in romantic relationships. *Journal of Psychology: Interdisciplinary and Applied, 134*, 337–341.
Diener, E. (2000). Subjective well-being: The science of happiness and a proposal for a national index. *American Psychologist, 55*, 34–43.
Downie, R. S. (1965). Forgiveness. *The Philosophical Quarterly, 15*, 128–134.
Eaton, J., Struthers, C. W., & Santelli, A. G. (2006). Dispositional and state forgiveness: The role of self-esteem, need for structure, and narcissism. *Personality and Individual Differences, 41*, 371–380.
Enright, R. D. (1994). Piaget on the moral development of forgiveness: Identity or reciprocity? *Human Development, 37*, 63–80.
Enright, R. D., Gassin, E. A., & Wu, C.-R. (1992). Forgiveness: A developmental view. *Journal of Moral Education, 21*, 99–114.
Fehr, R., Gelfand, M. J., & Nag, M. (2010). The road to forgiveness: A meta-analytic synthesis of its situational and dispositional correlates. *Psychological Bulletin, 5*, 894–914.
Fincham, F. D. (2000). The kiss of porcupines: From attributing responsibility to forgiving. *Personal Relationships, 7*, 1–23.
Fincham, F. D., Beach, S. R. H., & Davila, J. (2007). Longitudinal relations between forgiveness and conflict resolution in marriage. *Journal of Family Psychology, 21*, 542–545.
Fincham, F. D., Hall, J., & Beach, S. R. H. (2006). Forgiveness in marriage: Current status and future directions. *Family Relations, 55*, 415–427.
Fincham, F., & Beach, S. R. (2007). Forgiveness and marital quality: Precursor or consequence in well-established relationships? *Journal of Positive Psychology, 2*, 260–268.
Fleeson, W. (2001). Towards a structure- and process-integrated view of personality: Traits as density distributions of states. *Journal of Personality and Social Psychology, 80*, 1011–1027.
Girard, M., & Mullet, E. (1997). Propensity to forgive in adolescents, young adults, older adults, and elderly people. *Journal of Adult Development, 4*, 209–220.
Gordon, K. C., Hughes, F. M., Tomcik, N. D., Dixon, L. J., & Litzinger, S. C. (2009). Widening spheres of impact: The role of forgiveness in marital and family functioning. *Journal of Family Psychology, 23*, 1–13.
Gross, J. J., Richards, J. M., & John, O. P. (2006). Emotion regulation in everyday life. In D. K. Snyder, J. A. Simpson, & J. N. Hughes (Eds.), *Emotion regulation in couples and families: Pathways to dysfunction and health* (pp. 13–35). Washington, DC: American Psychological Association.
Hall, J. H., & Fincham, F. D. (2005). Self-forgiveness: The stepchild of forgiveness research. *Journal of Social and Clinical Psychology, 24*, 621–637.
Hill, P. L., Turiano, N. A., Mroczek, D. K., & Roberts, B. W. (2012). Examining concurrent and longitudinal relations between personality traits and social well-being in adulthood. *Social Psychological and Personality Science, 3*, 698–705.
Hill, P. L., & Allemand, M. (2011). Gratitude, forgivingness, and well-being in adulthood: Tests of moderation and incremental prediction. *Journal of Positive Psychology, 6*, 397–407.
Hill, P. L., Allemand, M., & Heffernan, M. E. (in press). Placing dispositional forgiveness within theories of adult personality development. *European Psychologist.*
Kachadourian, L. K., Fincham, F. D., & Davila, J. (2004). The tendency to forgive in dating and married couples: The role of attachment and relationship satisfaction. *Personal Relationships, 11*, 373–393.
Kearns, J. N., & Fincham, F. D. (2004). A prototype analysis of forgiveness. *Personality and Social Psychology Bulletin, 30*, 838–855.
Kurzynski, M. J. (1998). The virtue of forgiveness as a human resource management strategy. *Journal of Business Ethics, 17*, 77–85.

Lang, F. R., & Carstensen, L. L. (2002). Time counts: Future time perspective, goals, and social relationships. *Psychology and Aging, 17*, 125–139.

Lawler-Row, K. A., & Piferi, R. L. (2006). The forgiving personality: Describing a life well-lived? *Personality and Individual Differences, 41*, 1009–1020.

Macaskill, A. (2012a). A feasibility study of psychological strengths and well-being assessment in individuals living with recurrent depression. *Journal of Positive Psychology, 7*, 372–386.

Macaskill, A. (2012b). Differentiating dispositional and self-forgiveness from other-forgiveness: Associations with mental health and life satisfaction. *Journal of Social and Clinical Psychology, 31*, 28–50.

Maio, G. R., Thomas, G., Fincham, F. D., & Carnelley, K. B. (2008). Unraveling the role of forgiveness in family relationships. *Journal of Personality and Social Psychology, 94*, 307–319.

Maltby, J., Day, L., & Barber, L. (2005). Forgiveness and happiness. The differing contexts of forgiveness using the distinction between hedonic and eudaimonic happiness. *Journal of Happiness Studies, 6*, 1–13.

Marcia, J. E. (1980). Identity in adolescence. In J. Adelson (Ed.), *Handbook of adolescent psychology* (pp. 159–187). New York, NY: Wiley.

Mauger, P. A., Perry, J. E., Freeman, T., Grove, D. C., McBride, A. G., & McKinney, K. E. (1992). The measurement of forgiveness: Preliminary research. *Journal of Psychology and Christianity, 11*, 170–180.

McCullough, M. (2008). *Beyond revenge: The evolution of forgiveness*. San Francisco, CA: Jossey-Bass.

McCullough, M. E. (2000). Forgiveness as human strength: Theory, measurement, and links to well-being. *Journal of Social and Clinical Psychology, 19*, 43–55.

McCullough, M. E., & Witvliet, C. V. O. (2002). The psychology of forgiveness. In C. R. Snyder & S. J. Lopez (Eds.), *Handbook of positive psychology* (pp. 446–458). New York, NY: Oxford University Press.

McGary, H. (1989). Forgiveness. *American Philosophical Quarterly, 26*, 343–351.

Meeus, W., Iedema, J., Helsen, M., & Vollebergh, W. (1999). Patterns of adolescent identity development: Review of literature and longitudinal analysis. *Developmental Review, 19*, 419–461.

Paleari, F. G., Regalia, C., & Fincham, F. D. (2009). Measuring offence-specific forgiveness in marriage: The Marital Offence-Specific Forgiveness Scale (MOFS). *Psychological Assessment, 21*, 194–209.

Pansera, C., & La Guardia, J. (2012). The role of sincere amends and perceived partner responsiveness in forgiveness. *Personal Relationships, 19*, 696–711.

Parrott, W. G. (1993). Beyond hedonism: Motives for inhibiting good moods and for maintaining bad moods. In D. M. Wegner & J. W. Pennebaker (Eds.), *Handbook of mental control* (pp. 278–308). Englewood Cliffs, NJ: Prentice-Hall.

Paleari, F. G., Regalia, C., & Fincham, F. D. (2003). Adolescents' willingness to forgive their parents: An empirical model. *Parenting: Science and Practice, 3*, 155–174.

Rice, K. G., Cole, D. A., & Lapsley, D. K. (1990). Separation-individuation, family cohesion, and adjustment to college: Measurement validation and test of a theoretical model. *Journal of Counseling Psychology, 37*, 195–202.

Roberts, B. W. (2009). Back to the future: *Personality and assessment* and personality development. *Journal of Research in Personality, 43*, 137–145.

Roberts, B. W., Wood, D., & Caspi, A. (2008). The development of personality traits in adulthood. In O. P. John, R. W. Robins, & L. A. Pervin (Eds.), *Handbook of personality: Theory and research* (3rd ed., pp. 375–398). New York, NY: Guilford.

Roberts, R. C. (1995). Forgivingness. *American Philosophical Quarterly, 32*, 289–306.

Ross, S. R., Kendall, A. C., Matters, K. G., Rye, M. S., & Wrobel, T. A. (2004). A personological examination of self- and other-forgiveness in the five-factor model. *Journal of Personality Assessment, 82*, 207–214.

Sastre, M. T., Vinsonneau, G., Neto, F., Girard, M., & Mullet, E. (2003). Forgivingness and satisfaction with life. *Journal of Happiness Studies, 4*, 323–335.

Schneewind, K. A., & Gerhard, A.-K. (2002). Relationship personality, conflict resolution, and marital satisfaction in the first 5 years of marriage. *Family Relations, 51*, 63–71.

Schumann, K. (2012). Does love mean never having to say you're sorry? Associations between relationship satisfaction, perceived apology sincerity, and forgiveness. *Journal of Social and Personal Relationships, 30*, 997–1010.

Scobie, E. D., & Scobie, G. E. W. (1998). Damaging events: The perceived need for forgiveness. *Journal for the Theory of Social Behaviour, 28*, 373–402.

Specht, J., Egloff, B., & Schmukle, S. C. (2011). Stability and change on personality across the life course: The impact of age and major life events on mean-level and rank-order stability. *Journal of Personality and Social Psychology, 101*, 862–882.

Steiner, M., Allemand, M., & McCullough, M. E. (2011). Age differences in forgivingness: The role of transgression frequency and intensity. *Journal of Research in Personality, 45*, 670–678.

Steiner, M., Allemand, M., & McCullough, M. E. (2012). Do agreeableness and neuroticism explain age differences in the tendency to forgive others? *Personality and Social Psychology Bulletin, 38*, 441–453.

Tangney, J. P., Boone, A. L., & Dearing, R. (2005). Forgiving the self: Conceptual issues and empirical findings. In E. L. Worthington Jr. (Ed.), *Handbook of forgiveness* (pp. 143–158). New York, NY: Routledge.

Thompson, L., Snyder, C. R., Hoffman, L., Michael, S. T., Rasmussen, H. N., Billings, L. S., et al. (2005). Dispositional forgiveness of self, others, and situations. *Journal of Personality, 73*, 313–359.

Toussaint, L. L., Williams, D. R., Musick, M. A., & Everson, S. A. (2001). Forgiveness and health: Age differences in a US probability sample. *Journal of Adult Development, 8*, 249–257.

Toussaint, L., & Friedman, P. (2009). Forgiveness, gratitude, and well-being: The mediating role of affect and beliefs. *Journal of Happiness Studies, 10*, 635–654.

Wieselquist, J. (2009). Interpersonal forgiveness, trust, and the investment model of commitment. *Journal of Social and Personal Relationships, 26*, 531–548.

Wohl, M. J. A., DeShea, L., & Wahkinney, R. L. (2008). Looking within: Measuring state self-forgiveness and its relationship to psychological well-being. *Canadian Journal of Behavioural Science, 40*, 1–10.

Worthington, E. L., Jr. (Ed.). (2005). *Handbook of forgiveness*. New York, NY: Brunner-Routledge.

Worthington, E. L., Jr. (2013). *Moving forward: Six steps to forgiving yourself and breaking free from the past*. Colorado Springs, CO: Waterbrook Press.

Worthington, E. L., Jr., & Scherer, M. (2004). Forgiveness is an emotion-focused coping strategy that can reduce health risks and promote health resilience: Theory, review, and hypotheses. *Psychology & Health, 19*, 385–405.

Worthington, E. L., Jr., & Wade, N. G. (1999). The psychology of unforgiveness and forgiveness and implications for clinical practice. *Journal of Social and Clinical Psychology, 18*, 385–418.

Worthington, E. L., Jr., Witvliet, C. v. O., Pietrini, P., & Miller, A. J. (2007). Forgiveness, health, and well-being: A review of evidence for emotional versus decisional forgiveness, dispositional forgiveness, and reduced unforgiveness. *Journal of Behavioral Medicine, 30*, 291–302.

Part III
Factors Connecting Forgiveness and Health

Chapter 12
Sex, Forgiveness, and Health

Andrea J. Miller and Everett L. Worthington, Jr.

Sex Differences in Forgiveness

Two previous meta-analyses have addressed sex differences in forgiveness. Miller, Worthington, and McDaniel (2008) analyzed 70 research studies and found that, compared to males, females were slightly more forgiving ($d = .28$) and much less vengeful ($d = .83$). However, Fehr, Gelfand, and Nag (2010), as one part of a larger meta-analytic project, analyzed 53 research studies regarding sex and forgiveness and found no difference ($d = .02$). The discrepancy between these two meta-analyses is likely due to methodology such as different inclusion criteria for studies, different ways of handling non-significant sex findings, and whether missing statistics were imputed or not. For example, Miller et al. scoured method sections of articles that did not study sex differences as a focal variable; Fehr et al. tended to include a broad sample of forgiveness studies but only coded those for sex differences when sex was listed in title or abstract. This can be seen in the scope of the studies. Miller coded 33 % more studies than did Fehr et al, in spite of being published two years earlier. In the present review, we have included five studies on sex and forgiveness that have occurred since Fehr et al. When Fehr et al. and Miller et al. differed in their findings (which tended to be no sex difference for Fehr et al. and sex differences for Miller et al.), and when there were not relevant and more recent articles, we tended to give more weight to Miller et al. because they had higher statistical power to detect differences.

A.J. Miller (✉)
Hollins University, 7916 Williamson Road, Roanoke, VA 24020, USA
e-mail: milleraj2@hollins.edu

E.L. Worthington, Jr.
Department of Psychology, Virginia Commonwealth University, Richmond, VA, USA
e-mail: eworth@vcu.edu

L.L. Toussaint et al. (eds.), *Forgiveness and Health*,
DOI 10.1007/978-94-017-9993-5_12

Sex differences have been explored beyond asking whether males and females differ in levels of forgiveness and have examined *how* males and females differ in the forgiveness process. For instance, Konstam, Chernoff, and Deveney (2001) found that higher levels of guilt-proneness, anger reduction, and detachment predicted forgiveness for women while low pride and high shame-proneness predicted forgiveness for men.

In summary there appear to be some findings of sex differences in forgiveness, though different meta-analyses have differed on how large the differences are. Additionally, there is some evidence that how forgiveness occurs or what factors are important to facilitating forgiveness may be different for men and women.

Forgiveness and Health

Forgiveness has been associated with mental health including decreasing negative emotions such as depression, stress, and anger (Lawler et al., 2005; Toussaint & Webb, 2005). Forgiveness is related to physical health including cardiovascular health, blood pressure, number of physical symptoms reported, and medication use (Friedberg, Suchday, & Srinivas, 2009; Lawler, Younger, Piferi, Billington, et al., 2003; Lawler, Younger, Piferi, Jobe, et al., 2005; for a review, see Worthington, Witvliet, Pietrini, & Miller, 2007). Given sex differences in forgiveness and that there is a relationship between forgiveness and mental and physical health, it is possible that sex may play a role in the relationship between forgiveness and health.

Definitions and Scope

The current chapter addresses how sex (male or female) relates to forgiveness and mental and physical health. Both forgiveness of others and of self will be addressed. Trait forgivingness (i.e., relatively consistent forgiveness across time and situations) and state forgiveness (i.e., forgiveness of a specific transgression) will be discussed in relation to health and sex differences. Additionally, we discuss unforgiveness and health. Unforgiveness is considered a stress response and involves a combination of negative emotions such as resentment, hostility, anger, and bitterness towards a transgressor (Worthington, 2006).

Forgiveness in ongoing, close relationships is likely where there is the most impact on changing health-related outcomes because there is more emotional investment and commitment. In close relationships, forgiveness leads to lowered negative emotions (e.g., resentment, bitterness, hostility, hatred, anger, and fear) and increased positive emotions (e.g., empathy, sympathy, compassion) towards the offender (Worthington, 2006). However, it is possible that forgiveness in more casual relationships over time could affect health.

The term mental health includes specific disorders such as anxiety, depression, and PTSD, but also addresses constructs such as negative emotions and rumination. Physical health primarily addresses blood pressure and cardiovascular health, but a few general aspects of health such as number of physical complaints are included.

Although the terms sex and gender are often used interchangeably, we use sex to refer to biological factors that determine whether one is male or female while gender refers to one's socially constructed gender role or identity. Most research ostensibly on forgiveness and gender has only looked at biological sex. In fact, no studies were found that dealt with forgiveness, health, and gender as it is socially constructed. Therefore, for the current chapter, we use the term sex when discussing differences in forgiveness based on whether a person is male or female. However, when explaining why sex differences exist, gender socialization is often a theorized explanation. This is probably because it is assumed that gender is socialized based on whether one is biologically male or female.

The goal of the present chapter is to provide an overview of health and forgiveness research as it relates to sex. We also present a conceptual model that hypothesizes how sex may affect the forgiveness-health relationship. We discuss limitations of the current research as it relates to sex, forgiveness, and health and provide suggestions for future research. Finally, we make practical suggestions for how the information on forgiveness, health, and sex can be used to inform work with clients and interventions. Although previous reviews have also addressed the relationship between sex and forgiveness (e.g., Fehr et al., 2010; Miller et al., 2008), and the relationship between health and forgiveness (e.g., Worthington et al., 2007), the current review addresses, using a conceptual model, *how* sex differences in forgiveness may be related to health, which adds more understanding of reasons for differences to the literature than existed previously.

Conceptual Model to Explain How Sex May Affect the Forgiveness-Health Connection

We propose a basic conceptual model of what sex-related variables may be important in the forgiveness-health relationship. We do not believe this is an exhaustive list of variables that affect the forgiveness-health relationship, but we believe it is a starting point for theorizing how sex may be related to the forgiveness-health relationship. Many of these variables will be reviewed in the sections below in relation to sex, forgiveness, and health (See Fig. 12.1).

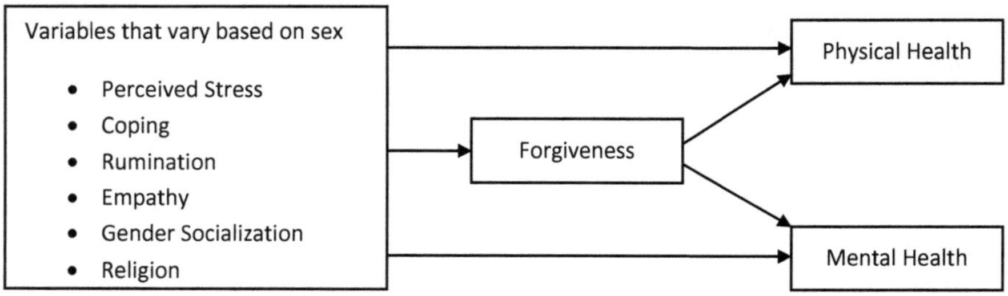

Fig. 12.1 Conceptual model for sex, forgiveness, health relationship

Literature Review of Sex, Forgiveness, and Health

Sex Differences in Forgiveness and Mental Health

State forgiveness and trait forgivingness are positively associated with mental health and negatively associated with mental health problems (for a review see Toussaint & Webb, 2005; for a recent review, see Griffin, Worthington, Lavelock, Wade, & Hoyt, Chap. 6, this volume). Forgiveness is also related to satisfaction with life and decreased negative emotions (Lawler et al., 2005). Forgiveness is negatively associated with depression (Toussaint & Webb, 2005), stress (Worthington, 2006), hostility, and anger (Berry et al., 2005). For instance, in a sample of participants with coronary artery disease, trait forgivingness was correlated with lower levels of anxiety, depression, and perceived stress (Friedberg et al., 2009). Unforgiveness has been positively associated with psychological disorders including depression, anxiety, and PTSD (Toussaint & Webb, 2005; Witvliet, Phipps, Feldman, & Beckham, 2004).

In relation to sex differences in mental health and forgiveness, Toussaint et al. (2008) examined trait forgivingness, depression, and sex differences in a community sample of over 1,400 participants. Forgiveness of others (when in the role of a victim) and forgiveness of self, forgiveness by God, and seeking forgiveness (when in the role of offender) were included. Females reported higher levels of forgiveness of others, forgiveness by God, and seeking forgiveness than did males. In addition, the role forgiveness played in risk for depressive episodes varied by sex. For females, forgiveness of others, self, and feeling forgiven by God were related to less risk for a depressive episode. However, for men, only forgiveness of self was related to decreasing risk for a depressive episode.

Additionally, sex differences in forgiveness in individuals with psychological diagnoses have been examined. For instance, how sex and willingness to forgive are related to specific diagnoses was investigated in a sample of 45 males and 55 females in outpatient treatment for mood and anxiety disorders (Ryan & Kumar, 2005). No sex difference in willingness to forgive was found. However, in males, higher state anxiety and higher symptom severity scores were correlated with less willingness to forgive. There was no relationship between these variables for women

(Ryan & Kumar, 2005). Therefore, it is possible that the importance of forgiveness may vary by both sex and disorder.

In summary, it is possible that specific types of forgiveness may play a more important role for certain mental disorders and may also vary by sex. For instance, self-forgiveness may be more important in determining mental health outcomes for males while forgiveness of others may be more important in determining mental health outcomes for females. Perhaps this is related to how men and women are socialized. Women are socialized to be more relational and more in tune interpersonally, but men are socialized to be more in tune to justice and consideration of fairness and equity (Agerström, Möller, & Archer, 2006). Therefore, women may more likely be affected by interpersonal stressors and the inability to forgive others. Men may be less likely to forgive interpersonally because they may feel that forgiveness does not fit with their sense of justice and fairness. Additionally, for men, who are socialized toward justice and fairness, they may be more prone to mental health complications related to mistakes and their inability to forgive themselves.

Sex Differences in Forgiveness and Physical Health

Sex Differences in Cardiovascular Health and Blood Pressure Forgiveness may be cardio-protective (Friedberg et al., 2009). In a sample of participants with coronary artery disease, trait forgivingness was correlated with cardiovascular risk, cholesterol total, and cholesterol LDL to HDL ratios (Friedberg et al., 2009). In a sample of over 100 college students, failing to forgive was related to a sustained period of cardiovascular reactivity when talking about a specific offense (Lawler et al., 2003). In addition, women with lower trait forgivingness have been found to have higher systolic blood pressure when recalling an interpersonal stressor than did men (Lawler-Row, Hyatt-Edwards, Wuensch, & Karremans, 2011). If women are experiencing increases in systolic blood pressure when experiencing or recalling interpersonal stressors, the wear and tear over time could affect cardiovascular health. Identifying women with low trait forgivingness who are experiencing high levels of stress may be a particular group that could benefit from forgiveness interventions. Another sex difference Lawler et al. (2003) found was that for women, state forgiveness was related to better systolic recovery while for men it was related to better diastolic recovery.

In summary, trait forgivingness appears to be related to positive health outcomes for blood pressure and cardiovascular health. The physical effects of forgiveness and forgivingness can differ according to sex.

Sex Differences in Stress, Rumination, and Physical Health Stress can cause negative emotions, which can lead to poor mental and physical health. Poor emotional health is related to a weakened immune system, which can lead to health problems (Svalina & Webb, 2012). Forgiveness can alleviate stress. Forgiveness can be considered an emotion-focused coping strategy that can decrease the effects of stress in reaction to a transgression (Worthington, 2006).

Males and females are affected by and cope with stress differently. In general, women tend to appraise the same events as more severe in level of stress than do men (Matheny, Ashby, & Cupp, 2005; Matud, 2004). Matheny et al. (2005) suggested women may be more susceptible to the negative effects of stressful events based, not on the events themselves, but on the appraisal of events as more stressful. Forgiveness is one way to cope with interpersonal stress and rumination. We tentatively suggest that it might be helpful for women, even if they are slightly more forgiving, to receive forgiveness training in order to buffer against the negative effects of more frequent perceptions of stress and rumination. Rumination, which can result from unforgiveness, can affect blood pressure (see Witvliet, Ludwig, & Vander Laan, 2001).

Forgiveness is also related to various physical health outcomes. For example, Lawler et al. (2005) found that, over the past month, both state forgiveness and trait forgivingness were correlated with number of physical symptoms indicated on a checklist, amount of medications taken, amount of fatigue, quality of sleep, and number of somatic complaints.

In summary, how each sex copes with stress, including perceived frequency and severity of stressors and rumination can affect cardiovascular health. Therefore forgiveness may be able to promote cardiovascular health for both men and women, but perhaps differently.

Sex Differences in Empathy, Forgiveness, and Health

Sex Differences in Dispositional Empathy, Forgiveness, and Health Forgiveness has been associated with state and trait empathy (Toussaint & Webb, 2005). Empathy can be important in facilitating forgiveness. For instance empathy, which entails the ability to understand, relate to, and treat another person as one would like to be treated, helps an individual be able to forgive others (Toussaint & Webb, 2005). Although dispositional empathy is an important variable in facilitating forgiveness, there is some evidence that it may be more important for the forgiveness process for men than for women. For instance, Toussaint and Webb (2005) found that dispositional empathy predicted whether men forgave, but did not predict whether women forgave. Additionally, Fincham, Paleari, and Regalia (2002) found that the effect of emotional empathy on forgiveness was stronger for husbands than for wives, suggesting empathy may have a greater impact on forgiveness for men than for women. Toussaint and Webb (2005) observe that women, who already have high levels of empathy, may not respond to empathy-based forgiveness interventions as well as men, who have lower levels of empathy. This might be because women already are practicing what the intervention promotes.

Socialization for Trait Empathy and the Impact on Forgiveness and Health Exline and Zell (2009) similarly suggest that, because women are typically socialized towards being empathic and relational, an additional empathic intervention might not have as much of an additive effect for women as for men. This suggests that, if physical and mental health are to be affected through forgiveness interventions, targeting empathy in men may have the largest potential for impacting health. Another suggested possibility is that because women are more likely to ruminate than are men, promoting empathy through self-reflection may trigger additional rumination in women, which could lead to negative emotional and (potentially) physical outcomes (Exline & Zell, 2009).

In summary, the role of empathy may vary in the process it plays in forgiveness for men and women. Empathy may vary in effectiveness for facilitating forgiveness based on sex.

Sex, Salience, and Age Differences in Forgiveness and Health

Whether sex differences are found may depend on factors such as the type of transgression or age. Furthermore, variables such as transgression and age may be moderators of the sex effect in the forgiveness-health relationship. For instance, there may be a 3-way interaction between age, sex, and forgiveness effects on health.

Sex Differences in Daily Salience of Forgiveness Ghaemmaghami, Allemand, and Martin (2011) examined state forgiveness across various age groups. They found that regardless of age, forgiveness was more salient in everyday life for women than for men. This might indicate that women may be more likely to participate in forgiveness interventions to promote health than will men because forgiveness is a topic they think about more frequently.

Sex Differences in Vengeance Generally, as people age, they become more willing to forgive, less vengeful, and report fewer angry memories (Ghaemmaghami et al., 2011). Therefore, if people wish to reap health benefits through forgiving, they would be well advised to seek forgiveness interventions in early and middle adulthood to prevent health problems later in adulthood. This may be especially challenging for young men who are more likely to not view forgiveness as desirable and seem more prone to responding to transgressions with vengeance. Ghaemmaghami et al. also found that sex differences in revenge motivations were more pronounced in younger adults than in middle-aged and older adults. Thus, there may be a complex interaction involving differential effects of forgiveness on health based on both age and sex. Sex effects may be more prevalent in younger age groups when health patterns are first established that might lead to health problems in middle and late adulthood.

Sex Differences in Types of Transgressions Reported Ghaemmaghami et al. (2011) also identified sex differences in types of transgressions reported. Men were more likely to report workplace transgressions as causing the most distress while women were more likely to report transgressions with romantic partners causing the most distress. Given that transgressions can occur either within continuing and valued relationships or between strangers or in relationships that one does not value or does not intend to continue, it is important that both men and women are bothered mostly by ongoing interactions that provide continuing opportunities to be hurt or offended—those that cannot easily be set aside, discontinued, or escaped from. Additionally, women were more likely than were men to report increased anger when dealing with unresolved interpersonal disagreements. Therefore, interventions for forgiveness aimed at improving health may be more beneficial in some settings relative to other settings. Men may gain more benefits from workplace forgiveness interventions especially if work groups are small and continued interactions with supervisors and co-workers are unavoidable rather than in large diffuse organizations in which it is possible to avoid contact with irritating and offending co-workers and supervisors. Women who report frequent transgressions with a romantic partner (to whom they are committed) might benefit more from interventions with the partner than with interventions that focus on workplace, friendship, elderly relatives, or more distant relationships.

In summary, how sex, forgiveness, and health are related may be moderated by age, type of transgression, and setting. This may inform who (men or women), how (type of transgression), where (what kinds of relationships), and when (young, middle age, older age) to target forgiveness interventions.

Sex Differences in Forgiveness Interventions

Sex differences in facilitating forgiveness through varying forgiveness prompts have been uncovered. These sex differences may be important when conducting forgiveness interventions to promote health. Root and Exline (2011) examined sex differences in the motives of goodwill (e.g., empathy, benevolence, and caring), moral obligation (i.e., societal expectations and ethics), and self-perceived benefit (i.e., self-preservation, personal control, and emotional relief) to facilitate forgiveness. For women, there were no differences between the control group and goodwill, moral obligation, and self-perceived benefit groups. However, for men all primes increased forgiveness, with the goodwill prime being the most effective. This suggests that it may be more difficult to promote forgiveness in women or that there is some unexamined variable that is important for facilitating forgiveness for women. Also men may respond best to goodwill motivations such as empathy, benevolence, and caring. In Study 2 women reported putting more time into the forgiveness process prior to any forgiveness prime (Root & Exline, 2011). This may explain why added motivation does not result in increases for women but does for men. In regards to interventions for improving health, it would be important to target men who may be more likely to need additional prompting to initiate the forgiveness process relative to women. In summary, the effectiveness of how forgiveness is facilitated may vary by sex.

Sex Differences in Self-Forgiveness

Dispositional self-forgivingness is the tendency to forgive the self when failures occur or when a person commits a transgression that causes harm to others (Hall & Fincham, 2005). Self-forgiveness is positively correlated with mental and physical health (Toussaint, Williams, Musick, & Everson, 2001) and negatively correlated with depression, anxiety, shame, anger, and hostility (Hall & Fincham, 2005). Thus, those with higher self-forgiveness may be less at risk for health problems.

Women generally tend to report more intense feelings of shame and guilt than do men (Rangganadhan & Todorov, 2010). Additionally, beginning in adolescence, females self-report being more empathic than men (e.g., Macaskill, Maltby, & Day, 2002; Rangganadhan & Todorov, 2010). Guilt, shame, and empathy are important variables related to self-forgiveness. More specifically, self-forgiveness is negatively correlated with guilt and empathic concern for others (Strelan, 2007; Rangganadhan & Todorov, 2010). Guilt can facilitate conciliatory behavior and empathy toward the victim, which can help relieve the guilt and facilitate self-forgiveness (Rangganadhan & Todorov, 2010). However, guilt can also increase other-oriented empathy, which can impede self-forgiveness (Macaskill, Maltby & Day, 2002). In a recent study examining self-forgiveness, shame, guilt, and empathy, women reported higher levels of shame, guilt, and empathic concern than did men (Rangganadhan & Todorov, 2010). The best predictors of inhibiting self-forgiveness were shame and personal distress empathy. It is possible that shame and focusing on the negative effects that one's behavior caused in someone else leads to more rumination and negative emotions, which then make it more difficult to forgive oneself. While empathy may facilitate forgiveness in others, it seems that too much empathy in self-forgiveness may trigger a set of negative emotions that then interferes with the self-forgiveness process. Therefore, women may be more likely to report difficulty with self-forgiveness. This is not to say that men are not at risk for health concerns due to lack of self-forgiveness, but given the pattern of females self-reporting more shame and empathic concern, females may be at an even higher risk.

In summary, self-forgiveness can affect mental and physical health. There have been no consistent sex differences in how self-forgiveness affects health. However, females are more likely to experience higher levels of variables related to inhibiting self-forgiveness. Therefore, it may be especially important to promote self-forgiveness in women. Additionally, self-forgiveness may need to be facilitated differently for men and women.

Synopsis of Key Findings

Overall, relatively little research has addressed how the forgiveness-health relationship varies by sex. However, a few key findings emerged. First, when sex differences in forgiveness are found, women are typically more forgiving than men and men are more vengeful than women (Miller et al., 2008). However, only two meta-analyses on sex and forgiveness have been conducted and they had conflicting results. Therefore, it has not clearly been demonstrated that there is a definitive sex difference in forgiveness. Additionally, how forgiveness is related to and affects mental health can vary by sex (e.g., Ryan & Kumar, 2005; Toussaint et al., 2008). However, there is not yet a clear consensus on whether mental health outcomes are more related to forgiveness for males or females. For instance, forgiveness was related more to mental health outcomes for males than for females based on research by Ryan and Kumar (2005) while Toussaint et al. (2008) found the opposite sex effect. Second, how forgiveness is related to and affects physical health can vary by sex (e.g., Hogan & Linden, 2004; Lawler et al., 2003; Lawler-Row et al., 2011; Whited et al., 2010). Third, forgiveness interventions aimed at improving mental and physical health may have some benefit in being tailored differently to men and women. We describe those in the final section of this chapter. We want to caution that sex differences should not be overemphasized. Sex is just one of many variables that likely affect the forgiveness-health relationship. However it is still important to acknowledge that sex differences can inform predictions of forgiveness-health outcomes and be utilized in interventions facilitating forgiveness.

Limitations of Current Research

Some of the findings in this review come from small sample sizes and have not been consistently replicated. Also, the sizes of the sex effects are generally small, and sex is just one of many variables that likely affect the forgiveness-health relationship. Additionally, many studies in this review examined different types of forgiveness and operationalized forgiveness slightly differently, which may have lead to variability in results. Therefore, we want to caution that sex differences should not be overemphasized and that the area of sex, forgiveness, and health is a relatively new area of study in need of much more work. However, it is still important to acknowledge that sex differences can tentatively inform predictions of forgiveness-health outcomes and be utilized in interventions facilitating forgiveness.

First, more research examines whether there are sex differences in forgiveness than how or why a sex difference in forgiveness may exist. The how and why is an important piece of the puzzle of the sex, forgiveness, and health relationship. Many variables have been identified that may explain sex differences in forgiveness such as how genders are socialized differently, rumination, perceived stress, religion, and even brain structures. However, there is little research evidence supporting these theoretical links. For example, there is some evidence that the differences in forgiveness are found in how forgiveness is processed in the brain. Pietrini et al. (2004) compared males' and females' thinking about forgiveness and unforgiveness while their brains were being scanned. They found females had more activation in the anterior cingulate cortex than did males when recalling hurtful events. Worthington, Witvliet, Pietrini, and Miller (2007) conclude that hurtful events may lead to more negative emotions in the processing of affective painful events in females than in males. This may account for some of the explanation in why women tend to report experiencing more negative emotions and rumination and how these variable affect forgiveness and health. This is just one example of research that has directly tried to uncover the why behind sex differences in forgiveness. More studies need to address possible explanations for why sex differences exist to better explain the significance of the forgiveness, sex, and health relationship.

Second, there are more complex questions of how, in which way, and under what contexts are there sex differences in forgiveness that need to be addressed. We must go beyond establishing whether there are sex differences; there clearly are. Several studies that found no sex differences have been subjected to more complex analyses and have found that the way forgiveness affects mental or physical health is different for men and women (e.g., Ryan & Kumar, 2005). For instance, sex differences may emerge in complex interactions of forgiveness and health based on variables such as age, type and severity of transgression, and type of relationship. Also, the effects of transgressions and forgiveness may have varying effects on males and females based on the type of mental or physical health problem.

Third, more research on forgiveness interventions aimed at improving health are needed to better understand the forgiveness, sex, and health relationship. For example, Waltman et al. (2009) conducted a pilot forgiveness intervention study with males diagnosed with coronary artery disease. After completing 10 individual therapy sessions focusing on forgiveness, self-reported forgiveness increased and anger-recall induced myocardial perfusion defects decreased in the intervention group relative to the control group. Results were maintained at a 10 week follow-up. Larger intervention studies like Waltman et al.'s, where sex can be compared to determine differences in specific health conditions, need to be done.

Fourth, little research has addressed sex differences in self-forgiveness and in the forgiveness-health relationship. Yet self-forgiveness appears to be important in mental and physical health. Therefore, there needs to be more focus on sex, self-forgiveness and health, and sex differences in self-forgiveness interventions aimed at impacting mental and physical health.

Fifth, although some research has tailored forgiveness interventions to specific medical conditions (e.g., Waltman et al., 2009), more research is needed. Factors that are important to increasing risk for certain chronic health conditions may vary by sex as well as interventions to promote forgiveness may vary by sex and chronic health condition.

Sixth, the majority of the research found in the current review involved samples from the United States with the exception of Rangganadhan and Todorov (2010) and Ghaemmaghami et al. (2011). Although past meta-analytic research did not find culture as a significant moderator in the sex and forgiveness literature (e.g., Miller et al., 2008), cultural variables still may be important in the sex, forgiveness, and health relationship.

Future Research Agenda

- Because most diseases and health effects take a long time to manifest, longitudinal studies are needed to examine the effects of forgiveness and health.
- More research is needed to understand why sex differences in forgiveness exist and how important they are for mental and physical health.
- More complex questions need to be addressed such as under what conditions (e.g., age, type of transgression, type of relationship) do sex differences in forgiveness emerge.
- More interventions examining sex differences in the health benefits of forgiveness are needed. Research must address (a) whether there are sex differences, (b) in what ways males and females may respond differently to health and forgiveness interventions, and (c) what types of forgiveness interventions promote better mental and physical health for which sex?
- More forgiveness interventions are needed to address forgiveness in specific populations diagnosed with chronic health problems. Specifically, anyone dealing with health problems who may blame themselves or others for their conditions could be helpful, such as individuals dealing with HIV/AIDS, chronic pain (which is more common in women), substance abuse, and injuries (which is more common in men).
- More self-forgiveness interventions are needed to address both mental and physical health and sex differences.
- There might be more forgiveness differences due to gender socialization than to sex.
- Culture needs to be examined in the study of sex, forgiveness, and health. For example, cultural differences in socialization, faith, or emotional expression may lead to differences in sex and forgiveness or the interpretation of mental or physical health outcomes related to sex and forgiveness.

Practical Implications

In closing, we suggest recommendations that may be helpful when working with male and female clients and patients. First, when screening for depression, based on Toussaint et al.'s (2008) research findings, it may be helpful to screen depressed clients for forgiveness of self and others. Women struggling with forgiveness of others may be at higher risk for a depressive episode, and men struggling more with forgiveness of self may be at higher risk for developing a depressive episode

(Toussaint et al., 2008). Second, women with low trait forgivingness who are also experiencing high levels of stress could especially benefit from forgiveness interventions. Similarly, because women tend to view more events as stressful and also tend to appraise events as more severe in level of stress than do men (Matheny et al., 2005; Matud, 2004), targeting forgiveness in women who are experiencing higher levels of overall stress and interpersonal stress may be particularly beneficial for women. Therefore, assessing interpersonal stress up front may result in better treatment recommendations for who would be more likely to have health benefits from forgiveness interventions. Third, based on Ryan and Kumar's (2005) research findings, males with anxiety or who report more severe symptoms may particularly benefit from individual counseling addressing forgiveness. Fourth, based on Hogan and Linden's (2004) work, men who frequently ruminate and use an avoidance response style of anger may particularly benefit from forgiveness interventions. This combination of coping has been related to by higher ambulatory diastolic and systolic blood pressure (Hogan & Linden, 2004). Promoting forgiveness may have cardiovascular benefits. In summary, assessing levels of forgiveness, stress, and coping along with mental health symptoms, may improve targeting of forgiveness interventions and maximize health benefits.

Recommendations that may facilitate forgiveness are described below. First, we summarize interventions for men, and then for women.

Interventions for Men Interventions specifically aimed at men might emphasize (a) including a discussion of issues related to fairness, justice, and restitution (Whited et al., 2010), (b) reducing vengeful acts or delaying them until anger subsides, (b) workplace interventions, (c) promoting empathy perhaps through having men recall how they might have inflicted a similar harm on someone, and (e) dealing with self-forgiveness that might arise after acting vengefully or otherwise offending a relationship partner or co-worker. Additional prompting to initiate forgiveness may be necessary for men relative to women (Root & Exline, 2011). Therefore, when discussing forgiveness, interventionists might need to spend more time explaining the reasons and benefits of forgiveness to men than women. Also, targeting health effects of chronic anger, notably cardiovascular effects, may be needed to motivate men to fully engage in forgiveness-promoting interventions (e.g., Waltman et al., 2009). Men have higher rates of mortality than do women (Matheny et al., 2005), so interventions may be more effective for men if they are pitched in terms of managing risks of long-term health problems or more serious health problems. For men, forgiveness interventions could be utilized as prevention for health problems. Facilitating forgiveness early on, especially in young men, may result in the best prevention of possible health problems (Ghaemmaghami et al., 2011). Interventions can be promoted during adolescence or young adulthood to maximize health benefits over time.

Interventions for Women Interventions specifically aimed at women might focus on (a) targeting home and family relationships and targeting forgiveness in friends, (b) seeking ways to manage long-term relational commitments that are frustrating to minimize offenses, (c) focusing on methods by which women can reduce rumination, (d) minimizing over-concern that manifests as shame or excessive empathic concern—such as directing women to focus on situational factors, (e) working on emotion regulation and emotional control, and (f) promoting self-forgiveness for failures, especially in important relationships. Women tend to have higher rates of illness and are more likely to engage in help-seeking behavior. Therefore, interventions may be effective if they are targeted at women who seek short-term improvements in health; women might be more willing to engage in forgiveness skill interventions as coping behaviors.

References

Agerström, J., Möller, K., & Archer, T. (2006). Moral reasoning: The influence of affective personality, dilemma content and gender. *Social Behavior and Personality, 34*, 1259–1276. doi:10.2224/sbp.2006.34.10.1259.

Berry, J. W., Worthington, E. L., Jr., O'Connor, L. E., Parrott, L., & Wade, N. G. (2005). Forgivingness, vengeful rumination, and affective traits. *Journal of Personality, 73*, 183–225. doi:10.1111/j.1467-6494.2004.00308.x.

Exline, J., & Zell, A. L. (2009). Empathy, self-affirmation, and forgiveness: The moderating roles of gender and entitlement. *Journal of Social and Clinical Psychology, 28*, 1071–1099. doi:10.1521/jscp.2009.28.9.1071.

Fehr, R., Gelfand, M. J., & Nag, M. (2010). The road to forgiveness: A meta-analytic synthesis of its situational and dispositional correlates. *Psychological Bulletin, 136*, 894–914. doi:10.1037/a0019993.

Fincham, F. D., Paleari, F. G., & Regalia, C. (2002). Forgiveness in marriage: The role of relationship quality, attributions, and empathy. *Personal Relationships, 9*, 27–37.

Friedberg, J. P., Suchday, S., & Srinivas, V. S. (2009). Relationship between forgiveness and psychological indices in cardiac patients. *International Journal of Behavioral Medicine, 16*, 205–211. doi:10.1007/s12529-008-9016-2.

Ghaemmaghami, P., Allemand, M., & Martin, M. (2011). Forgiveness in younger, middle-aged and older adults: Age and gender matters. *Journal of Adult Development, 18*, 192–203. doi:10.1007/s10804-011-9127-x.

Hall, J. H., & Fincham, F. D. (2005). Self-forgiveness: The stepchild of forgiveness research. *Journal of Social and Clinical Psychology, 24*, 621–637. doi:10.1521/jscp.2005.24.5.621.

Hogan, B. E., & Linden, W. (2004). Anger response styles and blood pressure: At least don't ruminate about it! *Annals of Behavioral Medicine, 27*, 38–49. doi:10.1207/s15324796abm2701_6.

Konstam, V., Chernoff, M., & Deveney, S. (2001). Toward forgiveness: The role of shame, guilt, anger, and empathy. *Counseling and Values, 46*, 26–39. doi:10.1002/j.2161-007X.2001.tb00204.x.

Lawler, K. A., Younger, J. W., Piferi, R. L., Billington, E., Jobe, R., Edmondson, K., & Jones, W. H. (2003). A change of heart: Cardiovascular correlates of forgiveness in response to interpersonal conflict. *Journal of Behavioral Medicine, 26*, 373–393. doi:10.1023/A:1025771716686.

Lawler, K. A., Younger, J. W., Piferi, R. L., Jobe, R. L., Edmondson, K. A., & Jones, W. H. (2005). The unique effects of forgiveness on health: An exploration of pathways. *Journal of Behavioral Medicine, 28*, 157–167. doi:10.1007/s10865-005-3665-2.

Lawler-Row, K. A., Hyatt-Edwards, L., Wuensch, K. L., & Karremans, J. C. (2011). Forgiveness and health: The role of attachment. *Personal Relationships, 18*, 170–183. doi:10.1111/j.1475-6811.2010.01327.x.

Macaskill, A., Maltby, J., & Day, L. (2002). Forgiveness of self and others and emotional empathy. *The Journal of Social Psychology, 142*, 663–665. doi:10.1080/00224540209603925.

Matheny, K. B., Ashby, J. S., & Cupp, P. (2005). Gender differences in stress, coping, and illness among college students. *Journal of Individual Psychology, 61*, 365–379.

Matud, M. (2004). Gender differences in stress and coping styles. *Personality and Individual Differences, 37*, 1401–1415. doi:10.1016/j.paid.2004.01.010.

Miller, A. J., Worthington, E. L., Jr., & McDaniel, M. A. (2008). Gender and forgiveness: A meta-analytic review and research agenda. *Journal of Social and Clinical Psychology, 27*, 843–876. doi:10.1521/jscp.2008.27.8.843.

Pietrini, P., Ricciardi, E., Gentili, C., Vanello, N., Sani, L., & Guazzelli, M. (2004). How the brain responds to hurtful events: Neural activity elicited by aggressive versus forgiving behavior in humans. *International Journal of Psychophysiology, 30*, 291–302. doi:10.1007/s10865-007-9105-8.

Rangganadhan, A. R., & Todorov, N. (2010). Personality and self-forgiveness: The roles of shame, guilt, empathy and conciliatory behavior. *Journal of Social and Clinical Psychology, 29*, 1–22. doi:10.1521/jscp.2010.29.1.1.

Root, B. L., & Exline, J. (2011). Gender differences in response to experimental forgiveness prompts: Do men show stronger responses than women? *Basic and Applied Social Psychology, 33*, 182–193. doi:10.1080/01973533.2011.568850.

Ryan, R. B., & Kumar, V. K. (2005). Willingness to forgive: Relationships with mood, anxiety and severity of symptoms. *Mental Health, Religion & Culture, 8*, 13–16. doi:10.1080/13674670410001666543.

Strelan, P. (2007). Who forgives others, themselves, and situations? The roles of narcissism, guilt, self-esteem, and agreeableness. *Personality and Individual Differences, 42*, 259–269.

Svalina, S. S., & Webb, J. R. (2012). Forgiveness and health among people in outpatient physical therapy. *Disability and Rehabilitation: An International, Multidisciplinary Journal, 34*, 383–392. doi:10.3109/09638288.2011.607216.

Toussaint, L., & Webb, J. R. (2005). Gender differences in the relationship between empathy and forgiveness. *Journal of Social Psychology, 145*, 673–685. doi:10.3200/SOCP.145.6.673-686.

Toussaint, L. L., Williams, D. R., Musick, M. A., & Everson, S. A. (2001). Forgiveness and health: Age differences in a U.S. probability sample. *Journal of Adult Development, 8*, 249–257. doi:10.1023/A:1011394629736.

Toussaint, L. L., Williams, D. R., Musick, M. A., & Everson-Rose, S. A. (2008). The association of forgiveness and 12-month prevalence of major depressive episode: Gender differences in a probability sample of U.S. adults. *Mental Health, Religion & Culture, 11*, 485–500. doi:10.1080/13674670701564989.

Waltman, M. A., Russell, D. C., Coyle, C. T., Enright, R. D., Holter, A. C., & Swoboda, C. M. (2009). The effects of a forgiveness intervention on patients with coronary artery disease. *Psychology & Health, 24*, 11–27. doi:10.1080/08870440801975127.

Whited, M. C., Wheat, A. L., & Larkin, K. T. (2010). The influence of forgiveness and apology on cardiovascular reactivity and recovery in response to mental stress. *Journal of Behavioral Medicine, 33*, 293–304. doi:10.1007/s10865-010-9259-7.

Witvliet, C. O., Phipps, K. A., Feldman, M. E., & Beckham, J. C. (2004). Posttraumatic mental and physical health correlates of forgiveness and religious coping in military veterans. *Journal of Traumatic Stress, 17*, 269–273. doi:10.1023/B:JOTS.0000029270.47848.e5.

Witvliet, C., Ludwig, T. E., & Vander Laan, K. L. (2001). Granting forgiveness or harboring grudges: Implications for emotion, physiology, and health. *Psychological Science, 12*, 117–123. doi:10.1111/1467-9280.00320.

Worthington, E. L., Jr. (2006). *Forgiveness and reconciliation: Theory and application*. New York, NY: Brunner-Routledge.

Worthington, E. L., Jr., Witvliet, C., Pietrini, P., & Miller, A. J. (2007). Forgiveness, health, and well-being: A review of evidence for emotional versus decisional forgiveness, dispositional forgivingness, and reduced unforgiveness. *Journal of Behavioral Medicine, 30*, 291–302. doi:10.1007/s10865-007-9105-8.

Chapter 13
Forgiveness of Others, Race/Ethnicity, and Health: A Nascent Area of Inquiry

Cheryl A. Smith and Michael J. McFarland

The past decade has witnessed a dramatic increase in research linking forgiveness to health and well-being. Forgiveness has been found to be associated with various health outcomes including: higher self-reported health, fewer symptoms of illness, less frequent use of medications (Lawler et al., 2005), improved cardiovascular functioning (Toussaint & Cheadle, 2009), and improved immune function (Seybold, Hill, Neumann, & Chi, 2001). Increased forgiveness is also associated with improved performance in physiological systems predictive of mortality risk (Miniño, Xu, & Kochanek, 2010). There is a dearth of research examining the differential impact of forgiveness on health for various race/ethnicities, with much of the work utilizing white samples.[1]

In this chapter we highlight race as one overlooked area of research in the forgiveness-health literature. We begin with broader arguments of why the forgiveness-health relationship may vary by race and emphasize the importance of considering how race is embedded within broader social and cultural context. We then focus exclusively on how the relationship between forgiveness and health differs for blacks and whites in the U.S. Overall, we conclude: (a) there are strong theoretical reasons to suspect the relationship between forgiveness and health varies by race; (b) there are pronounced black-white differences in levels of interpersonal forgiveness; (c) the role of race in the forgiveness-health connection as well as the

[1]From here forward we use the word "race" instead of the unwieldy term "race/ethnicity."

C.A. Smith, Ph.D. (✉)
Central Jersey Family Health Consortium, North Brunswick, NJ, USA
e-mail: cmcfarland@cjfhc.org

M.J. McFarland, Ph.D.
Department of Sociology, Florida State University, Tallahassee, FL, USA
e-mail: mmcfarland@fsu.edu

L.L. Toussaint et al. (eds.), *Forgiveness and Health*,
DOI 10.1007/978-94-017-9993-5_13

role of the broader social context have been woefully understudied and present a promising direction for future research.

While there is no agreed upon definition of forgiveness, we conceive of it as the process of releasing or letting go of negative affect directed toward an offender (Hargrave & Sells, 1997). Here we are concerned with forgiveness of others as an enduring trait that varies across situations and over time (Berry, Worthington, O'Connor, Parrot, & Wade, 2005). Forgiveness is not a static personality characteristic but a dynamic tendency that may follow different developmental trajectories. The literature largely acknowledges that the tendency to forgive can be cultivated, with important work using clinical and psychoeducational approaches (DiBlasio & Proctor, 1993). However, the research mostly focuses on an individual's motivation rather than the broader social and cultural context (Berry et al., 2005; McCullough, Worthington, & Rachal, 1997). This is particularly important because it suggests that the tendency to forgive and its potential beneficial effects do not exist in a vacuum and may be contingent on one's environment. In regards to the latter point, much of what we know regarding the beneficial role of forgiveness for health comes from experiments in controlled laboratories or convenience samples such as young college students (e.g., Wilson, Milosevic, Carrol, Hart, & Hibbard, 2008). In order to fully understand how forgiveness affects health, researchers must acknowledge that the broader social context in which forgiveness occurs may alter the nature of the forgiveness–health connection. Stated differently, by neglecting the role of race and the broader context in which people live their lives with regard to the forgiveness and health relationship, researchers are sacrificing external validity. Race represents an ascribed status that assigns particular social and cultural contexts and structures much of one's life including how, when and where forgiveness is appropriate and the benefits one garners from it. In other words, different races encounter different structural and cultural contexts that affect the propensity to forgive and the potential health benefits gained from forgiveness.

Why Is Race Pertinent to the Forgiveness and Health Relationship?

We assert that race is important for understanding the relationship between forgiveness and health based on five key points: (a) race structures the social and cultural context in which one lives; (b) the propensity to forgive varies by race; (c) the broader environment may react differently to forgiveness; (d) race structures exposure to stressors which can influence the effect of forgiveness; and (e) the effect of forgiveness will vary by race because different races have different levels of underlying biological risk. Taken together, these key arguments provide the impetus for a conceptual framework that aims to elucidate the role of race in the relationship between forgiveness and health.

First, race is an ascribed status that structures one's immediate social, economic and physical environment as well as assigning different forms of socialization congruent with broader familial and cultural orientations. These factors produce drastically different environments in which people of different races live their day-to-day lives. For example, Hispanics witness lower incomes and educational attainment, higher unemployment, and more physically demanding, stressful, and low paying jobs than their non-Hispanic white counterparts (Tienda & Mitchell, 2006). These structural factors organize the context in which interpersonal conflict and therefore forgiveness occurs.

One's race is interwoven with the race of their parents and therefore connected with specific cultural orientations and different patterns of socialization. These cultural orientations provide the scaffolding for how one views the world and their role in it. These orientations can be thought of as different constellations of knowledge that reflect a subset of past experiences. These constellations of knowledge or "cognitive schema" categorize relationships, scenarios, and events that either consciously or unconsciously shape people's behaviors and decisions such that belonging to a certain racial group provides shared common environments and experiences which produces common schemata within racial groups. For instance, there may be within race shared schema about the expectations regarding interpersonal forgiveness. The phenomenon of shared schema, therefore, provides an explanation as to how interpersonal forgiveness may develop differently vis-a-vis customs, norms, practices, and behaviors for people of different races. Overall, race situates the social, economic, physical, and cultural context in which individuals live their lives.

Second, the propensity toward forgiveness may vary systematically by race because of different types of socialization concerning forgiveness, social incentives to be forgiving (or not), and social sanctions concerning forgiveness. McCullough (2008) suggests that human beings possess the ability for both forgiveness and revenge. The ability to forgive or stay angry has developed over time in humans and the social context impacts when forgiveness (or revenge) is appropriate. The social milieu influences one's response to interpersonal conflict, the biological ability for forgiveness or revenge interacts with the broader social context to influence one's disposition to forgive. Thus, in order to understand the relationship between forgiveness and health among racial groups, the social context must be understood (McCullough, 2008).

Forgiveness may also vary across different racial groups based on the type of cultural orientations toward individualism and collectivism. Individualistic orientations are characterized by self-determination, pursuit of self-interest, and self-actualization with relatively little interest in group goals. This orientation is consistent with behaviors based on personal needs and goals with a larger focus on achieving personal goals rather than improving the greater good (Sandage & Williamson, 2005). A collectivist orientation is characterized by an emphasis on group goals, adhering to traditional authority, and maintaining harmony with groups

(Sandage & Williamson, 2005). Individuals with a collectivist orientation may be more forgiving of others because they feel more empathy toward transgressors and have a greater reason to forgive in order to prevent group conflict. Cross-cultural studies of forgiveness support these assertions. Takaku, Weiner, and Ohbuchi (2001) found that for both Americans and Japanese forgiveness was influenced by apology; however, Americans put more weight on the controllability of the transgression. Another study found that among collectivistic Indonesian students, the willingness to forgive was higher and long lasting resentment was lower compared to the more individualistic French students (Suwartono, Prawasti, & Mullet, 2007). Coon and Kemmelmeier (2001) suggest that collectivist and individualistic cultures exist within the U.S. and are racially patterned. In the U.S. whites tend to adhere to more individualistic motivations while people of color tend to be more collectivistic. To the extent to which racial groups differ in orientations toward individualism and collectivism, differences in the propensity toward forgiveness of others should also be pronounced.

Third, the environment that people live in may "respond" differently to forgiveness depending on the broader racially-shaped culture. The context in which forgiveness occurs is contingent on race such that the tendency to forgive or not to forgive influences the day-to-day lives within their environment. For racial minorities, being forgiving may be important in maintaining valuable social and interfamilial connections. When interpersonal conflict occurs within ethnic enclaves or in extended familial networks, forgiveness is needed to maintain these networks. The social and cultural context experienced by racial minorities may lead to the development of social norms regarding expectations of contrition and forgiveness that differ from whites. Hence being forgiving or not for a particular race or cultural context may elicit responses from others that impact social relationships. The neighborhood context is an example of an environment that may impact the forgiveness-health relationship. Forgiveness of others in most social environments reduces interpersonal conflict and allows for an individual to create and maintain social support networks essential for health and well-being. In more noxious environments, however, there is reason to expect that forgiveness will be harmful for health. In the most dilapidated neighborhoods, a predisposition to forgive others may be viewed as a weakness that decreases social status and opens one up to attack (Anderson, 1999). McCullough's (2008) argument that forgiveness is a function of a social and biological interaction suggests that forgiveness of others provides an evolutionary advantage in some social contexts but is harmful in others. If the social milieu sends signals to its residents that those who forgive others are weak and the residents internalize these messages, then the most forgiving of people will witness diminished social status and increases in interpersonal conflict because of others' perceptions that they make easy targets. Lower levels of status and higher levels of interpersonal conflict may lead to decreases in health. Indeed, social status is associated with functioning of adrenocortical, cardiovascular, and immune systems (Sapolsky, 2004). Similarly, interpersonal conflict can lead to weakening of the immune system (Cohen, Tyrell, & Smith, 1993).

Fourth, minorities are disproportionately likely to experience social risk factors that influence health, and the impact of forgiveness on health may vary because these stressors can either diminish or magnify the impact of forgiveness. For instance, a convincing literature shows that race shapes one's exposure to acute and chronic stressors as well as daily hassles such as financial strain, exposure to violence, and interpersonal conflict (Hatch & Dohrenwend, 2007; Thoits, 2010). These types of stressors are known to impact various dimensions of health including: self-reported health, number of serious health conditions, illness symptoms, functional impairments, and hypertension (Pearlin, Schieman, Fazio, & Meersman, 2005; Schoenthaler, Schwartz, Cassells, Tobin, & Brondolo, 2010). One's tendency to be forgiving, or not, may be protective or exacerbate the pernicious effects of these stressors. For instance, blacks disproportionately experience financial strain which can produce marital conflict. The tendency to forgive may minimize this marital conflict and allow individuals to utilize the social support provided by marriage rather than experiencing interpersonal conflict. Perhaps the health drawbacks associated with a lack of forgiveness are not as pronounced for the most advantaged as they possess a myriad of other social, economic, psychological, and physical resources that make forgiveness less salient to health.

Fifth, the relationship between forgiveness and health may differ because there are stark racial differences in the risk for disease and mortality (Williams, 2005). The relationship between stress and health may become progressively stronger with increasing biological risk (Krantz & McCeney, 2002) and to the extent that forgiveness is protective of stress, those with higher levels of biological risk will benefit more from forgiveness. Different races in the population are at different stages in the progression of disease as well as differing levels of under the skin non-clinical levels of biological risk. Because different racial groups are at different stages in the progression toward disease, the effect of forgiveness may differ by race. For instance, the protective influence forgiveness has on the repeated activation of the bodies' stress response may be especially protective of cardiovascular disease for those with atherosclerotic lesions, which are asymptomatic and vary in prevalence by race (Strong et al., 1999).

Figure 13.1 highlights the arguments laid out above, such that race structures numerous aspects of people's lives including: (a) the environment in which one lives; (b) cultural norms, expectations, and beliefs; (c) the overall tendency toward interpersonal forgiveness; (d) health; and (e) how beneficial forgiveness is for health. This latter point suggests that the extent to which forgiveness is beneficial for health is dependent on race because people of similar races share similar social, cultural, economic, and physical environments.

The underlying thrust of this framework is that the propensity for forgiveness, the process of forgiveness, and the benefits (or deficits) accrued from forgiveness do not occur in a vacuum. To understand the relationship between forgiveness and health requires an understanding of the macro (e.g. racial segregation), meso (e.g. group schema), and micro (e.g. biological risk) contexts in which people live their daily

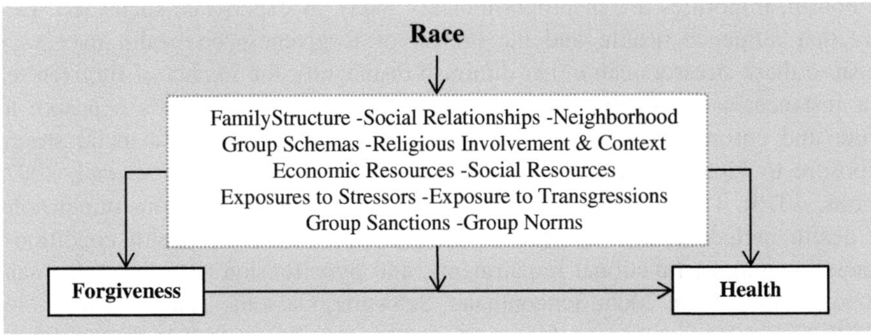

Fig. 13.1 Conceptual model

lives. Race, is one especially important dimension of life that structures from birth to death people's lives on multiple levels and may modify the relationship between forgiveness and health.

Black-White Differences in the Forgiveness and Health Relationship: A Case Study

The purpose of this chapter is to highlight the importance of race in the forgiveness and health relationship, and the remainder of this chapter focuses on synthesizing black-white differences in the influence of forgiveness on health. For the purposes of this chapter we argue for black-white differences, provide some preliminary empirical findings, and review the nascent literature in order to highlight an example of how our conceptual framework can be utilized to better understand the forgiveness and health relationship more generally. The black-white comparison example provides a case study, highlighting the relationship between race, forgiveness and health. There are four reasons for focusing on black-white differences: (1) blacks and whites experience different social environments; (2) blacks and whites have different cultural orientations; (3) blacks have a unique history in the U.S. characterized by racism, inequality, and adversity and these experiences are important when understanding how forgiveness is cultivated and the impact it has on health outcomes; and (4) the only published study to investigate race, forgiveness, and health examined whites and blacks (McFarland et al., 2012).

To understand the complex interplay between race, forgiveness and health, as well as the broader social context we consider two general propositions that are relevant to the notion of black-white differences in the forgiveness-health interplay: (a) blacks are more forgiving of others than their white counterparts; and (b) forgiveness has a more beneficial impact on health for blacks than whites.

Proposition 1: Blacks Are More Forgiving Than Their White Counterparts

Historically, exposure to discrimination and chronic adversity within the black communities has been ubiquitous and has influenced the development black culture. For this reason cultural tendencies for forgiveness may have also developed in ways that differ from whites. For instance, for blacks forgiveness may be of particular importance within extended familial and social networks and may have been cultivated within the black church.

Blacks tend to have large familial networks with multifaceted roles that may have emerged as an adaptation to deprivation (Edin & Kefalas, 2011). Family networks provide financial support, services, housing, and other exchanges of goods and services. Material support within extended families tends to be the prominent form of support with strong norms regarding reciprocity (Sarkisian & Gerstel, 2004). Black extended familial networks not only provide monetary and material services, but generally live with or within close proximity to one another and have frequent contact with each other (Taylor & Chatters, 1986). Within the black community, kin are more common members of social networks than non-kin and extended families are more prominent in the black community than among whites (Edin & Kefalas, 2011). Being part of these extended familial networks can protect individuals and provide them with support and emotional resources. However, this heightened level of interaction between family members and norms of reciprocity regarding support can lead to increased interpersonal conflict. Increases in interpersonal conflict among family members can lead to decreased levels of support and increased distress. Forgiveness likely plays a crucial role in maintaining extended familial networks. While blacks may need higher levels of forgiveness to maintain extended families, whites tend to live and interact with immediate family members. They are not as interconnected to extended families, and may not depend on family for material and emotional support to the same extent as black families. Whites may experience less interpersonal conflict due to their limited family network leading to less need for the cultivation for forgiveness.

The church also plays a central role for blacks and has direct connections with ideas surrounding interpersonal forgiveness. Forgiveness regardless of whether the transgressor shows acts of contrition is emphasized by church communities (Rye et al., 2000). Although all Christian traditions emphasis forgiveness at some level, there are several reasons that the black church may be especially suited to cultivate forgiveness among its members.

The black church originated and was maintained in oppressive social conditions. Historically the black church has offered tools and resources for coping with racism. In order to flourish they had to effectively deal with the suffering of its members due to these conditions. The black church is well-suited for addressing suffering, personal grievances, and oppression (Ellison, Musick, & Henderson, 2008). Support can include consolation, healing words, attempts to boost one's morale, and spiritual support (Krause, 2002; Taylor & Chatters, 1986); all of which can facilitate the cultivation of interpersonal forgiveness. Moreover, a tradition emphasizing collective worship activities including singing, dancing and other physical movement, vigorous preaching and shouting, and other dynamic jubilant services may have a cathartic effect that reduces anger and other negative emotions (Ellison et al., 2008). In a study of prayer group participation by blacks in New Haven, Griffith et al. (1980) finds that the spirit possession and testimony provides psychological support similar to the interaction in traditional forms of therapy. In addition, blacks have comparatively high levels of religious involvement and religious attendance is associated with higher levels of interpersonal forgiveness more broadly (Ellison & McFarland, 2013; Krause, 2012; Rye et al., 2000).

There are a limited number of studies that examined the relationship between forgiveness and race (Krause, 2012; McFarland et al., 2012; Stein et al., 2008). In a study of older blacks and whites, McFarland et al. found that blacks reported significantly higher levels of forgiveness than their white counterparts. In a comparison of older blacks, Mexican Americans, and whites, Krause (2012) found that blacks and Mexican Americans reported significantly higher levels of forgiveness than whites. Similarly, in a study conducted in South Africa, Stein et al. (2008) found that forgiveness was significantly associated with being black. Although Stein's work may not be applicable to U.S. populations, blacks in South Africa have experienced discrimination and racism that is similar if not more severe to blacks in the U.S. These results suggest that there is reason to believe that racial differences in forgiveness exist.

Building from previous empirical evidence, we attempt to replicate these findings by utilizing data from three national surveys. Specifically, we highlight racial differences in forgiveness using the Religion, Aging, and Health Survey, the 1998 General Social Survey, and the American's Changing Lives Survey. In order to test the relationship we conduct independent samples t-tests to determine if there is a significant difference in mean forgiveness scores for black and white respondents participating in each survey. Although forgiveness is being measured in different ways in each survey, they are all tapping into the tendency to forgive others.

The Religion, Aging, and Health Survey is a national sample of older non-institutionalized white and black Americans (See Krause, 2006). Forgiveness of others was measured by a 4-item scale centered on zero ($\alpha = .68$). The questions were "How often do you forgive others for things they have done to you?, How often do you hold a grudge?, How often do you feel resentful toward others for things they have done?, How hard is it for you to forgive others?" The coding of each question was never, once in a while, fairly often, and very often.

The General Social Survey is a nationally representative cross-sectional sample of adults in the U.S. that is conducted bi-annually (See Smith, Mardsen, Hout, & Kim, 2012). In 1998, several questions about religion and forgiveness were included in a sub-sample of the survey. A total of 1,391 respondents were interviewed, and were asked "Because of your religious or spiritual beliefs have you always, almost always, often, seldom, or never felt the following ways: I have forgiven those who hurt me."

Table 13.1 Testing for differences in levels of forgiveness for whites and blacks (mean (std))

	Blacks	Whites	*t* test by race
RAHS Forgiveness t = 1[a]	0.12 (0.51)	−0.13 (0.56)	6.35***
RAHS Forgiveness t = 2	0.11 (0.55)	−0.09 (0.76)	5.44***
GSS Forgiveness[b]	3.41 (0.82)	3.29 (0.78)	1.95*
ACLS Forgiveness[c]	3.46 (0.90)	3.40 (0.83)	1.23
ACLS Grudges[d]	3.45 (0.94)	3.33 (0.93)	2.05*

[a]The sample size for RAHS is n = 436 blacks and n = 500 whites
[b]The sample size for GSS is n = 189 blacks and n = 1,071 whites
[c]The response rate for the forgiveness question in ACLS is n = 403 blacks and n = 1,220 whites
[d]The response rate for grudges question in ACLS is n = 402 blacks and n = 1,222 whites
$p \leq 0.05$, $^{**}p \leq 0.01$, $^{***}p \leq 0.001$

The third dataset is the American's Changing Lives Survey (See House, 2010). Like the Religion, Aging, and Health Survey, the American's Changing Lives Survey is a nationally representative longitudinal survey that collects various information including questions regarding holding grudges and forgiving offenders for various offenses. Forgiveness questions were asked during Wave 4. Respondents were told: "Now I have a few questions about how you feel when things go wrong. For each statement please tell me whether you agree strongly, agree somewhat, disagree somewhat, or disagree strongly." The forgiveness question states: "I have forgiven those who have hurt me." The grudge question asks: "I have grudges that I have held onto for months or years." A total of 1,668 respondents participated in Wave 4.

Table 13.1 shows the results suggest that blacks generally report higher levels of forgiveness of others than whites. This pattern was most pronounced among the RAH survey participants, possibly because forgiveness was measured with four items and because the sample consisted of older adult and age is positively associated with forgiveness (Toussaint, Williams, Musick, & Everson, 2001). However, the pattern was not evident in the American Changing Lives survey when respondents were asked how often they forgave others who had hurt them, although blacks reported higher levels of forgiveness the findings were not statistically significant. Based on previous research and the findings presented above, we find that proposition one is plausible such that blacks report higher levels of forgiveness than their white counterparts. We caution that these results are preliminary and more in-depth studies are needed to take into account potential selection issues. For instance, black men are disproportionately likely to be incarcerated and incarcerated individuals are not included in these data. Perhaps the least forgiving black but not white individuals were not included in these studies due to different rates of incarceration. Nonetheless, given this pattern was replicated across three data sets with different sample designs the results should not be discounted.

Proposition 2: Blacks Benefit More from Forgiveness Than Whites

The social and economic environments are often very different for blacks and whites in the U.S. and these environments provide the context in which forgiveness occurs and may moderate how beneficial forgiveness is for health. Blacks experience a pernicious reality of discrimination including: racism, segregation, employment discrimination, and interpersonal maltreatment (Feagin & Sikes, 1994; Jackson, Thoits, & Taylor, 1995). There is mounting evidence of anti-black racism including studies that report racial disadvantage in access to resources and discrimination in the economic and institutional arenas is especially pronounced (Ellison et al., 2008; Pager & Shepherd, 2008). Racial discrimination and stressors lead to poorer health outcomes (Pascoe & Smart Richman, 2009; Williams & Mohammed, 2009).

Although the link between health and forgiveness is well established, the relationship between race, forgiveness, and health is largely unknown. Moreover, the research on forgiveness and health is largely limited to white populations, with investigations of blacks being limited. However, the pathways by which forgiveness impacts health may be especially important for blacks. Thoresen et al. (2000) propose several pathways by which forgiveness may influence health outcomes which serve as the backdrop for understanding the role of race: (a) a decrease in chronic blaming, hostility, and anger, (b) decreases in sympathetic nervous system (SNS) hyper arousal and allostatic load, (c) increases in optimism and positive self-evaluative thoughts, (d) increases in self-efficacy, (e) increases in social and emotional support, and (f) increases in transcendent consciousness (greater religious or spiritual well-being). Based on the pathways proposed by Thorensen et al., there are at least four reasons why blacks might benefit more from forgiveness than their white counterparts.

First, blacks have large social networks in which they go to for support. Blacks have high rates of intergenerational homes, they tend to live in racially segregated communities, and frequently attend religious services. These extended social networks provide both tangible and intangible support, which has been shown to impact health (Uchino, 2006). Forgiveness is essential for maintaining extended social networks. Within large social networks, there is a high probability for conflict to arise; this interpersonal conflict may reduce available social support. The ability to forgive may reduce the negative effects of interpersonal conflict, thereby expanding the social supports available and hence garnering the health benefits from forgiveness.

Second, blacks have witnessed social and economic adversity which can lead to a process of biological weathering. Severe adversity leads to higher levels of physiological stress. Experiencing chronic stress can lead to a dysregulation of the body's biological stress response system. This dysregulation leads to stress-related health disorders and accounts for a large portion of disparities in health and mortality found among minorities in the U.S (Geronimus et al., 2006). Moreover, unforgiveness has neuro-physiological consequences similar to anger where in states of unforgiveness the brain demonstrates decreased cognitive activity in the prefrontal cortex and increases in limbic activity (Worthington & Scherer, 2004). These increases correspond with glucocorticoid secretion consistent with a stress response. Forgiveness may be more beneficial for blacks because it is a coping mechanism that can aid in dealing with disproportionate exposure to interpersonal conflict and social stress (Worthington & Scherer, 2004). Issues of discrimination, racism, and economic adversity are negative forces present in the social lives of blacks; however, emotion-focused coping mechanisms like forgiveness may yield a positive result when problem focused approaches are not available (Ysseldyk, Matheson & Anisman, 2009). Forgiveness of others also decreases chronic blaming, which may decrease the sensitivity of the stress response (Thoresen et al., 2000); decrease involvement in harmful health behaviors (Toussaint & Webb, 2005); and improve health (McFarland et al., 2012).

The adversity witnessed by blacks may create higher levels of interpersonal conflict during their day-to-day lives. Blacks report higher levels of daily tensions, self appraisal of stress associated with interpersonal conflict or arguments, and negative affect (Birditt, Cichy, & Almeida, 2011). Several studies report that not only do blacks experience higher levels of these stressors, they respond to conflict with more confrontational behaviors and negative affect than do whites (Kochman, 1981; Mackey & O'Brien, 1998). Interpersonal conflict, in turn, can create anger which has a pernicious effect upon health. In a study of blacks and Latinos, daily interpersonal conflict was associated with increased blood pressure (Schoenthaler et al., 2010). Forgiveness may prove to be a useful tool in counteracting the negative impacts of adversity. Forgiveness is thought to bring about higher levels of optimism and self-efficacy which are both positively related to health (Lawler et al., 2005). Forgiveness reduces anger and negative affect which may serve as an advantageous coping mechanism in these stressful situations. Decreasing the negative response to stressors through forgiveness may thereby decrease the negative health response to such stressors.

Third, forgiveness is associated with higher levels of positive emotions (e.g., optimism) and lower levels of negative emotions (e.g., anger; Lawler et al., 2005). While forgiveness is associated with positive health benefits, anger is associated with a host of deleterious health outcomes (Scheiman, Pearlin & Meersman, 2006). Blacks are exposed to stressors that have long-lasting effects on physical and mental health. Responding to stressors with anger and other forms of negative emotions can lead to a host of negative health outcomes. Given the benefits of positive emotions, the tendency to forgive may act as a buffer for negative emotions that lead to poor mental and physical health. For blacks experiencing chronic exposure to adversity, the availability of forgiveness as a coping mechanism can alleviate some of the negative health effects stressors can have.

Fourth, there is strong evidence to suggest that religious involvement can improve health and well-being (Hummer, Rogers, Nam, & Ellison, 1999; Koenig, 2008; Koenig et al., 2001). The religion-forgiveness-health connection may be more pronounced for blacks. On average, blacks tend to be more religious than whites on virtually all indicators of religiosity (Ellison & McFarland, 2013). Studies have also found a beneficial effect of religious attendance on blood pressure and related cardiovascular disease among blacks (Koenig et al., 1998; Luskin, 2000). The impact religion has on health for blacks may be mediated by levels of forgiveness. Recent work by Lutjen et al. (2012) uses path models to test this relationship and finds that religion improves health through the mediating pathway of increasing forgiveness and decreasing hostility. In another study, Lawler-Row (2010) found that forgiveness of others partially mediated the religion-health relationship. Currently, very few studies have investigated the relationship between forgiveness and health for blacks.

Toussaint and Williams (2003) investigated the relationship between forgiveness and resting blood pressure and cortisol levels among blacks and whites. Using an interview-based study of 100 residents in a Midwestern community, they found that forgiveness of others was associated with lower diastolic blood pressure and basal cortisol for low SES blacks while there was no relationship between forgiveness and these health measures for whites or high SES blacks. In a more recent study, McFarland et al. (2012) found that forgiveness shared a stronger relationship with health for blacks compared to whites. They found that for blacks, forgiveness was significantly associated with self-reported health, but not among whites. The effect of forgiveness on the number of chronic health conditions was different for whites and blacks. Forgiveness was shown to be associated with fewer chronic conditions for blacks, but there was no significant association for whites. Overall, these two studies provide preliminary evidence to support our assertion that race plays an integral role in the forgiveness and health relationship.

Conclusions

Research on forgiveness largely explores the cultivation of forgiveness or social and psychological factors that enhance or diminish the use of forgiveness (Enright, 1996). The research implicitly assumes that factors influencing forgiveness are the same across all people. Although, a few studies have moved beyond this framework to include explorations of age and sex differences in forgiveness (Girard & Mullet, 1997; Miller et al., 2008; Toussaint et al., 2001), until recently, racial differences in forgiveness have been ignored (Krause, 2012; McFarland et al., 2012). Overlooking the influence race has on forgiveness is surprising considering race impacts various dimensions of life including family structure, social relationships, neighborhood, group schemas, religious involvement, economic resources, social resources, exposures to stressors, exposure to interpersonal transgressions, group sanctions, and group norms. The goal of this chapter was to move the field of forgiveness research forward by discussing racial differences in forgiveness and health generally and specifically with a case study comparing blacks with whites. In this chapter, we provided arguments as to why blacks would be more forgiving than whites, provided evidence from three data sets that this argument is correct, provided arguments as to why blacks would benefit more from forgiveness, and provided evidence from the nominal literature supporting this latter argument.

There are several potential directions on race-informed forgiveness and health research. First, future research should examine the relationship between forgiveness and health for other racial and ethnic groups in the U.S. For instance, based on a cultural orientation of more collectivist mentality, the impact of forgiveness may be especially important for Asians. Second, future research should test the differential social and cultural mechanisms by which forgiveness operates differently by race. Because race structures the social, economic, and cultural aspects of people's lives including social, economic, and psychosocial resources that may substitute for forgiveness, the pathways by which forgiveness operates should also vary by race.

Third, researchers should incorporate measures of biological risk that represent risk for disease and mortality as racial differences in biological risk are especially pronounced (Seeman et al., 2008) and may make the protective influence of forgiveness greater for some groups than others. Fourth, because the extent of racial disparities differs by the dimension of health, the impact of forgiveness for various health outcomes may also vary by race. Future research should incorporate a number of health outcomes to test for racial differences in the magnitude of the influence of forgiveness for differing dimensions of health. Finally, future research should consider the role of race in different countries as race structures the lives of people in drastically different ways around the world.

Incorporating the role of race into forgiveness and health research represents a potentially fruitful area for understanding the complex ways in which forgiveness impacts health. While we have argued that race may be important for understanding how forgiveness impacts health, a dearth of research on this topic precludes us from making any definitive claims. Nonetheless, without assessing the role of race as well as the broader environment in which people live, researchers remain vulnerable to problems of external validity.

References

Anderson, E. (1999). *Code of the street. Decency, violence, and the moral life of the inner city*. New York, NY: Norton.

Berry, J. W., Worthington, E. L., O'Connor, L. E., Parrott, L., & Wade, N. G. (2005). Forgiveness, vengeful rumination, & affective traits. *Journal of Personality, 73*, 183–225.

Birditt, K. S., Cichy, K. E., & Almeida, D. (2011). Age differences in exposure and reactivity to interpersonal tensions among black and white individuals across adulthood. *Race and Social Problems, 3*, 225–239.

Cohen, S., Tyrell, D. A. J., & Smith, A. P. (1993). Negative life events, perceived stress negative affect, and susceptibility to the common cold. *Journal of Personality and Social Psychology, 64*, 131–140.

Coon, H. M., & Kemmelmeier, M. (2001). Cultural orientations in the United States (re) examining differences among ethnic groups. *Journal of Cross-Cultural Psychology, 32*(3), 348–364.

DiBlasio, F. A., & Proctor, J. H. (1993). Therapists and the clinical use of forgiveness. *American Journal of Family Therapy, 21*(2), 175–184.

Edin, K., & Kefalas, M. (2011). *Promises I can keep: Why poor women put motherhood before marriage*. Berkeley, CA: University of California Press.

Ellison, C. G., Musick, M. A., & Henderson, A. K. (2008). The Balm of Gilead: Racism, religious involvement, and psychological distress among African American adults. *Journal for the Scientific Study of Religion, 47*, 291–309.

Ellison, C. G., & McFarland, M. J. (2013). The social context of religion and spirituality in the United States. In K. I. Pargament (Editor-in-Chief), J. J. Exline, & J. W. Jones (Associate Eds.), *APA handbook of psychology, religion, and spirituality* (Vol. 1, pp. 21–51).

Enright, R. D. (1996). Counseling within the forgiveness triad: On forgiving, receiving forgiveness, and self-forgiveness. *Counseling and Values, 40*(2), 107–126.

Feagin, J. R., & Sikes, M. P. (1994). *Living with racism: The black middle-class experience*. Boston, MA: Beacon.

Geronimus, A. T., Hicken, M., Keene, D., & Bound, J. (2006). "Weathering" and age patterns of allostatic load scores among blacks and whites in the United States. *American Journal of Public Health, 96*, 826–833.

Girard, M., & Mullet, E. (1997). Forgiveness in adolescents, young, middle-aged, and older adults. *Journal of Adult Development, 4*, 209–220.

Griffith, E. E., English, T., & Mayfield, V. (1980). Possession, prayer, and testimony: Therapeutic aspects of the Wednesday night meeting in a Black church. *Psychiatry: Journal for the Study of Interpersonal Processes, 43*(2), 120–128.

Hargrave, T. D., & Sells, J. N. (1997). The development of a forgiveness scale. *Journal of Marital and Family Therapy, 23*, 41–64.

Hatch, S. L., & Dohrenwend, B. P. (2007). Distribution of traumatic and other stressful life events by race/ethnicity, gender, ses and age: A review of the research. *American Journal of Community Psychology, 40*(3–4), 313–332.

House, J. S. (2010). *Americans' changing lives: Waves I, II, III, and IV, 1986, 1989, 1994, and 2002*. Ann Arbor, MI: Inter-university Consortium for Political and Social Research.

Hummer, R. A., Rogers, R. G., Nam, C. B., & Ellison, C. G. (1999). Religious involvement and US adult mortality. *Demography, 36*(2), 273–285.

Jackson, P. B., Thoits, P. A., & Taylor, H. F. (1995). Composition of the workplace and psychological well-being: The effects of tokenism on America's Black elite. *Social Forces, 74*(2), 543–557.

Kochman, T. (1981). *Black and white styles in conflict*. Chicago, IL: The University of Chicago Press.

Koenig, H. G. (2008). *Medicine, religion, and health: Where science and spirituality meet*. West Conshohocken, PA: Templeton Foundation Press.

Koenig, H. G., George, L. K., Hays, J. C., Larson, D. B., Cohen, H. J., & Blazer, D. G. (1998). The relationship between religious activities and blood pressure in older adults. *The International Journal of Psychiatry in Medicine, 28*(2), 189–213.

Koenig, H. G., Larson, D. B., & Larson, S. S. (2001). Religion and coping with serious medical illness. *The Annals of Pharmacotherapy, 35*(3), 352–359.

Krantz, D. S., & McCeney, M. K. (2002). Effects of psychological and social factors on organic disease: A critical assessment of research on coronary heart disease*. *Annual Review of Psychology, 53*(1), 341–369.

Krause, N. (2002). Exploring race differences in a comprehensive battery of church-based social support measures. *Review of Religious Research, 44*, 126–149.

Krause, N. (2006). *Religion, aging, and health survey, 2001, 2004*. Ann Arbor, MI: Inter-university Consortium for Political and Social Research.

Krause, N. (2012). Studying forgiveness among older whites, older blacks, and older Mexican Americans. *Journal of Religion, Spirituality & Aging, 24*(4), 325–344.

Lawler, K. A., Younger, J. W., Piferi, R. L., Jobe, R. L., Edmondson, K. A., & Jones, W. H. (2005). The unique effects of forgiveness on health: An exploration of pathways. *Journal of Behavioral Medicine, 28*, 157–167.

Lawler-Row, K. A. (2010). Forgiveness as a mediator of the religiosity-health relationship. *Psychology of Religion and Spirituality, 2*(1), 1–16.

Luskin, F. (2000). Review of the effect of spiritual and religious factors on mortality and morbidity with a focus on cardiovascular and pulmonary disease. *Journal of Cardiopulmonary Rehabilitation and Prevention, 20*(1), 8–15.

Lutjen, L. J., Silton, N. R., & Flannelly, K. J. (2012). Religion, forgiveness, hostility and health: A structural equation analysis. *Journal of Religion and Health, 51*(2), 468–478.

Mackey, R. A., & O'Brien, B. A. (1998). Marital conflict management: Gender and ethnic differences. *Social Work, 43*(2), 128–141.

McCullough, M. E. (2008). *Beyond revenge: The evolution of the forgiveness instinct*. San Francisco, CA: Jossey-Bass.

McCullough, M. E., Worthington, E. L., Jr., & Rachal, K. C. (1997). Interpersonal forgiving in close relationships. *Journal of Personality, 73*, 321–336.

McFarland, M. J., Smith, C. A., Toussaint, L., & Thomas, P. A. (2012). Forgiveness of others and health: Do race and neighborhood matter? *The Journals of Gerontology. Series B, Psychological Sciences and Social Sciences, 67*(1), 66–75.

Miller, A. J., Worthington, E. L., Jr., & McDaniel, M. A. (2008). Gender and forgiveness: A meta-analytic review and research agenda. *Journal of Social and Clinical Psychology, 27*(8), 843–876.

Miniño, A. M., Xu, J., & Kochanek, K. D. (2010). Deaths: Preliminary data for 2008. *National Vital Statistics Reports, 59*, 1–72.

Pager, D., & Shepherd, H. (2008). The sociology of discrimination: Racial discrimination in employment, housing, credit, & consumer markets. *Annual Review of Sociology, 34*, 181.

Pascoe, E. A., & Smart Richman, L. (2009). Perceived discrimination and health: A meta-analytic review. *Psychological Bulletin, 135*(4), 531.

Pearlin, L. I., Schieman, S., Fazio, E. M., & Meersman, S. C. (2005). Stress, health, and the life course: Some conceptual perspectives. *Journal of Health and Social Behavior, 46*(2), 205–219.

Rye, M. S., Pargament, K. I., Ali, M. A., Beck, G. L., Dorff, E. N., Hallisey, C., . . . , & Williams, J. G. (2000). Religious perspectives on forgiveness. In *Forgiveness: Theory, research, and practice* (pp. 17–40). New York, NY: Guilford Press.

Sandage, S. J., & Williamson, I. (2005). Forgiveness in the cultural context. In *Handbook of forgiveness* (pp. 41–56). New York, NY: Routledge.

Sapolsky, R. M. (2004). Social status and health in humans and other animals. *Annual Review of Anthropology, 33*, 393–418.

Sarkisian, N., & Gerstel, N. (2004). Kin support among blacks and whites: Race and family organization. *American Sociological Review, 69*, 812–837.

Schieman, S., Pearlin, L. I., & Meersman, S. C. (2006). Neighborhood disadvantage and anger among older adults: Social comparisons as effect modifiers. *Journal of Health and Social Behavior, 47*, 156–172.

Schoenthaler, A. M., Schwartz, J., Cassells, A., Tobin, J. N., & Brondolo, E. (2010). Daily interpersonal conflict predicts masked hypertension in an urban sample. *American Journal of Hypertension, 23*(10), 1082–1088.

Seeman, T., Merkin, S. S., Crimmins, E., Koretz, B., Charette, S., & Karlamangla, A. (2008). Education, income and ethnic differences in cumulative biological risk profiles in a national sample of US adults: NHANES III (1988–1994). *Social Science & Medicine, 66*(1), 72–87.

Seybold, K. S., Hill, P. C., Neumann, J. K., & Chi, D. S. (2001). Physiological and psychological correlates of forgiveness. *Journal of Psychology and Christianity, 20*, 250–259.

Smith, T. W., Marsden, P. V., Hout, M., & Kim, J. (2012). *General social surveys, 1972–2012*. Chicago, IL: NORC.

Stein, D. J., Seedat, S., Kaminer, D., Moomal, H., Herman, A., Sonnega, J., & Williams, D. R. (2008). The impact of the truth and reconciliation commission on psychological distress and forgiveness in South Africa. *Social Psychiatry and Psychiatric Epidemiology, 43*(6), 462–468

Strong, J. P., Malcom, G. T., McMahan, C. A., Tracy, R. E., Newman, W. P., III, Herderick, E. E., & Cornhill, J. F. (1999). Prevalence and extent of atherosclerosis in adolescents and young adults. *JAMA, the Journal of the American Medical Association, 281*(8), 727–735.

Suwartono, C., Prawasti, C. Y., & Mullet, E. (2007). Effect of culture on forgivingness: A Southern Asia-Western Europe comparison. *Personality and Individual Differences, 42*, 513–523.

Takuku, S., Weiner, B., & Ohbuchi, K. (2001). A cross-cultural examination of the effects of apology and perspective taking on interpersonal forgiveness. *Journal of Language and Social Psychology, 20*, 144–166.

Taylor, R. J., & Chatters, L. M. (1986). Church-based informal support among elderly blacks. *The Gerontologist, 26*(6), 637–642.

Thoits, P. A. (2010). Stress and health major findings and policy implications. *Journal of Health and Social Behavior, 51*(1 suppl), S41–S53.

Thoresen, C. E., Harris, A. H. S., & Luskin, F. (2000). Forgiveness and health: An unanswered question. In *Theory, research, and practice* (pp. 254–280). New York, NY: Guilford Press.

Tienda, M., & Mitchell, F. (Eds.). (2006). *Hispanics and the future of America*. Washington, DC: National Academies Press.

Toussaint, L. L., Williams, D. R., Musick, M. A., & Everson, S. A. (2001). Forgiveness and health: Age differences in a U.S. probability sample. *Journal of Adult Development, 8*, 249–257.

Toussaint, L., & Cheadle, A. C. D. (2009). Unforgiveness and the broken heart: Unforgiving tendencies, problems due to unforgiveness, and 12-month prevalence of cardiovascular health conditions. In E. D. Walker (Ed.), *Religion and Psychology*. New York, NY: Nova Publishers.

Toussaint, L., & Webb, J. R. (2005). Theoretical and empirical connections between forgiveness, mental health, and well-being. In *Handbook of forgiveness* (pp. 207–226). New York, NY: Routledge.

Toussaint, L. L., & Williams, D. R. (2003). *Physiological correlates of forgiveness: Findings from a racially and socioeconomically diverse sample of community residents*. Presented at A Campaign for forgiveness research conference, Atlanta, GA.

Uchino, B. N. (2006). Social support and health: A review of physiological processes potentially underlying links to disease outcomes. *Journal of Behavioral Medicine, 29*(4), 377–387.

Williams, D. R. (2005). The health of U.S. racial and ethnic populations. *Journal of Gerontology Social Sciences, 60B*, 53–62.

Williams, D. R., & Mohammed, S. A. (2009). Discrimination and racial disparities in health: Evidence and needed research. *Journal of Behavioral Medicine, 32*(1), 20–47.

Wilson, T., Milosevic, A., Carroll, M., Hart, K., & Hibbard, S. (2008). Physical health status in relation to self-forgiveness and other-forgiveness in healthy college students. *Journal of Health Psychology, 13*, 798–803.

Worthington, E. R., & Scherer, M. (2004). Forgiveness is an emotion- focused coping strategy that can reduce health risks and promote health resilience: Theory, review, and hypotheses. *Psychology & Health, 19*, 385–405.

Ysseldyk, R., Matheson, K., & Anisman, H. (2009). Forgiveness and the appraisal-coping process in response to relationship conflicts: Implications for depressive symptoms. *Stress: The International Journal on the Biology of Stress, 12*, 152–166.

Chapter 14
Aging, Forgiveness, and Health

Neal Krause and R. David Hayward

One of the most persistent themes in the literature on successful aging involves the importance of developing and maintaining close interpersonal relationships with advancing age (e.g., Rowe & Kahn, 1998). So if social relationships become increasingly important as people grow older, it is essential that researchers identify the factors that enhance the quality of interpersonal ties in late life. There is evidence that forgiveness may play a significant role in this respect (Worthington & Scherer, 2004). The purpose of this chapter is to examine the relationships among aging, forgiveness, and health. Although any number of issues could be examined within this context, we focus on five that have either not received sufficient attention or that are especially salient in the field. First, we discuss evidence for age differences in forgiveness, the association of forgiveness with health and well-being, and whether there are also age differences in the relationship between forgiveness and health. Second, we explain why it is important to distinguish between age, cohort, and life course influences in the aging and forgiveness literature. Third, we briefly review conceptual and theoretical perspectives that provide insight into why people may become more forgiving as they grow older. Fourth, we discuss a number of constructs that explain why forgiveness may be associated with health in late life. Fifth, we identify factors that may reduce the willingness and ability of older people to forgive. Finally, on the basis of these observations, we highlight elements that may be instructive for those seeking to develop clinical applications for forgiveness in older adulthood.

N. Krause (✉) • R.D. Hayward
Department of Health Behavior and Health Education, School of Public Health, University of Michigan, 1415 Washington Heights, Ann Arbor, MI, 48109-2029 USA
e-mail: nkrause@umich.edu

L.L. Toussaint et al. (eds.), *Forgiveness and Health*,
DOI 10.1007/978-94-017-9993-5_14

Age Variations in Forgiveness and Health

As it currently stands, the literature on aging, forgiveness, and health is comprised of two main bodies of research. Findings from the first body of work indicate that people who are currently older are more likely than individuals who are presently younger to forgive others for the things they have done (e.g. Allemand, 2008; Girard & Muller, 1997; Steiner, Allemand, & McCullough, 2012). However, researchers have not reached consensus on this issue. For example, a recent meta-analysis uncovered only negligible effects of age on forgiveness of others (Fehr, Gelfand, & Nag, 2010). A few studies have also been devoted to assessing age differences in other types of forgiveness. This research reveals that older people are also more likely than younger individuals to feel they have been forgiven by God (e.g., Toussaint, Williams, Musick, & Everson, 2001).

The second main body of research is concerned with the relationship between forgiveness and health in samples of older people. This research reveals that trait forgivingness is associated with better physical health (McFarland, Smith, Toussaint, & Thomas, 2012), better mental health (e.g., Krause & Ellison, 2003), and a lower mortality risk (Toussaint, Owen, & Cheadle, 2012).

In addition to these widely replicated findings, research further indicates that there appears to be age differences in this relationship, forgivingness and health. More specifically, a study by Toussaint and his colleagues indicates that potentially beneficial effects of forgiving others on physical and mental health are stronger for middle and older age adults than for younger people (Toussaint et al., 2001).

There are, however, at least two significant shortcomings in research on aging, forgivingness, and health. First, with the exception of a few studies (e.g., McFarland et al., 2012), research in this field has largely been conducted with cross-sectional data. As we discuss in the next section, working with cross-sectional data glosses over a number of important issues. Second, most of the empirical studies on aging and forgivingness have focused on forgiving others, while considerably less attention has been devoted to the other types of forgiveness.

One way to address this issue involves assessing whether the various dimensions of forgiveness are correlated highly. The following example illustrates the rationale behind this approach. If forgiving others increase with age and feeling forgiven by God is correlated highly with forgiving others, then perhaps feeling forgiven by God increases with age, as well. We evaluated this reasoning by analyzing data on forgiveness from a nationwide survey of older adults ($N = 1,500$) by Krause (2002). This unpublished research reveals the following correlations among the different types of forgiveness: forgiveness of others and being forgiven by God ($r = .225$: $p < .01$); forgiveness of others and forgiveness of self ($r = .157$; $p < .01$); forgiveness of others and being forgiven by others ($r = .159$; $p < .01$); forgiveness by God and forgiveness of self ($r = .212$; $p < .01$); forgiveness by God and being forgiven by others ($r = .158$; $p < .01$); and forgiveness of self and being forgiven by others ($r = .172$; $p < .01$). The average correlation between these indicators of forgiveness is only .178, indicating that the various dimensions of forgiveness are significantly shaped by different causal forces.

Variations Within Late Life, Cohort, and Life Course Issues

The problems that arise when assessing age differences in forgiveness with cross-sectional data mask three complex problems that have yet to be fully resolved in the literature: (a) in addition to differences that emerge between younger and older people, there may be variation *within* old age, as well; (b) variations in forgiveness that are observed across different age groups may really reflect cohort effects; and (c) it is also important to keep life course influences in mind.

Variations Within Late Life

A potentially significant problem with the literature on age differences in forgiveness arises from the way late life is typically construed. The wide majority of researchers assess age differences in forgiveness by comparing all people 65 years of age and older with individuals who are younger. However, investigators who employ this strategy implicitly assume that there are no variations in forgiveness beyond age 65. This seems unlikely because late life lasts from age 65 to increasingly older ages. In fact, people age 85 and over are the fastest growing segment of the older population (Federal Interagency Forum on Aging Related Statistics, 2012). Moreover, living to age 100 is becoming much more common. This means that it is not unusual for late life to encompass a period of approximately 35 years. It is difficult to believe that psychosocial development ceases during this time.

Empirical support for the notion that there may be age differences in forgiveness within late life is found in a recent study of people age 66 and over by Hayward and Krause (2013). These investigators conducted a series of individual growth curve analyses to estimate trajectories of forgiveness over a 7-year period. They observed increases over time in forgiveness of others, forgiveness of self, forgiveness by God, and being forgiven by others. These findings are consistent with the notion that developmental differences in forgiveness may not cease when individuals reach age 65.

Cohort Differences

Unfortunately, researchers have yet to fully address cohort effects in the process of studying age differences in forgiveness. Whereas age differences refer to changes that are associated with typical biological, psychological, and social maturation, cohort differences arise from unique historical experiences that were shared by people who were born in close proximity of each other. Although researchers have yet to agree on how to operationally define cohorts, many consider people who were born in the same decade to be in the same cohort. But regardless of how they are defined, cohort effects should be taken into account because historical events that are shared by individuals in the same cohort can have a significant impact on their world views. For example, many people who were born between 1910 and 1920 came of age during the Great Depression. And as Elder (1999) discusses in his widely cited volume, *Children of the Great Depression*, growing up during trying economic times left an enduring mark on the way the members of this cohort view the world.

Cohort effects were also evaluated in the study by Hayward and Krause (2013) that were discussed above. These investigators found that compared to older cohorts, members of younger cohorts are less likely to forgive themselves, they are less likely to feel they were forgiven by God, and they are less likely to feel forgiven by other people. Because so little is known about cohort differences in late life it was difficult for these researchers to pinpoint the precise historical events that may explain these findings.

In order to properly disentangle age and cohort effects, researchers must have data from a number of different cohorts that have been assessed at multiple points in time. Unfortunately, the study by Hayward and Krause (2013) was not based on this type of data. Clearly, obtaining the appropriate data should be a high priority in future research.

Life Course Influences

The issue of distinguishing between age and cohort effects may be even more challenging because life course influences should be taken into account, as well. Evidence of life course effects may be found in the work of Vaillant (2002). In this volume, Vaillant sums up all he learned from the Harvard Study of Adult Development, which is a study of Harvard graduates who were followed from their undergraduate years through age 75. He found four factors that emerged earlier in life that were protective of health and well-being in old age. One of these factors is the capacity for gratitude and forgiveness.

The findings reported by Vaillant (2002) may be interpreted in at least two ways. First, forgiveness early in life may exert a direct effect on health in late life. Second, forgiveness early in life may shape forgiveness late in life which may, in turn, affect health in old age. Unfortunately, Vaillant did not explore these different mechanisms in his empirical analysis. But regardless of this problem, the basic point still stands: practices that emerge earlier in life may have influences that span the entire life course.

Taken as a whole, the literature that has been discussed in this section suggests that the seemingly straightforward question regarding age differences in forgiveness quickly becomes mired in complex issues involving age, cohort, and life course effects. In order to move the literature forward, these vexing issues must be met head-on.

Theoretical Perspectives on Age Differences in Forgiveness

Although the picture provided by empirical studies of age differences in forgiveness is murky, greater consensus may be found in theoretical frameworks that have been devised by developmental psychologists. As the discussion that is provided below will reveal, many of these theorists did not discuss forgiveness explicitly. Even so, they identified a number of age-related qualities that make it easy to argue that the willingness and ability to forgive increases with age.

Evidence of this may be found in Tornstam's (2005) theory of gerotranscendence. According to Tornstam, as people enter late life, they experience significant changes in their lives, including a marked decrease in self-centeredness, a higher degree of altruism, a sense of having closer ties with previous generations, a decline in the importance of material things, and an increase in the importance of close relationships. It is not difficult to see why a person who experiences these changes might also be more likely to forgive others.

Like Levenson (1996), Tornstam (2005) discusses a series of age-related changes that appear to provide especially fertile ground for the development of forgiveness in late life. More specifically, he maintains that as people grow older, they lose ego-centric views of the self and reach out to others in an effort to forge closer relationships with them. These efforts are fueled in part by increases in compassionate regard for others. This is important because a number of researchers have argued that people who are more compassionate are also more forgiving (Worthington & Scherer, 2004).

In her widely-cited theory of aging, Carstensen (1992) argues that as people enter late life, they become more aware that they have relatively less time to live and as a result, they initiate a significant shift in their priorities. More specifically, they tend to trim more casual social ties and attach greater importance to a relatively smaller circle of relationships that are emotionally close. If older people become increasingly concerned with building emotionally close relationships, then it seems that the capacity for forgiveness would be an important asset in reaching this goal.

Of all the theorists that are discussed in this section, the work of Butler (1963) speaks more directly to issues involving forgiveness. Butler's begins by arguing that due in part to a growing awareness of death, older people engage in a deliberate review of their life experiences. He points out that in the process of making this review, older adults often experience a "... resurgence of unresolved conflicts" (Butler, 1995, p. xvii). He goes on to point out that a number of positive outcomes can emerge from this life review, including the "righting of old wrongs" and "reconciliation with enemies." Themes of forgiving others and forgiving oneself are clearly evident in his work.

The observations of Butler (1995) are consistent with the experiences of therapists who work with older people. For example, Hargrave and Anderson (1992) report that one of the prominent issues confronting older clients involves feelings of guilt that have arisen from longstanding family conflicts. This is one reason why Butler's (1995) work has played a role in developing a therapeutic technique for older clients that is known as reminiscence therapy (Haight & Webster, 1995).

A final conceptual explanation for why there may be age differences in forgiveness cannot be traced to the work of any specific theorist but instead emerges from an extensive body of research on changes in religious involvement over the life course. Although the issue is far from resolved, a significant number of studies indicate that people may become more religious as they grow older (see Krause, 2008a, for a review of this research). This is important because, as many researchers point out, virtually every major faith tradition in the world places an emphasis on forgiveness (Lundberg, 2010). So if people become more religious with age and if a heavy emphasis is placed in religion on forgiveness, then it follows that people should become more forgiving as they grow older.

From Correlation to Explanation

As the literature continues to develop, researchers have shifted the focus of their work from assessing the relationships among aging, forgiveness, and health to deriving explanations of how these potential health-related benefits arise. Although a host of explanatory mechanisms have been proposed, we focus on four that are ripe for further exploration and elaboration.

Acts of Contrition

The first set of mediators in research on forgiveness and health involve acts of contrition. Acts of contrition involve conciliatory behaviors that a transgressor may perform in order to be forgiven by a victim. Among the acts of contrition that a transgressor may perform are explicitly recognizing the hurtful act, apologizing for it, promising not to commit the offense again, and providing restitution whenever possible.

Two perspectives are found in the literature on the health-related implications of performing acts of contrition (Lang, 1994; Scobie & Scobie, 1998). The first perspective suggests that performing acts of contrition is beneficial because it gets the hurt out into the open where it can be discussed and resolved. In contrast, the second perspective specifies that a transgressor need not engage in acts of contrition because he or she is forgiven unconditionally (i.e., automatically). Doing so is thought to get the hurtful act quickly behind both parties. Moreover, requiring others to perform acts of contrition may set new problems in motion because a transgressor may, for example, not provide the kind of restitution a victim was expecting or a transgressor may not offer an apology that is as sincere as the victim desires. As a result, these new problems may initiate further cycles of recrimination and revenge, thereby intensifying the potentially noxious effect of the transgression.

A study by Krause and Ellison (2003) represents one of the few to examine these competing views empirically. Their work suggests that compared to victims who forgive unconditionally, victims who require transgressors to perform acts of contrition experience a diminished sense of psychological well-being.

So far, most of the empirical studies have focused on acts of contrition between a transgressor and a victim. However, at least one study has also assessed the role that acts of contrition may play in the process of seeking forgiveness from God. Research by Krause and Hayward (2015) suggests that performing acts of contrition in order to be forgiven by God is associated with a greater sense of well-being (i.e., diminished death anxiety).

The contrast between the findings from these two studies raises an interesting question: Why might requiring other people to perform acts of contrition have detrimental effects while performing acts of contrition in order to be forgiven by God have the opposite effect?

Clearly, the focal person is the victim in the first scenario while he or she is the transgressor in the second. Viewing the findings in this way makes it possible to take advantage of the general literature on self-consistency and dissonance reduction (Stone & Cooper, 2001). Although their theoretical framework is not explicitly cast in terms of contrition and forgiveness, it nevertheless can be easily adapted to this issue. Stone and Cooper (2001) argue that people maintain an internal set of self-standards. When an individual commits an act that violates these self-standards, they experience feelings of dissonance that arise from the painful realization that they are not the type of person they set out to become. This dissonance motivates compensatory behavior that helps restore a sense of self-consistency. Cast with the context of our discussion, their work suggests that acts of contrition help reassure the transgressor and the victim that future actions will be consistent with positive self-standards. And in the process, acts of contrition reduce the painful dissonance. Moreover, by performing acts of contrition, the transgressor avoids downplaying or minimizing the importance of the transgression and instead minimizes the extent to which the transgression is diagnostic of the self.

The views of Stone and Cooper (2001) can be extended in another potentially important way. The more costly and painful the transgression, the more effective acts of contrition may be in reducing the dissonance that it creates. More specifically, the more elaborate the acts of contrition become, the more rapid and more completely the dissonance associated with the transgression may be dispelled.

Returning to the contradictory findings that are described above, our adaptation of the work of Stone and Cooper (2001) suggests that performing acts of contrition for one's own transgressions are beneficial because they alleviate painful feelings of dissonance. But when someone else is the transgressor, this beneficial function is no longer possible.

This is just one of a host of issues that researchers need to address in the largely overlooked domain of acts of contrition. For example, Cooper (2003) maintains that requiring a transgressor to perform acts of contrition may impede the process of forgiveness because only in the context of unconditional forgiveness can a transgressor lay down his or her self-righteous defenses and freely enter into a responsible effort at resolution. In addition, only when these defenses have been dropped can the transgressor engage in the kind of introspection that will lead to a sincere apology, a firm resolution to avoid further hurtful acts, and a heartfelt effort to provide restitution.

The insights provided by Cooper (2003) are thought-provoking because they provide a different view of the interface between acts of contrition and unconditional forgiveness. These constructs are typically juxtaposed in the literature: either a transgressor must perform acts of contrition or they are forgiven unconditionally. But if Cooper is correct, then the two may take place in tandem. Letting a transgressor know that he or she is forgiven unconditionally makes it possible for a transgressor to perform acts of contrition more sincerely, thereby helping the transgressor forgive himself or herself for the hurtful act he or she has committed. Viewed in a more general way, Cooper's work brings an element of timing to the foreground. And as Hall and Fincham (2008) maintain, much more empirical research on the timing and sequencing of the steps in the process of forgiveness is clearly needed.

Focusing on acts of contrition also provides a way to bring aging related issues to the foreground. If people are more likely to forgive others as they grow older, then perhaps they are able to do so because they are more likely to forgive unconditionally. Surprisingly, the study by Hayward and Krause (2013) that was discussed earlier further reveals that over time, older people appear to be more likely to require transgressors to perform acts of contrition. One potential explanation for this anomalous finding may be that as older adults deepen their engagement in the process of forgiveness, they also give more thought and reflection to the conditions that make forgiveness possible. Alternatively, this trend may reflect changes in the scope of the types of behavior viewed as evidence of contrition. However, data provided by people from a wider range of ages is needed to resolve this issue conclusively.

Relationship Histories and Forgiveness

The process of forgiveness is also likely to be shaped by nature of the relationship between the victim and the transgressor. Although this overlooked aspect of forgiveness can be approached in a number of ways, we extend the insights that can be derived from it by contrasting forgiveness of individuals whom a victim knows well with forgiveness of strangers.

Recall that a core tenet of socioemotional selectivity theory specifies that as people grow older, they shed more casual social ties in order to devote their time and effort to relationships that are more close emotionally (Carstensen, 1992). We suspect that relationships that are more emotionally close are likely to have been maintained by older people for some time, perhaps for decades. This means that as people grow older, they are likely to turn to those with whom they have a long history. Perhaps this is one reason why empirical research by Carstensen (1992) suggests that the closest others are often family members.

These insights are important for the following reason. Some time ago, Jackson and Antonucci (1992) formulated the notion of the support bank. They devised this perspective in order to explain the nature of the relationship between parents and their children over the life course. Jackson and Antonucci maintain that when children are young, parents do virtually everything for them. But in the process of doing so, parents are depositing credits in the support bank. Depositing credits in the support bank is important because the nature of the social support process changes significantly with age. As parents reach late life, the balance of support tips and their grown children now provide a disproportionately greater amount of support to them. But this imbalance in social exchanges does not create tension because elderly parents are merely cashing in the credits from their support banks. The same principle may explain the process of forgiveness in the long-standing relationships that people tend to prefer in late life: if parents forgive children when they were young, then once children reach adulthood, they may be more likely to forgive their parents should the need arise.

All people have shortcomings and as a result, they are likely to hurt those they love whether they intend to or not. However, if a relationship has survived for a long period of time, both parties are likely to have forgiven each other numerous times. So when a new hurtful act is perpetrated, the transgressor should be able to draw on the credits that he or she has accrued in their "forgiveness bank": the victim will be less likely to seek retribution for a hurtful act because the transgressor has forgiven them in the past. Moreover, because of their history with transgressors, victims will be more likely to forgive, knowing they may likely find themselves in a future situation where they will need the current transgressor's forgiveness, as well.

The discussion that has been provided up to this point suggests that the process of forgiveness may unfold in specific ways within relationships with long histories. But it is instructive to shift to the opposite extreme and consider relationships that have little or no history because individuals may also be hurt by people they do not know. Being the victim of a random crime is an obvious example. Focusing on forgiveness involving strangers makes it possible to derive additional principles and insights into the process of forgiveness.

As the discussion that has been provided up to this point suggests, people can forgive individuals they love or they can forgive individuals they either do not know at all or do not know well. The Christian Bible is clear about the importance of this difference. In the Sermon on the Mount, Jesus spoke directly to the payoff of dealing only with people whom one knows well: "For if ye love them which love you, what reward have ye? Do not even the publicans do the same?" (Matthew 5:46, KJV). Applying this basic religious precept to the study of forgiveness suggests that the spiritual benefits of forgiving strangers may differ from those that are associated with forgiving loved ones. In order to see why this may be so, it is helpful to return to the insights of Jackson and Antonucci (1992). As we argued above, strangers have no credits in their "forgiveness bank" and as a result, forgiving them typically requires considerably more effort. Moreover, doing so does not hold out the promise of reciprocity on the part of the transgressor in the future. Even so, perhaps deep lessons in life are learned as the victim finds that he or she has developed a broader capacity for forgiveness in the process.

Forgiveness and Meaning in Life

As we discussed earlier, virtually every major faith tradition in the world extols the virtue of forgiveness (Lundberg, 2010). Researchers also frequently maintain that one of the primary functions of religion is to help people derive as sense of meaning in life (Hood, Hill, & Spilka, 2003). This raises the possibility that forgiveness may somehow help people derive a deeper sense of meaning in life. However, the reason why the two might be related is not clear. The purpose of the discussion in this section is to explain why this may be so.

The quality of interpersonal relationships serves as the linchpin that links forgiveness with meaning in life. Although the issue is often overlooked in the literature, there is some evidence that forgiveness may maintain, and perhaps enhance, the quality of a social relationship after the process of forgiveness is complete. More specifically, as an experimental study by Karremans and Van Lange (2004) indicates, "... forgiveness is related to smoother interactions between relationship partners, which ultimately may result in greater relationship satisfaction" (p. 223).

The notion that forgiveness may bolster the long-term efficacy of personal relationships is important because researchers have argued for decades that strong interpersonal ties form the basis for deriving a sense of meaning in life. The essence of this view is captured in Berger and Pullberg's (1965) discussion of meaning (i.e., world building): "... *men together* engage in constructing a world, which then becomes their common dwelling ... (this) world must be confirmed and reconfirmed *by others*" (p. 201, emphasis in the original). Support for the notion that stronger social ties promote a greater sense of meaning in life may be found in two studies by Krause (2007, 2008b). So if forgiveness promotes stronger social relationships and stronger social relationships, in turn, foster a deeper sense of meaning in life, it follows that forgiveness affects meaning indirectly through close interpersonal ties.

There are two reasons why the emphasis on meaning in life is justified. First, a growing body of research suggests that a stronger sense of meaning is associated with better physical health (Krause, 2004), better mental health (Wong, 2012), and a lower mortality risk (Krause, 2009). Second, strong sense of meaning takes on added importance as people reach late life. Evidence of this may be found, for example, in Erikson's (1959) theory of human development. He divides the life span into eight stages, each of which poses a unique developmental challenge. The final stage, which arises in late life, is characterized by the crisis of integrity versus despair. This is a time of deep introspection where an individual attempts to reconcile the inevitable gap between what they set out to do in life and what they were actually able to accomplish. If this crisis is resolved successfully, the individual is thought to derive a deep sense of meaning in life. But if it is not resolved successfully, they are likely to slip into despair. Empirical support for the notion that a sense of meaning becomes increasingly important as people grow older is provided by Steger, Oishi, and Kashdan (2009).

Taken as a whole, the insights that in this section form the foundation for a potentially useful conceptual model in which religious involvement promotes forgiveness, forgiveness bolsters and maintains the quality of interpersonal relationships, close interpersonal ties foster a deeper sense of meaning in life, and a stronger sense of meaning enhances health and well-being.

Factors that Disrupt the Process of Forgiveness

Although a number of psychosocial factors may facilitate the process of forgiveness, other factors may make it either more difficult to forgive or they may impede progress toward a full and complete reconciliation. It is important to consider this issue because doing so provides a more balanced view of the literature. Three potentially detrimental factors are discussed below.

Barriers to Forgiving Others – Religious

The first detrimental factor has to do with forgiving others out of fear of retribution by God. A close variant of this issue is found with people who believe that God will not forgive them unless they first forgive others (Exline, 2008; Krause & Ingersoll-Dayton, 2001). These two closely-related themes share a common conceptual base: people may forgive others out of a sense of duty. There is some evidence that forgiving others out of a sense of duty may not convey the health-related benefits that are typically associated with this virtue. Evidence of this may be found, for example, in the work of Vaillant (2008). He reports that, "Forgiveness imposed by religious duty increases blood pressure; forgiveness mediated by empathy and love does not" (Vaillant, 2008, p. 138; see also Huang & Enright, 2000). There are two possible explanations for this finding. First, individuals who only forgive out of a sense of duty may say they forgive a transgressor but fail to do so in a sincere or heart-felt way. Consequently, they may never let go of the underlying hurt completely. Second, if a person believes that God requires them to forgive others they may overlook elements that are intrinsic to the transgression, such as whether a transgressor deserves to be forgiven. And failure to take this issue into account may invite repeated hurtful acts in the future.

Barriers to Forgiving Others – Personality Traits

The second factor that may inhibit forgiveness in late life may be found by turning to the literature on change and stability in personality traits as a point of departure. Writing over a century ago, Williams James observed that, "… in most of us, by the age of 30, the character has set like plaster, and will never soften again" (1892/1961, p. 11). A remarkably similar conclusion is reached by McCrae and Costa (2003) in their exhaustive review of research on personality change over the life course. These investigators wrap up their review by stating that, " … the take-home message is that, after age 30, the mean levels of personality traits change little" (McCrae & Costa, 2003, p. 81). These insights are important because a number of studies indicate that willingness and ability to forgive are influenced significantly by personality traits. Evidence of this may be found, for example, a recent meta-analysis of the literature by Riek and Mania (2012). These investigators conclude that greater agreeableness is associated with a greater willingness to forgive whereas greater neuroticism is associated with diminished willingness to forgive. So if personality traits change little after age thirty and if some personality traits inhibit the process of forgiveness, then it follows that encouraging some older individuals to become more forgiving may be a difficult task. But as the discussion in the next section will show, this is only one of several factors that may complicate the process of forgiveness in late life.

Barriers to Feeling Forgiven by Others

Recall that Erikson's life review suggests that when people reach old age, they look back over the course of their lives and try to reconcile what has happened in the past. This suggests that they may revisit decades old transgressions and feel a growing sense of urgency to lay them to rest. Butler's (1995) discussion of the life review speaks directly to this issue.

Unfortunately, it may be more difficult to initiate and successfully complete the process of forgiveness when a victim died years ago. Victims cannot confront them with what they have done and if acts of contrition are in order, they are obviously in no position to engage in them.

Researchers also need to see if the same similar challenges arise when older people try to forgive themselves for transgressions that are long past. Once again, it seems that often little, if anything, can be done about the hurtful act. Nelissen and Zeelenberg (2009) provide some insight into this issue in their study of guilt. They begin by noting that guilt motivates compensatory pro-social behavior to repair social bonds. But they go on to argue that when opportunities for compensation are not present, guilt may lead to self-punishment including self-denied pleasure and other self-enforced penalties. Cast within the context of the current discussion, this study suggests that unlike younger people, older adults may have fewer opportunities to engage in acts of contrition. And when this happens, the guilt they feel for the transgressions they have committed may lead to self-punishment, which may have undesirable consequences.

But the situation may not necessarily be this bleak. Earlier, we noted that one of the primary goals of religion is forgiveness. While this often involves forgiving others, it also pertains to forgiving oneself. Perhaps the role that religion plays in self-forgiveness is especially beneficial when little can be done to correct the transgression. This may be accomplished by specific religious rituals that provide the opportunity for atonement. For example, the Catholic Church institutes the practice of confession and provides a formal day of atonement. A day of atonement is also found in the Jewish faith tradition, as well. Studies are needed to provide greater insight into how the potentially beneficial effects of these religious rituals operate.

Conclusions

One advantage of studying forgiveness arises from the fact that this research has direct applications in clinical practice. Evidence of this may be found, for example, in the work of Allemand, Steiner, and Hill (2012). However, the majority of this work has involved younger people. Although significant headway has been made in the clinical work with older adults (e.g., Hargrave & Anderson, 1992), there are two straightforward reasons why more interventions are needed with individuals who are at this point in the life course. First, the incidence of physical health problems escalates rapidly as people enter and move through late life (Federal Interagency Forum on Aging Related Statistics, 2012). Second, although the incidence of clinical mental disorders may decline with age, there is considerable evidence that there is a sharp upturn in depressive symptoms around age 60 or so (see Krause, 1999, for a review of this research). So if forgiveness promotes better physical and mental health, and if physical health problems and certain mental health problems increase markedly with age, then placing a greater emphasis on interventions with a focus on forgiveness holds out the promise of reducing health care costs.

Although a good deal of the research that has been done so far is preliminary, five themes that have emerged from our discussion may help shape intervention efforts. First, clinicians should be more mindful of the diversity that exists within our aging population. This is especially true with respect to cohort differences within late life. Second, fostering unconditional forgiveness rather than focusing on acts of contrition may provide a useful point of departure for promoting forgiveness of others, but not the perception of being forgiven by God. Third, encouraging meaning-making through the process of reminiscence is a strategy that is worthy of further consideration. Fourth, a good deal of patience may be required when efforts are made to encourage initiating forgiveness because significant push-back may be encountered among some older people with certain deeply ingrained personality traits. Fifth, for older people who are so inclined, encouragement to engage in religious rituals may also prove to be beneficial.

Although it is sometimes challenging to work with older people, it is helpful to keep Nuland's (2007) observations in mind. In the process of discussing successful aging, he offers the following encouragement: "The repair of severed relationships has no 'use by" date. It is never too late to reach out and forgive others, and to forgive ourselves" (Nuland, 2007, p. 177).

References

Allemand, M. (2008). Age differences in forgiveness: The role of future time perspective. *Journal of Research on Personality, 42*, 1137–1147.

Allemand, M., Steiner, M., & Hill, P. L. (2012). Effects of a forgiveness intervention for older adults. *Journal of Counseling Psychology, 60*, 279–286.

Berger, P. L., & Pullberg, S. (1965). Reification and sociological critique of consciousness. *History and Theory, 4*, 196–211.

Butler, R. N. (1995). Forward: The life review. In B. K. Haight & J. D. Webster (Eds.), *The art and science of reminiscing: Theory, research, methods, and applications* (pp. xvii–xxi). Washington, DC: Taylor & Francis.

Butler, R. N. (1963). The life review: An interpretation of reminiscence in the aged. *Psychiatry, 26*, 65–76.

Carstensen, L. L. (1992). Social and emotional patterns in adulthood: Support for socioemotional selectivity theory. *Psychology and Aging, 7*, 331–338.

Cooper, T. D. (2003). *Sin, pride, & self-acceptance*. Downers Grove, IL: Intervarsity Press.

Elder, G. H. (1999). *Children of the great depression: Social change and life experience*. Bouolder, CO: Westview.

Erikson, E. (1959). *Identity and the life cycle*. New York, NY: International University Press.

Exline, J. J. (2008). Beliefs about God and forgiveness in a Baptist church sample. *Journal of Psychology and Christianity, 27*, 131–139.

Federal Interagency Forum on Age Related Statistics. (2012). *Older Americans 2012: Key indicators of well-being*. Washington, DC: U. S. Government Printing Office.

Fehr, R., Gelfand, M. J., & Nag, M. (2010). The road to forgiveness: A meta-analytic synthesis of its situational and dispositional correlates. *Psychological Bulletin, 136*, 894–914.

Girard, M., & Muller, E. (1997). Forgiveness in adolescents, young, middle-aged, and older adults. *Journal of Adult Development, 4*, 209–220.

Haight, B. K., & Webster, J. D. (1995). *The art and science of reminiscing: Theory, methods, and applications*. New York, NY: Taylor & Francis.

Hall, J. H., & Fincham, F. D. (2008). The temporal course of self-forgiveness. *Journal of Social and Clinical Psychology, 27*, 174–202.

Hargrave, T. D., & Anderson, W. T. (1992). *Finishing well: Aging and reparation in the intergenerational family*. New York, NY: Brunner/Mazel.

Hayward, R. D., & Krause, N. (2013). Trajectories of change in dimensions of forgiveness among older adults and their association with religious commitment. *Mental Health, Religion & Culture, 16*, 643–659.

Hood, R. W., Hill, P. C., & Spilka, B. (2003). *The psychology of religion: An empirical approach* (4th ed.). New York, NY: Guilford Press.

Huang, S. T., & Enright, R. D. (2000). Forgiveness and anger-related emotions in Taiwan: Implications for therapy. *Psychotherapy: Theory, Research, Practice, Training, 37*, 71–79.

Jackson, J. S., & Antonucci, T. C. (1992). Social support processes in health and effective functioning for the elderly. In M. L. Wykle, E. Kahana, & J. Kowal (Eds.), *Stress and health among the elderly* (pp. 72–95). New York, NY: Springer.

James, W. (1892/1961). *Psychology: The briefer course.* New York, NY: Harper & Row.

Karremans, J. C., & Van Lange, P. A. (2004). Back to caring after being hurt: The role of forgiveness. *European Journal of Social Psychology, 34*, 207–227.

Krause, N. (1999). Mental disorder in late life: Exploring the influence of stress and socioeconomic status. In C. S. Aneshensel & J. C. Phelan (Eds.), *Handbook of the sociology of mental health* (pp. 183–208). New York, NY: Plenum.

Krause, N. (2002). Exploring race differences in a comprehensive battery of church-based social support measures. *Review of Religious Research, 44*, 126–149.

Krause, N. (2004). Stressors in highly valued roles, meaning in life, and the physical health status of older adults. *Journal of Gerontology: Social Sciences, 59B*, S287–S297.

Krause, N. (2007). A longitudinal study of social support and meaning in life. *Psychology and Aging, 22*, 456–469.

Krause, N. (2008a). *Aging in the church: How social relationships affect health.* West Conshohocken, PA: Templeton Foundation Press.

Krause, N. (2008b). The social foundations of religious meaning in life. *Research on Aging, 30*, 395–427.

Krause, N. (2009). Meaning in life and mortality. *Journal of Gerontology: Social Sciences, 64B*, 517–527.

Krause, N., & Ellison, C. G. (2003). Forgiveness by God, forgiveness of others, and psychological well-being in late life. *Journal for the Scientific Study of Religion, 42*, 77–93.

Krause, N., & Ingersoll-Dayton, B. (2001). Religion and the process of forgiveness in late life. *Review of Religious Research, 42*, 252–276.

Krause, N., & Hayward, R. D. (2015). Acts of contrition, forgiveness by God, and death anxiety among older Mexican Americans. Under review at the *International Journal for the Psychology of Religion, 25*, 57–73.

Lang, B. (1994). Forgiveness. *American Philosophical Quarterly, 31*, 105–117.

Levenson, M. R. (1996). Three models of adult development. *Human Development, 39*, 135–149.

Lundberg, C. D. (2010). *Unifying truths of the world's religions.* New Fairfield, CT: Heavenlight Press.

McCrae, R. R., & Costa, P. T. (2003). *Personality in adulthood: A five-factor theory perspective.* New York, NY: Guilford Press.

McFarland, M. J., Smith, C. A., Toussaint, L. L., & Thomas, P. A. (2012). Forgiveness of others and health: Do race and neighborhood matter? *Journal of Gerontology: Social Science, 67B*, 66–75.

Nelissen, R. M., & Zeelenberg, M. (2009). When guilt evokes self-punishment: Evidence of a Dobby effect. *Emotion, 9*, 118–122.

Nuland, S. B. (2007). *The art of aging.* New York, NY: Random House.

Riek, B. M., & Mania, E. W. (2012). The antecedents and consequences of interpersonal forgiveness: A meta-analytic review. *Personal Relationships, 19*, 304–325.

Rowe, J. W., & Kahn, R. L. (1998). *Successful aging.* New York, NY: Pantheon.

Scobie, E. D., & Scobie, G. E. (1998). Damaging events: The perceived need for forgiveness. *Journal for the Theory of Social Behavior, 28*, 373–401.

Steger, M. F., Oishi, S., & Kashdan, T. B. (2009). Meaning in life across the life span: Levels and correlates of meaning in life from emerging adulthood to older adulthood. *The Journal of Positive Psychology, 4*, 43–52.

Steiner, M., Allemand, M., & McCullough, M. E. (2012). Do agreeableness and neuroticism explain age differences in the tendency to forgive others? *Personality and Social Psychology Bulletin, 38*, 441–453.

Stone, J., & Cooper, J. (2001). A self-standards model of cognitive dissonance. *Journal of Experimental Social Psychology, 37*, 228–243.

Tornstam, L. (2005). *Gerotranscendence: A developmental theory of positive aging*. New York, NY: Springer.
Toussaint, L. L., Owen, A. D., & Cheadle, A. (2012). Forgive to live: Forgiveness, health, and longevity. *Journal of Behavioral Medicine, 35*, 375–386.
Toussaint, L. L., Williams, D. R., Musick, M. A., & Everson, S. A. (2001). Forgiveness and health: Age differences in a U.S. probability sample. *Journal of Adult Development, 8*, 249–257.
Vaillant, G. E. (2002). *Aging well*. Boston, MA: Little, Brown, and Company.
Vaillant, G. E. (2008). *Spiritual evolution: A scientific defense of faith*. New York, NY: Broadway Books.
Wong, T. P. (2012). *The human quest for meaning: Theories, research, and applications*. New York, NY: Routledge.
Worthington, E. L., Jr., & Scherer, M. (2004). Forgiveness in an emotion-focused coping strategy can reduce health risks and promote resilience: Theory, review, and hypotheses. *Psychology & Health, 19*, 385–405.

Chapter 15
Culture, Forgiveness, and Health

Mark M. Leach and Stephanie Parazak

Our current understanding of forgiveness has been largely decontextualized, meaning that it has been considered within a culture-free context for much of its short life. This is unfortunate given the undeniable role that culture plays in almost every aspect of human behavior and dynamics. The examination of culture can be considered from multiple perspectives, both national and international, the latter of which is the focus of this chapter. Despite the proliferation of forgiveness research over the past two decades, comparatively little is understood about forgiveness from non-US-based perspectives.

There are at least two means of considering the international forgiveness literature. First, there is research conducted solely in countries outside of the US, and this type comprises the majority of the literature. Several articles and chapters have been written about various forms of forgiveness in a few countries, primarily European and Asian countries. Second, we can consider the cross-cultural forgiveness literature, comparing forgiveness constructs in two or more countries. There are few multinational studies, including those comparing forgiveness in the US with other countries. For ease of reading, the term "international" will be used to include both types of research, unless specified. When discussing international research, the overlap between the country under investigation and the myriad of cultures within the country is concerning. Culture can be considered from multiple frames, (Carter & Qureshi, 1995) but for the sake of this chapter we will equate country with culture, noting strongly that the authors understand the perils of equating the two.

M.M. Leach (✉)
University of Louisville, Louisville, KY, USA
e-mail: m.leach@louisville.edu

S. Parazak
University of Cincinnati, Cincinnati, OH, USA
e-mail: stephanie.parazak@gmail.com

L.L. Toussaint et al. (eds.), *Forgiveness and Health*,
DOI 10.1007/978-94-017-9993-5_15

The Necessity of Including Culture into Forgiveness Work

Forgiveness as a process is contextually-based, though it is often discussed from a decontextualized perspective. While some components of forgiveness show consistency when compared from an international perspective, further research is necessary to discern their universality. For example, McCullough and Witvliet (2002) found apology and intentionality as consistent predictors of forgiveness across cultures. Related, Takaku, Weiner, and Ohnuchi (2001) compared Japanese and US university students on apology acceptance and found similarities in both countries. Namely, when people increased their perspective-taking by considering their own past misdeeds, it increased the likelihood that they would forgive another person. Despite some consistencies, some differences have also been established across various countries. For example, the two Big Five personality traits, Neuroticism and Agreeableness, are often considered predictors of forgiveness in Western cultures (e.g., McCullough, Bellah, Kilpatrick, & Johnson, 2001), but these may not be valid in non-Western cultures. Fu, Watkins, and Hui (2004) found that personality constructs related to forgiveness, such as self-esteem and anxiety, often found in individualistic societies were not significantly related to forgiveness in China, whereas other factors like harmony and relationship orientation were considered more influential.

Since Sandage and Williamson's (2005) well-constructed introduction to the field, there has been a significant increase in the international forgiveness literature. In order to make the chapter manageable, it is delineated into sections consistent with the type of forgiveness often found in the international literature, namely lay conceptualizations of forgiveness, dispositional forgivingness, interpersonal forgiveness, and group forgiveness. International literature on self-forgiveness and other types of forgiveness could not be found. In order to offer theoretical context to this chapter we will begin with an overview of national values, followed by research in the four forgiveness areas.

National Values Overview

National values reflect what a country typically considers noble and attractive (Schwartz, 1997) and are reflected in shared norms, practices, and rituals (Sagiv & Schwartz, 2007). By extension, theories developed from studies of national values have been used to predict international experiences and behaviors at the individual, group, and organizational levels (see Hofstede, 2001). The role of national values holds particular promise for international forgiveness research. Though beyond the scope of this chapter much work has been accomplished examining national cultural values such as (a) Individualism-Collectivism (a worldview addressing the relationship between the individual and the group or society), (b) Power Distance (relationships to authority and legitimate power), (c) Uncertainty avoidance, the degree to a society tolerates risk and feels uncomfortable or comfortable with ambiguity and uncertainty), (d) Masculinity/Femininity (related to traits such as determination, relationships, and flexibility), (e) Long-term versus Short-Term Orientation, (whether individuals are primarily focused on the past, present, or future), and (f) Indulgence versus restraint, (the degree to which people are allowed self-expression, life control, and pursuit of leisure). The relationship of national values to forgiveness has only recently received acknowledgement, though readers are encouraged to delve into the national values literature to better appreciate the foundations from which they are conceptualized and understood.

National Values and Forgiveness

The most frequent cultural value included in the international forgiveness literature is individualism-collectivism. While easy to conceptualize, forgiveness is actually a complex cultural dynamic. Countries and cultures stressing collectivistic worldviews conceptualize identity in a relational and interdependent manner. Accordingly, forgiveness is viewed as a social obligation in order to maintain social harmony, and is closely tied to, although conceptually distinct from, reconciliation. Reconciliation is tied to behaviors often associated with forgiveness, but the two can be distinct. Fundamental questions include how culture influences the two and what cultural components may influence the alignment of the two more closely than other cultures? Other community members may be involved with the process since personal boundaries are more fluid; thus in collectivistic cultures (e.g., Hmong; Sandage, Hill, & Vang, 2003), community rituals may be part of the forgiveness process.

Cross-cultural studies on forgiveness are relatively scarce and increasingly complex as we consider types of intrapersonal forgiveness (decisional vs. emotional), types of general forgiveness (e.g., group forgiveness), and cultural values (e.g., individualism and collectivism). The following sections will present a review of the current English language international forgiveness literature. National values, largely individualism-colllectivism, will be contextualized within conceptualizations of forgiveness, forgivingness, interpersonal forgiveness, and intergroup forgiveness.

Conceptualizations of Forgiveness

Conceptualizations of forgiveness refer to how forgiveness is defined and the processes involved, and a literature has developed assessing lay conceptualizations of forgiveness. There is inconsistency between lay individuals and professionals regarding conceptualizations of forgiveness, and these are influenced by culture. Among professionals in individualistic cultures forgiveness and reconciliation are generally considered distinct categories with different processes. However, Friesen and Fletcher (2007) found that almost 70 % of US college students believed that reconciliation was a necessary component of forgiveness. It is likely that there are a range of processes that influence forgiveness in different cultures, so it is important to also gain an understanding of lay conceptualizations of forgiveness. However, while important to understand how lay individuals understand forgiveness it should not dramatically influence the scientific definition or process of forgiveness, as misconceptions abound about psychological processes.

International studies on lay conceptualizations of forgiveness are scarce, but the current evidence points to some key inconsistencies in the way people of different national origin and culture consider it. To illustrate, there is growing evidence that collectivistic cultures view forgiveness interpersonally, linking it with group harmony and reconciliation (e.g., Hook, Worthington, Utsey, Davis, & Burnett, 2012). Kadiangandu, Gauché, Vinsommeau, and Mullet (2007) compared French and Congolese samples, the latter considered collectivistic. The authors tested the hypothesis that individualistic and collectivistic cultures would differ in forgiveness conceptualizations because collective cultures would consider forgiveness as an interpersonal construct instead of an individualistic, intrapersonal construct. Differences occurred between the countries, including the Congolese view that forgiveness could be extended beyond the dyadic relationship to include unknown individuals, groups, and the deceased. The Congolese were also more positive about forgiveness and more willing to forgive in general than the French, leading the researchers to conclude that forgiveness may be more characteristic of collectivistic than individualistic cultures. They concluded that forgiveness opportunities may be more abundant in collectivistic cultures due to closer and broader relationships found in collectivistic cultures.

Similar results were found in a comparison of Latin American and French participants, (Bagnulo, Muňoz-Sastre, & Mullet, 2009). Finally, using a sample of US individualist and collectivist participants, Hook et al. (2012) demonstrated that an interpersonal perspective of forgiveness can reap benefits, especially if one continues the relationship with the transgressor. In sum, there is a small but growing literature examining the effects of beliefs about forgiveness on relationship and societal enhancement, as well as cross-cultural processes that offer multiple worldview perspectives on forgiveness. Overall, initial evidence indicates that conceptualizations of forgiveness are not consistent internationally and culture strongly influences views of the relationship between forgiveness and reconciliation.

Forgivingness

Forgivingness (or willingness to forgive, or dispositional forgiveness), has been a topic of investigation for approximately a decade, and must be differentiated from forgiveness. Forgivingness is an overall disposition to forgive and can be manifested across different domains and life events (Suwartono, Prawasti, & Mullet,

2007) whereas forgiveness applies to specific circumstances, such as a specific transgression. A variety of US studies have investigated personality traits thought to be associated with forgivingness such as the Big Five personality factors of Neuroticism, Extraversion, and Agreeableness (e.g., Brose, Rye, Lutz-Zois, & Ross, 2005). Other personality variables such as anger, cynicism, and guilt have also been shown to be related to forgivingness (Walker & Gorsuch, 2002).

Few international or cross-cultural studies have been conducted examining forgivingness. In a recent study Idemudia and Mahri (2011) attempted to determine the role of gender, religion, age, and the three-factor personality model on willingness to forgive in a South African sample. Only Extraversion and an education variable were related. Thus, Extraversion appears to have some cross-cultural consistency. Fu, Watkins, and Hui (2004) conducted a personality-based study in China, using four emic group solidarity-based subscales (reflective of Chinese culture) of the Chinese Personality Assessment Inventory (CPAI-2), along with Western concepts of personality. As expected, individual personality constructs such as anxiety and self-esteem were not related to forgivingness whereas relationship orientation, personal harmony, and saving face were significantly correlated (see also Hui & Bond, 2009). In essence, a collectivistic worldview which includes social harmony and group solidarity influenced the way the Chinese view forgiveness more strongly than Western conceptions.

Finally, a dispositional forgiveness study comparing French, individualistic students and Indonesian, collectivistic students confirmed that Indonesian students were more sensitive to social circumstances, report lower resentment scores, and were more willing to forgive in order to maintain social harmony (Suwartono, Prawasti, & Mullet, 2007). Interestingly, the primary difference between the two countries was that Indonesian students showed lower levels of long-term resentment than the French students, perhaps reflecting the idea that individuals in collectivistic cultures may have to give up resentment faster to speed the process of reconciliation when compared with individualistic countries. Related, Kadiangandu, Mullet, and Vinsonneau (2001) found that Congolese participants were less willing to seek revenge than French participants, though in other studies dispositional forgiveness and lasting resentment did not differ among Chinese and French participants (Paz, Neto, & Mullet, 2008).

The role of religion a related to willingness to forgive has received limited but growing international interest, though it should be noted that these studies have not teased out the intersection of religion and other cultural variables. In South Africa, Idemudia and Mahri (2011) examined religious affiliation of Christians versus Muslims as predictors of willingness to forgive. Religious affiliation, defined dichotomously (Christian or Muslim) was not a significant predictor of willingness to forgive in their sample. While research in American samples generally indicated that religiousness, religious involvement, and religious belief predict broad forgivingness (e.g., McCullough & Worthington, 1999), this study painted a different picture. One way of interpreting these contradictions could be the distinction between religious affiliation and religiousness, religious involvement, and/or religious belief; the study in South Africa compared dichotomous groups based on religious affiliation, whereas American studies have examined religion in a more fluid, continuous variable. Comparatively, the same study that examined the similar Buddhist and Christian conceptualizations of forgiveness in China (Paz, Neto, & Mullet, 2007) found a difference in willingness to forgive between Buddhist and Christian participants, with Buddhist participants significantly less forgiving and more resentful than Christian participants, in addition to other differences found. Finally, Hui, Watkins, Wong, & Sun (2006) compared forgivingness of Christian and non-religious individuals in China, finding that Christians were significantly more willing to forgive than non-Christians.

Each of these studies speaks to the limits of not directly assessing individualism-collectivism, not including other values that may offer a finer understanding of forgivingness, and not including religion as important components of forgivingness. Not directly assessing these within a country offers broad strokes and does not assess the nuances of the constructs.

Interpersonal Forgiveness

Empirical study of interpersonal forgiveness has undergone a substantial increase over the past two decades in the US. Internationally, comparatively little empirical research has been conducted examining forgiveness between individuals in close personal relationships. In perhaps the largest study of this type, Karremans et al. (2011) surveyed participants from three individualist, two collectivist, and one mixed (individualist and collectivist) country to determine the association between relationship closeness (previously found to facilitate forgiveness, see Finkel, Rusbult, Kumashiro, & Hannon, 2002) and interpersonal forgiveness, as well as assessing for trait forgiveness. Karremans et al. (2011) indicated that relationship closeness was related to interpersonal forgiveness across all countries, consistent with an evolutionary functional analysis perspective which states that forgiveness evolved in humans to maintain survival and our reproductive benefits (McCullough, 2008). In the collective countries, the relationship between closeness and forgiveness was weaker than individualist countries, perhaps giving credence to the idea that collective cultures are less likely to distinguish between close and non-close relationships and are more likely to forgive due to cultural norms of maintaining harmony.

Decisional and emotional forgiveness and its relationship to collectivism received support in a Nepalese sample. Watkins et al. (2011) found that collectivism was associated with decisional rather than emotional forgiveness, conciliatory behaviors, and avoidance of revenge motivations. Interestingly, collective individuals have also been shown to display more negative affect (e.g., Huang & Enright, 2000). Chi, Du, and Lam (2011) evaluated decisional and emotional forgiveness for Hong Kong individuals whose partners had extramarital affairs, finding that those with high decisional forgiveness and low emotional forgiveness reported higher life satisfaction, and those high on both types reported less rumination. Because only these two studies have delineated decisional from emotional forgiveness, there appears to be promise for future researchers.

Interpersonal forgiveness has been examined in connection with religiousness in some international literature. Jose and Alfons (2007) examined the role of religiousness in forgiveness in a sample of Belgian adults. Religiousness significantly predicted broadly defined interpersonal forgiveness; interestingly, age, years in marriage, number of children, and being female were also positively correlated with religiousness, highlighting the intersectionality of multiple aspects of culture and demographics in forgiveness. These findings were consistent with an earlier forgiveness study conducted in a Western European sample of predominantly Catholic participants (Mullet, Barros, Frongia, Usai, & Shafighi, 2003). Together, these findings not only lend evidence to a connection between forgivingness and religiousness across cultures, but also highlight the effects of intersecting aspects of culture in understanding forgiveness across various demographics.

Intergroup Forgiveness

Intergroup conflict has been the topic of social psychological research for decades and there is a large literature examining related constructs such as intergroup hostility, prejudice, and ingroup-outgroup bias (e.g., Noor, Brown, Gonzalez, Manzi, & Lewis, 2008). These studies typically examine negative psychological processes, but there has been increased interest examining the processes that lead from negative to positive outcomes, and forgiveness research has become more prominent at the group level within the context of intergroup conflict, intergroup relations, and reconciliation (Myers, Hewstone, & Cairns, 2009). Much of this work has been accomplished in high conflict areas such as Northern Ireland, Rwanda, Chile, Bosnia and Herzegovenia, and Congo, as well as literature on specific issues such as group apologies and truth commissions (see a forthcoming meta-analysis by Van Tongeren, Burnette, O' Boyle, Worthington, & Forsyth, 2014),

Two fundamental questions are whether one group can forgive another group, and whether one individual can forgive a group. Thoughtful consideration of these questions leads to other questions such as to whom should forgiveness be directed? Is intergroup forgiveness reasonable when another group has or has not asked for forgiveness? Who speaks for the group? (Neto, da Conceição Pinto, & Mullet, 2004). Forgiveness has been traditionally considered to occur between two people directly connected with a transgression. Only recently has intergroup forgiveness been considered a reasonable area of study. Recent research indicates that when considering ethnopolitical conflicts it may be better served to consider forgiveness and reconciliation as closely related (Cairns & Hewstone, 2011).

Intergroup forgiveness differs qualitatively from interpersonal forgiveness in that the former must include a reduction in negative feelings toward a group rather than an individual, even though each member of the group has not harmed the individual (Myers et al., 2009). Early studies of forgiveness in sociopolitical contexts failed to consider that offenses are committed against groups and not individuals. Genocides in Rwanda and Bosnia-Herzegovenia, for example, were not directed against specific individuals but against ethnic groups, though individuals were certainly perpetrators and victims of acts of violence. Thus, transgressions are collective and forgiveness is collective (for more information interested readers may want to consult Digeser, 2001) in addition to individuals' experiences. A number of national governments have apologized for previous atrocities to a subsection of their populations, such as those in Australia and South Africa, provoking questions of whether these apologies result in group attitudinal and behavioral differences.

A few studies from different geographic regions (e.g., Congo, Timor) have assessed whether individuals believe group forgiveness is possible, and the majority of individuals believe it is possible and societally beneficial (e.g., Kadiangandu & Mullet, 2007; Neto, da Conceição Pinto, & Mullet, 2004). The process of doing so, however, remains quite complex, as illustrated by the difficulties experienced by the Truth and Reconciliation Commission in South Africa in practically promoting group forgiveness.

Truth and Reconciliation commissions (TRC) have occurred in North, Central, and South America, Africa, Asia, Oceania, and Europe (often with different aims such as reconciliation or retributive or restorative justice), but the South Africa (SA) TRC has had perhaps the greatest amount of research associated with it. Chapman (2007) analyzed SA TRC transcripts and found that members of the TRC had difficulty conceptualizing intergroup forgiveness and reconciliation, and instead moved toward individual victim and transgressor relationships. Victims (and their families) were not proactive or receptive to forgiving their perpetrator, and the perpetrators were often reluctant to apologize or express regret. This is consistent with other literature finding that 80 % of sampled human rights victims in SA reported not forgiving their perpetrator, though over half said that they had begun the forgiving process (Allan, Allan, Kaminer, & Stein, 2006). Kaminer, Stein, Mbanga, and Zungu-Dirwayi (2001) found that participants in the SA TRC showed no significant difference in depression, PTSD, and anxiety rates among individuals who gave public, private, or no testimony. In other geographic regions Touze, Silove and Zwi (2005) found that while there were benefits for the majority of TRC participants in East Timor, a minority continued to experience significant distress related to anger, largely due to perceived immunity given to many perpetrators who fled to neighboring countries. In Sierre Leone forgiveness differences were noted based on age, gender, and trauma exposure (Doran, Kalayjian, Toussaint, & DeMucci, 2012).

Schaal, Weierstall, Dusingizemungu, and Elbert (2012) assessed both imprisoned perpetrators and community survivors of the Rwandan genocide. Survivors found positive reconciliation attitudes to act as a protective factor against further psychological issues whereas it was a risk factor for psychological issues for non-killing perpetrators (see also Cardozo, Kaiser, Gotway, & Agani, 1995). It should be noted that due to the exceptionally high number of deaths in Rwanda the TRC process comprised largely of village-based gacaca trials in which coercion and reprisals were common.

Perhaps the region with the largest amount of empirical research on intergroup forgiveness is Northern Ireland. Research has consistently shown higher rates of mental health problems in Northern Ireland than those in surrounding areas (e.g., Myers et al., 2009). Huyse (2005) argued that at the group level active reconciliation is necessary to alleviate mental health concerns rather than just the cessation of violence, and forgiveness is an essential component of reconciliation (Myers et al., 2009).

In one of the earlier studies, McLernon, Cairns, Hewstone, and Smith (2004) found that secondary school Catholic females in Ireland were reluctant to forgive for past perceived hurts. Their finding is consistent with other literature stating that younger individuals are less likely to forgive another group than older individuals, and that engagement in intergroup forgiveness may be more difficult than in interpersonal forgiveness.

Other studies assessing forgiveness in this region have tested the contact hypothesis, with mixed results. Contact was positively associated with interdenominational mixing, outgroup attitudes, empathic perspective-taking, and trust (Hewstone, Cairns, Voci, Hamberger, & Niens, 2006). However, other results indicated that contact was influential (i.e. reduced hostility) for individuals who did not identify strongly with their religious/cultural group, but increased hostility for those highly committed to their group (Cairns, Tam, Hewstone, & Niens, 2005). Moeschberger, Dixon, Niens, and Cairns (2005) found that intergroup forgiveness may be influenced by factors consistent with those involved with interpersonal forgiveness, namely empathy, other-community contact, rumination, and indirectly via religiousness and trait hope.

In one of the few studies specifically investigating intergroup forgiveness as it relates to mental health, Myers et al. (2009) found that collective guilt (which can motivate relationship repair and group-level forgiveness) mediated the relationship between ethnopolitical conflict and mental health at the group level. Their findings highlight the uniqueness of these group variables from interpersonal forgiveness and guilt. Readers interested in the inclusion of guilt in intergroup research can also consult other authors regarding Northern Ireland (e.g., Huyse, 2005) and Chile (Manzi & González, 2007). In sum, research on individual healing through forgiveness after national traumas is becoming more prominent in the forgiveness literature, and researchers would do well to include culturally-relevant variables that may help explain some unexpected results. Overall, truth commissions cannot substitute for therapeutic interventions for human rights abuse survivors, and forgiveness may be a predictor of reduced psychiatric risk.

Foundations for Future Research

As is evident when reviewing the present literature, much of the research on international forgiveness has relied on or implied Hofstede's individualism-collectivism dimensional construct, as it has become a foundation from which to compare various constructs in different countries. However, its current use in the forgiveness literature gives rise to some important concerns. First, individualism-collectivism is not assessed directly or is misapplied as a binary, global concept; countries are described as individualistic or collectivistic though in actuality this is a rather arbitrary distinction, as countries lie on a cultural continuum. Perhaps more importantly, future research could focus on the level of an individual's idiocentrism-allocentrism, the degree to which a specific individual holds "individualistic-collectivistic" attitudes (Triandis, 1996). Moving beyond the larger distinction of individualism-collectivism on the national level toward assessing individual differences in values within countries holds great promise for further research and a more nuanced understanding of how national values and individual differences intersect in their relationship with various dimensions of forgiveness.

Including other national value variables could result in richer, more meaningful research results. For example, Triandis (1996) spoke of tight versus loose cultures, which refers to the strength of social norms and the degree to which deviant behavior is accepted (Gelfand, Nishii, & Raver, 2006). It is part of a complex, multilevel system that comprises issues such as distal historical and ecological threats (e.g., territorial conflict, resource scarcity) and psychological issues (e.g., need for structure). Related, Schwartz (1994) developed a hierarchical versus egalitarian dimension, assessing the degree to which social systems ascribe to assigned roles or believe in equal worth and deservingness within its citizenry. These are two ripe examples of national value constructs that have promise to enrich our understanding of forgiveness internationally. By assessing forgiveness based on a multilevel systems approach our insights into forgiveness experiences can become much more refined.

In addition to the examination of national values in forgiveness literature, other theories could help lay the foundation for further expansion of the international forgiveness literature. Ho and Fung (2011) presented an informative article that includes a variety of theories that could be tested internationally, and add a forgiveness process model of their own based on emotion regulation theory. Emotion regulation theory states that individuals regulate their emotional responses following a transgression, and this emotion modulation can cause stress. This process is often highly related to cultural factors, as some cultures are more likely than others to express and suppress their emotions (e.g., Mesquita & Albert, 2007). Ho and Fung (2011) also discussed the role of dialectical thinking culturally as well as causal attribution theory, socially (dis)engaged emotions, and approach and avoidance motivations. This application of well-formed psychological theory to forgiveness processes would be an excellent springboard for expanding this research into the international realm.

Additionally, Noor, Brown, and prentice (2008a) examined intergroup forgiveness within the context of social identity theory (Tajfel & Turner, 1986), which states that an individual does not have one "self" but many selves, or social identities, and that these memberships provoke "ingroup" and "outgroup" thinking. Noor et al. (2008a) linked this concept to forgiveness processes by positing that differences in interpersonal and intergroup forgiveness are related to social identity such that the more one identifies with a group, the more the group influences the likelihood of forgiving a member(s) of an outgroup. Noor and colleagues included multiple models to consider in this light (e.g., Common Ingroup Identity Model (CIIM); Gaertner et al., 2000; trust models, and competitive victimhood, (Noor et al., 2008a, 2008b). Across multiple cultures and countries they found evidence of the importance of these variables when investigating intergroup forgiveness.

Beyond the models presented here, additional theoretical factors have been presented in the literature and warrant further investigation in future research. For example, intergenerational trauma and collective memories have been put forward as a means to understand the additive continuing hurt found in some cultures, such as that in Northern Ireland and South Africa where generations of hurt and trauma must be considered when assessing forgivingness (Cairns & Roe, 2003). Relatedly, psychological factors such as embitterment and collective guilt may contribute to personal and national healing. This provides yet another lens through which future research can examine forgiveness with a focus on important cultural and historical factors.

International Forgiveness and Health Research Possibilities

Little research has been accomplished integrating international forgiveness research with health. Countries vary in current and historical conflict, and this has undoubtedly taken its toll on health and well-being. As researchers consider multiple ways to better understand forgiveness internationally does the possibility of encouraging forgiveness offer especially important benefits for health for those countries that have turbulent pasts or even present conflictual circumstances. Some research suggests that positive affect and health benefits are strongest for the poorest countries (Pressman, Gallagher, & Lopez, 2013), and questions arise as to whether this might also apply to forgiveness. Other questions include, (1) What is the role of emotion regulation on forgiveness for countries previously engaged in decades long conflict, and how does it relate to health? (2) Are their greater health benefits in regions in which forgiveness and reconciliation closely tied rather than in regions in which they are less connected? (3) Are their greater health benefits for types of forgiveness (e.g., decisional versus emotional) depending on culture and national values? (4) Do qualitative differences exist among cultures with a long history of atrocities versus those more recent? Overall, our knowledge of the relationship of health and forgiveness is in need of significant research when considered internationally, and readers are in a unique opportunity to develop their own research agendas that can hold great promise.

Summary

The forgiveness literature has exploded in the United States, but is clearly still in its infancy from an international perspective. This chapter has offered a glimpse of the international literature stemming from four research angles: conceptualizations of forgiveness, forgivingness, interpersonal forgiveness, and intergroup forgiveness. Though this literature is growing, it is hindered by a lack of theoretical foundation. The authors recommend that national values be considered more specifically when considering cross-national, and even interpersonal, forgiveness. Other relevant theoretical foundations include emotional regulation, causal attribution, and ingroup identity theories, as well as psychological issues such as intergenerational trauma and collective guilt. Delineating decisional and emotional forgiveness in future research also holds great promise due to the theoretical association between the process of forgiveness and reconciliation. Forgiveness research on the international stage holds great promise and can benefit from an inter-professional perspective. Colleagues in sociology and political science, among others, can offer perspectives in order to gain a robust understanding of the antecedents and processes of forgiveness. Doing so will assist in concentrating important factors relevant to our understanding of forgiveness across culturally diverse individuals and groups.

References

Allan, A., Allan, M., Kaminer, D., & Stein, D. J. (2006). Exploration of the association between apology and forgiveness amongst victims of human rights violations. *Behavioral Sciences and the Law, 24*, 673–682.

Bagnulo, A., Muñoz-Sastre, M., & Mullet, E. (2009). Conceptualizations of forgiveness: A Latin America-Western Europe comparison. *Universitas Psychologica, 8*, 673–682.

Brewer, M. P. (1999). The psychology of prejudice: Ingroup love or outgroup hate? *Journal of Social Issues, 55*, 429–444.

Brose, L. A., Rye, M. S., Lutz-Zois, C., & Ross, S. R. (2005). Forgiveness and personality traits. *Personality and Individual Differences, 39*, 35–46.

Cairns, E., & Hewstone, M. (2011). Embitterment and forgiveness in the context of the conflict in Northern Ireland. In M. Linden & A. Maercker (Eds.), *Embitterment: Societal, psychological, and clinical perspectives* (pp. 220–229). New York, NY: Springer.

Cairns, E., & Roe, M. D. (Eds.). (2003). *The role of memory in ethnic conflict*. London: Palgrave/MacMillan.

Cairns, E., Tam, T., Hewstone, M., & Niens, U. (2005). Forgiveness in northern Ireland. In E. L. Worthington (Ed.), *Handbook of forgiveness* (pp. 461–476). New York, NY: Brunner/Routledge.

Cardozo, B. L., Kaiser, G., Gotway, C. A., & Agani, F. (1995). Mental health, social functioning, and feelings of hatred and revenge of Kosovar Albanians one year after the war in Kosovo. *Journal of Traumatic Stress, 16*, 351–360.

Carter, R. T., & Qureshi, A. (1995). A typology of philosophical assumptions in multicultural counseling and training. In J. G. Ponterotto, C. J. Manuel, L. A. Suzuki, & C. M. Alexander (Eds.), *Handbook of multicultural counseling* (pp. 239–262). Thousand Oaks, CA: Sage.

Chapman, A. R. (2007). Truth commissions and intergroup forgiveness: The case of the South African Truth and Reconciliation Commission. *Peace and Conflict: Journal of Peace Psychology, 13*, 51–69.

Chi, P., Du, H., & Lam, D. (2011). Mental health following partner's extramarital involvement: Role of decisional forgiveness and emotional forgiveness. *Chinese Journal of Clinical Psychology, 19*, 331–334.

Digeser, P. (2001). *Political forgiveness*. Ithaca, NY: Cornell University Press.

Doran, J. M., Kalayjian, A., Toussaint, L., & DeMucci, J. (2012). The relationship between trauma and forgiveness in post-conflict Sierra Leone. *Psychological Trauma: Theory, Research, Practice, and Policy, 4*, 614–623.

Emmons, R. A. (2000). Personality and forgiveness. In M. E. McCullough, K. I. Pargament, & C. E. Thoresen (Eds.), *Forgiveness: Theory, research, and practice* (pp. 156–175). New York, NY: Guilford Press.

Finkel, E. J., Rusbult, C. E., Kumashiro, M., & Hannon, P. A. (2002). Dealing with betrayal in close relationships: Does commitment promote forgiveness? *Journal of Personality and Social Psychology, 82*, 956–974.

Friesen, M. D., & Fletcher, G. J. O. (2007). Exploring the lay representation of forgiveness: Convergent and discriminant validity. *Personal Relationships, 14*, 209–223.

Fu, H., Watkins, D., & Hui, E. K. P. (2008). Forgiveness and personality in a Chinese cultural context. *IFE Psychologia: An International Journal, 16*, 1–15.

Fu, H., Watkins, D., & Hui, E. P. (2004). Personality correlates of the disposition towards interpersonal forgiveness: A Chinese perspective. *International Journal of Psychology, 39*, 305–316.

Gaertner, S. L., Dovido, J. F., Nier, J. A., Banker, B. S., Ward, C. M., Houletter, M., & Loux, S. (2000). The common ingroup identity model for reducing intergroup bias: Progress and challenges. In D. Capozza & R. Brown (Eds.), *Social identity processes: Trends in theory and research* (pp. 133–148). Thousand Oaks, CA: Sage.

Gelfand, M. J., Nishii, L. H., & Raver, J. L. (2006). On the nature and importance of cultural tightness-looseness. *Journal of Applied Psychology, 91*, 1225–1244.

Hewstone, M., Cairns, E., Voci, A., Hamberger, J., & Niens, U. (2006). Intergroup contact, forgiveness, and experience of 'The Troubles' in Northern Ireland. *Journal of Social Issues, 62*, 99–120.

Ho, M. Y., & Fung, H. H. (2011). A dynamic process model of forgiveness: A cross-cultural perspective. *Review of General Psychology, 15*, 77–84.

Hofstede, G., Hofstede, G. J., & Minkov, M. (2010). *Cultures and organizations: Software of the mind* (3rd ed.). New York, NY: McGraw-Hill.

Hofstede, G. (2001). *Culture's consequences: Comparing values, behaviors, institutions and organizations across nations*. Thousand Oaks, CA: Sage.

Hook, J. N., Worthington, E. L., Jr., Utsey, S. O., Davis, D. E., & Burnette, J. L. (2012). Collectivistic self-construal and forgiveness. *Counseling and Values, 57*, 109–124.

Hook, J. N., Worthington, E. L., Jr., & Utsey, S. O. (2009). Collectivism, forgiveness, and social harmony. *The Counseling Psychologist, 37*, 821–847.

Huang, S., & Enright, R. D. (2000). Forgiveness and anger-related emotions in Taiwan: Implications for therapy. *Psychotherapy: Theory, Research, Practice, Training, 37*, 71–79.

Hui, E. K. P., Watkins, D., Wong, T. N. Y., & Sun, R. C. F. (2006). Religion and forgiveness from a Hong Kong Chinese perspective. *Pastoral Psychology, 55*, 183–195.

Hui, V., & Bond, M. (2009). Target's face loss, motivations, and forgiveness following relational transgression: Comparing Chinese and US cultures. *Journal of Social and Personal Relationships, 26*, 123–140.

Huyse, L. (2005). Theory and practice. In G. Kelly & B. Hamber (Eds.), *Reconciliation: Rhetoric or relevant?* (pp. 1–59). Belfast, UK: Democratic Dialogue.

Idemudia, E. S., & Mahri, S. (2011). Can gender, religion, education, age and personality predict willingness to forgive? *Gender & Behaviour, 9*, 3765–3781.

Jose, O. A., & Alfons, V. (2007). Religiousness and forgiveness among first-married and remarried adults. *Mental Health, Religion, & Culture, 10*, 379–394.

Kadiangandu, J. K., Gauché, M., Vinsonneau, G., & Mullet, E. (2007). Conceptualizations of forgiveness: Collectivist-Congolese versus individualist-French viewpoints. *Journal of Cross-Cultural Psychology, 38*, 432–437.

Kadiangandu, J. K., & Mullet, E. (2007). Intergroup forgiveness: A Congolese perspective. *Peace and Conflict: Journal of Peace Psychology, 13*, 37–49.

Kadiangandu, J. K., Mullet, E., & Vinsonneau, G. (2001). Forgivingness: A Congo-France comparison. *Journal of Cross-Cultural Psychology, 32*, 504–511.

Kaminer, D., Stein, D. J., Mbanga, I., & Zungu-Dirwayi, N. (2001). The Truth and Reconciliation Commission in South Africa: Relation to psychiatric status and forgiveness among survivors of human rights abuses. *British Journal of Psychiatry, 178*, 373–377.

Karremans, J. C., Regalia, C., Paleari, F. G., Fincham, F. D., Cui, M., Takada, N., ..., & Uskul, A. K. (2011). Maintaining harmony across the globe: The cross-cultural association between closeness and interpersonal forgiveness. *Social Psychological and Personality Science, 2*, 443–451.

Manzi, J., & González, R. (2007). Forgiveness and reparation in Chile: The role of cognitive and emotional intergroup antecedents. *Peace and Conflict: Journal of Peace Psychology, 13*, 71–91.

McCullough, M. E. (2008). *Beyond revenge: The evolution of the forgiveness instinct*. San Francisco, CA: Jossey-Bass.

McCullough, M. E., Bellah, C. G., Kilpatrick, S. D., & Johnson, J. L. (2001). Vengefulness: Relationships with forgiveness, rumination, well-being, and the Big Five. *Personality and Social Psychology Bulletin, 27*, 601–610.

McCullough, M. E., & Witvliet, C. V. O. (2002). The psychology of forgiveness. In C. R. Snyder & S. J. Lopez (Eds.), *Handbook of positive psychology* (pp. 446–458). New York, NY: Oxford University Press.

McCullough, M. E., & Worthington, E. L., Jr. (1999). Religion and the forgiving personality. *Journal of Personality, 67*, 1141–1164.

McLernon, F., Cairns, E., Hewstone, M., & Smith, R. (2004). The development of intergroup forgiveness in Northern Ireland. *Journal of Social Issues, 60*, 587–601.

Mesquita, B., & Albert, D. (2007). The cultural regulation of emotions. In J. J. Gross (Ed.), *Handbook of emotion regulation* (pp. 486–503). New York, NY: Guilford Press.

Moeschberger, S. L., Dixon, D. N., Niens, U., & Cairns, E. (2005). Forgiveness in Northern Ireland: A model for peace in the midst of the 'Troubles'. *Peace and Conflict: Journal of Peace Psychology, 11*, 199–214.

Mullet, E., Barros, J., Frongia, L., Usaï, V., & Shafighi, S. R. (2003). Religious involvement and the forgiving personality. *Journal of Personality, 71*, 1–19.

Myers, E., Hewstone, M., & Cairns, E. (2009). Impact of conflict on mental health in Northern Ireland: The mediating role of intergroup forgiveness and collective guilt. *Political Psychology, 30*, 269–290.

Neto, F., da Conceição Pinto, M., & Mullet, E. (2004). Perdão intergrupal: Uma perspectiva Timorense = Intergroup forgiveness: A Timorese viewpoint. *Psicologia Educação Cultura, 8*, 263–288.

Noor, M., Brown, R., Gonzalez, R., Manzi, J., & Lewis, C. A. (2008). On positive psychological outcomes: What helps groups with a history of conflict to forgive and reconcile with each other? *Personality and Social Psychology Bulletin, 34*, 819–832.

Noor, M., Brown, R. J., & Prentice, G. (2008a). Precursors and mediators of intergroup reconciliation in Northern Ireland: A new model. *British Journal of Social Psychology, 47*, 481–495.

Noor, M., Brown, R. J., & Prentice, G. (2008b). Prospects for intergroup reconciliation: Social-psychological predictors of intergroup forgiveness and reparation in Northern Ireland and Chile. In A. Nadler, T. E. Malloy, & J. D. Fisher (Eds.), *The social psychology of intergroup reconciliation* (pp. 97–114). New York, NY: Oxford University Press.

Paz, R., Neto, F., & Mullet, E. (2007). Forgivingness: Similarities and differences between Buddhists and Christians living in China. *The International Journal for the Psychology of Religion, 17*, 289–301.

Paz, R., Neto, F., & Mullet, E. (2008). Forgiveness: A China-Western Europe comparison. *Journal of Psychology: Interdisciplinary and Applied, 142*, 147–157.

Pressman, S. D., Gallagher, M. W., & Lopez, S. J. (2013). Is the emotion-health connection a 'first-world problem'? *Psychological Science, 24*, 544–549.

Sagiv, L., & Schwartz, S. H. (2007). Cultural values in organizations: Insights for Europe. *European Journal of International Management, 1*, 176–190.

Sandage, S. J., Hill, P. C., & Vang, H. C. (2003). Toward a multicultural positive psychology: Indigenous forgiveness and Hmong culture. *Counseling Psychologist, 31*, 564–592.

Sandage, S. J., & Williamson, I. (2005). Forgiveness in cultural context. In E. L. Worthington Jr. (Ed.), *Handbook of forgiveness* (pp. 41–55). New York, NY: Routledge.

Schaal, S., Weierstall, R., Dusingizemungu, J. P., & Elbert, T. (2012). Mental health 15 years after the killings in Rwanda: Imprisoned perpetrators of the genocide against the Tutsi versus a community sample of survivors. *Journal of Traumatic Stress, 25*, 446–453.

Schwartz, S. H. (1997). Values and culture. In D. Munro, J. F. Schumaker, & S. C. Carr (Eds.), *Motivation and culture* (pp. 69–84). New York, NY: Routledge.

Schwartz, S. H. (1994). Beyond individualism/collectivism: New cultural dimensions of values. In U. Kim, H. C. Truandis, C. Kâğitçibaşi, S. C. Choi, & G. Yoon (Eds.), *Individualism and collectivism: Theory, method, and applications* (pp. 85–119). Thousand Oaks, CA: Sage.

Staub, E. (1999). The origins and prevention of genocide, mass killing, and other collective violence. *Peace and Conflict: Journal of Peace Psychology, 5*, 303–336.

Suwartono, C., Prawasti, C. Y., & Mullet, E. (2007). Effect of culture on forgivingness: A Southern Asia-Western Europe comparison. *Personality and Individual Differences, 42*, 513–523.

Tajfel, H., & Turner, J. C. (1986). An integrative theory of intergroup conflict. In S. Worchel & W. Austin (Eds.), *Psychology of intergroup relations* (pp. 2–24). Chicago, IL: Nelson-Hall.

Takaku, S., Weiner, B., & Ohbuchi, K. I. (2001). A cross-cultural examination of the effects of apology and perspective taking on forgiveness. *Journal of Language and Social Psychology, 20*, 144–166.

Touze, D., Silove, D., & Zwi, A. (2005). Can there be healing without justice? Lessons from the commission for reception, Truth and Reconciliation in East Timor. *Intervention: International Journal of Mental Health, Psychosocial Work & Counselling in Areas of Armed Conflict, 3*, 192–202.

Triandis, H. C. (1996). The psychological measurement of cultural syndromes. *American Psychologist, 51*, 407–415.

Van Tongeren, D. R., Burnette, J. L., O' Boyle, E., Worthington, E. L., & Forsyth, D. (2014). A meta-analysis of intergroup forgiveness. *Journal of Positive Psychology, 9*, 81–95.

Walker, D. L., & Gorsuch, R. L. (2002). Forgiveness within the big five personality model. *Personality and Individual Differences, 32*, 1127–1138.

Watkins, D. A., Hui, E. K. P., Luo, W., Regmi, M., Worthington, E. L., Jr., Hook, J. N., & Davis, D. E. (2011). Forgiveness and interpersonal relationships: A Nepalese investigation. *The Journal of Social Psychology, 151*, 150–161.

Watkins, D., & Regmi, M. (2004). Personality and forgiveness: A Nepalese perspective. *Journal of Social Psychology, 144*, 539–540.

Part IV
Applications Regarding Forgiveness and Health

Chapter 16
Forgiveness and Health in Nonmarried Dyadic Relationships

Jody L. Davis, Jeffrey D. Green, Chelsea A. Reid, Jaclyn M. Moloney, and Jeni Burnette

Transgressions occur in all types of relationships, romantic or otherwise. Any dyadic relationship characterized by interdependence inevitably provides opportunities for a partner's behavior to offend, setting the stage for the granting or withholding of forgiveness. In the context of nonmarried dyadic relationships, forgiveness research primarily has focused on dating relationships, with comparatively sparse research on other relationships such as friendships or work relationships. Across these relationship contexts, research elucidates a range of physical, mental, and relationship health benefits of forgiveness that largely parallels benefits present in the context of marital relationships. Based upon existing research, it is unclear the extent to which health implications of forgiveness may vary depending upon the distal context of the forgiveness – the type of relationship in which the forgiveness occurs (e.g., friendships vs. dating relationships vs. marital relationships); however, characterizing relationships in terms of their proximal processes – psychological mechanisms underlying forgiveness – may be a fruitful strategy for exploring differences in health outcomes. Three foundational relationship theories (investment model of commitment, evolutionary theory, and attachment theory) provide a framework for identifying important proximal moderators of the link between forgiveness and health that may supersede relationship type and provide a blueprint for future research.

J.L. Davis (✉) • J.D. Green • J.M. Moloney
Virginia Commonwealth University, 820 W Franklin St, Richmond, VA 23284, USA
e-mail: jldavis@vcu.edu; jdgreen@vcu.edu; moloneyjm@vcu.edu

J. Burnette
North Carolina State University, 640 Poe Hall, Box 7650, Raleigh, NC 27695, USA
e-mail: jlburne5@ncsu.edu

C.A. Reid
College of Charleston, 66 George Street, Charleston, SC 29424, USA
e-mail: reidca@cofc.edu

L.L. Toussaint et al. (eds.), *Forgiveness and Health*,
DOI 10.1007/978-94-017-9993-5_16

Forgiveness involves transforming negative thoughts, feelings, and behavior towards a perpetrator into more positive thoughts, feelings, and behavior (e.g., McCullough, Fincham, & Tsang, 2003). From this perspective, forgiveness is intraindividual, prosocial change toward a perpetrator (McCullough, Pargament, & Thoresen, 2000) that involves reducing motivation to retaliate as well as increasing motivation for conciliation and goodwill. Trait and state level forgiveness both are linked to health. *Trait forgivingness* transcends relationships, time, and situations and is defined as a dispositional tendency to grant forgiveness, whereas *state forgiveness* unfolds within the context of specific transgressions and perpetrators.

Three Domains of Health

Physical Health In the aftermath of transgressions, forgiveness can protect physical health by reducing stress and rumination. Cardiovascular reactivity can be associated with physical health; the ability to quickly return to baseline blood pressure and heart rate levels after a stressor is an indication of physiological hardiness and the ability to cope successfully with stress (Dienstbier, 1989). Among individuals who discussed a past conflict that they had with a friend, parent, or romantic partner, greater trait forgivingness was associated with lower blood pressure, and greater state forgiveness was associated with lower blood pressure as well as lower heart rate (Lawler et al., 2003). In addition, failure to forgive was associated with a longer period of cardiovascular reactivity, particularly among individuals who were lower in trait forgivingness or who discussed a conflict with a parent (vs. friend or romantic partner). Failure to forgive also was associated with stress and hostility as well as self-reported illness. A similarly-designed study took into account attachment style (i.e., the quality of the emotional bond between individuals) and revealed that securely (vs. insecurely) attached individuals exhibited greater trait forgivingness and state forgiveness (Lawler-Row, Younger, Piferi, & Jones, 2006). In addition, insecurely (vs. securely) attached individuals had greater diastolic blood pressure and mean arterial pressure during the recovery period as well as greater systolic blood pressure during the discussion and recovery periods.

Importantly, not all forgiveness may buffer equally against stress. Motivations to forgive can focus on obligation (yielding to pressure from others such as a religious authority to forgive) or on love (Huang & Enright, 2000). Individuals who forgave friends, spouses, or coworkers out of obligation (vs. love) held onto more residual anger and had higher blood pressure while describing an interpersonal conflict. In a related vein, a rare investigation of forgiveness and health in a workplace setting (Cox, Bennett, Tripp, & Aquino, 2012) validated five motives for forgiving and found that forgiveness does not always correlate positively with reduced stress and increased health. For example, those who forgave because it was the morally correct thing to do experienced less stress (but not better health), whereas those who forgave because they felt they had no other alternative (given the nature of the workplace relationship) had greater stress and worse physical health. These different motivations may relate to Worthington's (2003) decisional versus emotional forgiveness; this is a particularly promising area for future investigation.

Other research has more explicitly examined the role of stress in the link between forgiveness and health. Stress activates the neural, neuroendocrine, and neuroendocrine-immune mechanisms that collectively are termed the *allostatic systems*. When allostatic systems are overstimulated, the condition is referred to as high allostatic load (McEwen, 2004). Impaired immunity, obesity, and atrophy of nerve cells in the brain are some of the physical consequences of high allostatic load from chronic stress. Conflict in close relationships may be a particularly toxic source of stress, but forgiveness can protect against the deleterious effects of conflict. For example, college students recalled being hurt or betrayed by a close friend or relationship partner and reported their stress, symptoms of physical illness, and trait forgivingness and state forgiveness (Lawler et al., 2005). Those who reported greater forgiveness – particularly greater state forgiveness – reported better health. Moreover, the link between state forgiveness and health was partially accounted for by reduced stress, and the link between trait forgivingness and health was fully accounted for by reduced stress. Forgiveness appears to protect physical health in a manner beyond cardiovascular reactivity by reducing longer-term stress; "letting go" via forgiveness appears to entail unloading a stress burden.

Additional research has examined amount of salivary cortisol as a measure of stress reactivity. Research using cortisol measurement has revealed that acute physiological stress is associated with poorer quality romantic relationships. Individuals in happy or unhappy romantic relationships thought about typical interactions with their partners, and those in unhappy relationships exhibited increased cortisol production (Berry & Worthington, 2001). Moreover, individuals who were higher in trait anger and lower in trait forgivingness were more likely to report being in lower quality relationships, which accounted for their stress reactivity. Other research has revealed that cortisol is associated with a tendency to ruminate about a past transgression (McCullough, Orsulak, Brandon, & Akers, 2007); after interpersonal transgressions, victims often ruminate. To the extent that individuals reported having ruminated about a transgression a great deal during the previous two weeks, their cortisol reactivity levels were higher. Rumination also plays a role in the link between both state forgiveness and trait forgivingness and sleep quality. Individuals who were more forgiving of a transgression reported less anger rumination, which in turn predicted less negative affect and ultimately better sleep quality (Stoia-Caraballo et al., 2008). Thus, both relationship quality and the tendency to ruminate were associated with stress reactivity and healthy behavior.

Other research has used alternative measures of stress. In a particularly well-designed study, individuals imagined unforgiving responses to past transgressions (e.g., betrayal of trust, lies) as well as forgiving responses to the same transgressions several times for 16 s each (Witvliet, Ludwig, & Vander Laan, 2001). Their physiological responses were continuously measured throughout the imagery and recovery periods. While imagining unforgiving responses, individuals experienced greater facial tension at the brow muscle region, greater sympathetic nervous system arousal, and greater cardiovascular reactivity. These results extended into the recovery period, suggesting that the effects of not forgiving take some time to quell.

In summary, when it comes to physiological processes often associated with physical health, there are protective effects of forgiveness and reactive effects of unforgiveness. The extent to which individuals who experience transgressions in non-marital close relationships are likely to experience a cascade of unforgiveness, stress, and negative health outcomes depends upon individual differences (e.g., attachment style, tendency to ruminate, level of trait forgivingness), the nature of the forgiveness (e.g., love vs. obligation), and relationship quality.

Mental Health Forgiveness also is linked to mental health. The vast majority of research on forgiveness and mental health in nonmarried dyads has examined negative outcomes of unforgiveness. That is, most work on mental health has focused on clinical diagnoses or subclinical symptoms, particularly symptoms regarding anxiety disorders (e.g., post-traumatic stress disorder) and depression. Only a few have addressed potential positive benefits of forgiveness such as subjective well-being.

An investigation of infidelity in dating relationships (Kluwer & Karremans, 2009) found that unforgiving motivations (i.e., revenge and avoidance) were associated with more negative affect and less positive affect. Importantly, this link was stronger when individuals were highly committed to the unfaithful other. In another study, individuals imagined forgiveness and unforgiveness (Witvliet et al., 2001) and reported their feelings of anger, sadness, arousal, empathy, and perceived control during each imagery period. When imagining unforgiveness (vs. forgiveness), they experienced greater anger, sadness, and arousal, but less empathy and less control. Though it is unclear how brief imagery relates to long-term health, such reactions may occur immediately after a transgression as well as later when the transgression is recalled.

The link between state forgiveness and depressive symptoms has been studied in undergraduate women who had experienced abuse in their romantic relationship, and undergraduate women and men who had experienced a recent conflict or break-up in their relationship (Ysseldyk, Matheson, & Anisman, 2009). Appraisals of threat and of control accounted for the link between forgiveness and depressive symptoms in both samples, perhaps because forgiveness facilitates a reappraisal of past transgressions and perpetrators. That is, unforgiveness was associated with greater depressive symptoms in both samples, and this was partially accounted for by appraisals of reduced control and greater threat. Such appraisals have a storied history in research on stress and health (e.g., Strelan & Covic, 2006; Worthington, 2006; Worthington & Scherer, 2004).

Unforgiveness appears to be related to anxiety symptoms in addition to depressive symptoms. One study examined college students who had experienced significant traumas (e.g., sexual assault, childhood abuse; perpetrators included dating partners and friends but also family members and strangers) and subsequently felt extreme fear, helplessness, or powerlessness (Orcutt, Pickett, & Pope, 2008). To the extent that individuals forgave the perpetrator, they experienced fewer PTSD symptoms. In a longitudinal study of a similar set of variables, forgiveness of a transgression at one time period reduced distress (i.e., depressive symptoms, anxiety, stress) at a second time period (36 weeks later on average; Orcutt, 2006). Given that individuals tend to report a linear decline in unforgiveness in the weeks following relational transgressions (McCullough et al., 2003), it seems possible that the simple passage of time reduced distress symptoms, which then led to increased forgiveness.

Forgiveness interventions allow for stronger causal conclusions regarding the effect of forgiveness on health outcomes (for a review see Worthington, Jennings, & DiBlasio, 2010). One study of college women who had been seriously wronged in a romantic relationship (e.g., 50 % reported infidelity, 38 % emotional or verbal abuse, 24 % physical abuse or threat) randomly assigned women to one of two forgiveness interventions (secular vs. religious, but no differences were found between these two intervention types) or a control wait-list (Rye & Pargament, 2002). The interventions consisted of six weekly, 90-min sessions. Although no significant differences were found on some negative affect items such as anxiety and hostility, the interventions did lead to somewhat fewer depressive symptoms, and, notably, higher ratings of existential well-being. Another study of individuals who reported transgressions by coworkers randomly assigned individuals to forgiveness training or job satisfaction training. The forgiveness intervention consisted of social motivation training designed to encourage victims to analyze their perceptions of a transgression. Those who experienced the forgiveness intervention reported improved self-image (Struthers, Dupius, & Eaton, 2005). Both of these studies included rare assessments of positive psychological functioning. Outside the context of marital relationships, there is modest research supporting the efficacy of other forgiveness interventions on health outcomes (e.g., Coyle & Enright, 1997; Rye et al., 2005. The practical limitations of laborious interventions invite research on briefer (e.g., one-session, online) interventions.

In summary, research on nonmarital dyads has addressed forgiveness of a variety of transgressions, particularly serious transgressions (e.g., infidelity). However, operationalizations of mental and emotional health largely have focused on subclinical symptoms of anxiety and depression. Very few have assessed positive outcomes such as subjective well-being or hardiness. (A recent meta-analysis by Riek and Mania (2012) of outcomes of forgiveness—examining all relationship types—confirmed that forgiveness reduces depression, anxiety, stress and negative affect and increases life satisfaction and positive affect.) Forgiveness, at least of serious transgressions, reduces anxiety and depressive symptoms. However, future research on these populations should investigate mild transgressions, study friendships and work relationships in particular, and assess a wider variety of positive mental health outcomes. For example, might forgiveness foster increased resilience, gratitude, or savoring in particular contexts? That is, would a habit of forgiving others lead to less reactivity when experiencing future offenses, or even gratitude for the relationship in spite of inevitable conflicts? Additional experimental work, including different types of interventions, also is necessary. Finally, mediators of the link between forgiveness and mental health should continue to be studied.

Relationship Health In addition to contributing to physical and mental health, forgiveness also affects relationship health. Forgiveness of a friend or romantic partner is linked to a stronger likelihood of resolving a betrayal (Hannon, Rusbult, Finkel, & Kumashiro, 2010) and maintaining rather than terminating the relationship (Morse & Metts, 2011). Relationship stability likely is enhanced by several post-forgiveness pro-relationship responses by perpetrators and victims. For example, individuals who recalled a past transgression that they had forgiven (vs. not forgiven) were more likely to sacrifice (i.e., eschew valued activities) for their partner, and they were more likely to cooperate with their partner on a social task. Similarly, individuals who recalled a forgiven (vs. unforgiven) transgression engaged in greater levels of accommodation (i.e., inhibiting negative impulses and responding constructively rather than destructively following a partner's destructive act). That is, individuals were more likely to respond to hypothetical scenarios in which their partner engaged in a destructive behavior (e.g., "the other suddenly yells at you") by endorsing constructive (e.g., "you think 'never mind,' probably the other had a bad day") rather than destructive (e.g., "you yell back at the other") actions (Karremans & Van Lange, 2004).

Forgiveness of transgressions also predicts greater relationship satisfaction (Braithwaite, Selby, & Fincham, 2011; Wieselquist, 2009). Couples (whose marital status was not indicated) who reported an emotional injury in their relationship and then underwent an emotion-focused couple's therapy intervention for resolving emotional injuries showed improvements in trust and satisfaction compared to wait-list participants (Greenberg, Warwar, & Malcolm, 2010). Other research revealed that to the extent that romantic partners had greater levels of trait forgivingness, they reported greater relationship satisfaction due to exerting greater relationship effort and experiencing less negative conflict. In other words, individuals who tended to be more forgiving were more likely to regulate their behavior with the goal of enhancing relationship quality by engaging in less negative and more positive communication. These behaviors in turn produced greater levels of relationship satisfaction (Braithwaite et al., 2011). Interestingly, forgiveness not only promotes greater relationship satisfaction for the victim, but for the perpetrator as well. Being forgiven by a romantic partner bolstered perpetrators' trust in the partner and ultimately led to greater relationship satisfaction on the part of the perpetrator (Wieselquist, 2009).

Where relationship satisfaction goes, relationship commitment typically follows; thus, it is unsurprising that forgiveness also predicts relationship commitment. In a longitudinal study examining severe transgressions, unforgiveness of a dating partner resulted in a decline in relationship commitment, but forgiveness attenuated the decline (Ysseldyk & Wohl, 2012). Similarly, in research examining the relationship over time among three subtypes of forgiveness and relationship commitment, undergraduates reported increased levels of closeness and commitment to the perpetrator to the extent that they reported less avoidance and revenge and more benevolence (Tsang, McCullough, & Fincham, 2006). In addition, when victims forgave the perpetrator, perpetrators reported increased commitment to the relationship, demonstrating again that forgiveness benefits relationship health for both parties (Wieselquist, 2009).

In summary, forgiveness yields protective benefits by promoting resolution of betrayals and pro-relationship processes such as accommodation, willingness to sacrifice, and positive communication. Ultimately, forgiveness enhances relationship trust, satisfaction, commitment, and relationship stability.

Linking Domains of Health Most research has examined only one of the types of health reviewed (i.e., physical, mental, or relationship health); however, these different types of health obviously are intertwined. For example, relationship health positively influences both physical and mental health in numerous ways, though the relation may be bidirectional in particular instances (e.g., anxiety disorder symptoms affecting relationship quality), and there may be occasional tradeoffs (e.g., forgiving when it is less warranted may improve relationship health but reduce mental health; Luchies, Finkel, McNulty, & Kumashiro, 2010). Some research indicates that post-forgiveness intrapersonal markers of health (e.g., psychological well-being) are in part due to interpersonal markers of health (e.g., relationship quality). For example, trait forgivingness was associated with interpersonal adjustment (i.e., ability to establish positive relationships with others and receive support), which in turn predicted psychological well-being (i.e., lower depression and greater positive affect, optimism, and self-efficacy; Tse & Yip, 2009). Future work should address the integration of these domains of health, but should do so within a solidly grounded theoretical context. The next section recommends three particularly promising theoretical orientations to guide future research.

Three Theories to Guide Research

Are the predictors and consequences of forgiveness different in friendships and nonmarried romantic relationships relative to married relationships? Generally, research examining links between forgiveness and health has revealed parallel findings whether forgiveness is examined in the context of friendship, nonmarried romantic relationships, or married relationships, and because researchers tend not to report direct comparisons among relationship types (and often do not even report the relationship type of their research participants), no meta-analysis has addressed the question of whether there are relationship type effects. Nevertheless, a more productive approach may be to consider three relationships theories—investment model of commitment, attachment theory, and evolutionary theory—that can provide theory-based insight into the likely nature of any relationship-relevant differences. Put another way, these relationship theories proffer proximal explanations for forgiveness-health effects that likely are more powerful and theoretically rich compared to examining the more distal context of relationship type (e.g., married vs. not).

Investment Model of Commitment According to the investment model of commitment (Rusbult, 1980), individuals who have high satisfaction (i.e., benefits received in the relationship), high investments (i.e., resources tied to the relationship), and low alternatives (i.e., options for receiving benefits without the current relationship) experience greater commitment to their relationship, which is conceptualized as a combination of psychological attachment, long-term orientation, and intent to persist in the relationship. A meta-analysis revealed that the three theorized bases robustly predict commitment across a variety of interpersonal relationships including romantic relationships (marital, dating, exclusive, nonexclusive, homosexual, heterosexual, short duration, and long duration) as well as friendships (Le & Agnew, 2003). Importantly, to the extent that individuals are committed to their relationship, they are likely to engage in a host of relationship maintenance behaviors such as forgiveness (Finkel, Rusbult, Kumashiro, & Hannon, 2002). Future research could examine the extent to which variations in the bases of commitment link to forgiveness and associated health outcomes.

For example, individuals' level of investments in their relationship could influence the likelihood of forgiving their partner and associated health outcomes. Investments can be tangible (e.g., a shared home mortgage) or intangible (e.g., sacrifices made for the partner). Legal marriage and its associated tangible investments may lead married couples to persist in a relationship even in the presence of unforgiveness of severe transgressions, whereas nonmarried couples may be quicker to leave such a relationship. It seems plausible that such persistence could result in a detrimental cumulative effect of stress due to unforgiveness. In addition, individuals who are prevented from marrying (e.g., homosexual couples in certain states) may consequently have fewer tangible investments in a relationship or their investments may be less powerful predictors of commitment (Lehmiller, 2010) and thus forgiveness and associated health outcomes. In addition, the extent to which commitment and therefore forgiveness is driven by tangible versus intangible investments could have varying implications for health outcomes.

In addition, the extent to which individuals perceive that they have high quality alternatives to their current relationship may affect the likelihood of forgiving their partner and experiencing corresponding health outcomes. For example, when individuals are dependent on their partner for their well-being and perceive that they would be unable to meet their needs without the partner, the partner has corresponding greater power in the relationship. Such a dynamic could lead individuals to persist in relationships even when their partners transgress and are not forgiven, and such situations seem likely to be particularly stressful and unhealthy for individuals who feel trapped in a relationship due to lack of alternatives. In addition, whereas most individuals have a primary and exclusive romantic relationship, they tend to have a network of friends. Therefore, it is likely that individuals would perceive greater quality of alternatives to their friendships than to their romantic relationships, and there are likely to be fewer negative health effects of unforgiveness to the extent that the benefits received from one friendship can be replaced by others. Relatedly, the degree to which individuals are dependent on friends may be affected by whether they are in a romantic relationship; relationship experiences with a best friend predicted individuals' happiness only when they did not have a romantic partner (Demir, 2010). In summary, examining the bases of commitment to a particular relationship could predict the likelihood of forgiveness as well as potential health effects of forgiveness and unforgiveness.

Evolutionary Theory An evolutionary perspective on forgiveness suggests that an optimally functioning forgiveness system selectively processes information that enables adaptive decisions that, under ancestral conditions, would have led to fitness-maximizing trade-offs (Duchaine, Cosmides, & Tooby, 2001). That is, individuals would consider the trade-off between the fitness-enhancing value of deterrence (e.g., revenge) and the potential value of benevolence (e.g., forgiveness). The trade-off should, on most occasions, lead to fitness-enhancing resources. Specifically, an evolved forgiveness system examines information relevant to estimating (a) exploitation risk, or the probability of incurring costs to oneself in the future; and (b) relationship value, or the probability of fitness gains for oneself from re-establishing or continuing an association with the perpetrator (Burnette, McCullough, Van Tongeren, & Davis, 2012). After weighing the exploitation risk and relationship value, an individual's forgiveness system should generate a subjective "forgiveness index," which indicates whether forgiveness is an adaptive decision (Petersen, Sell, Tooby, & Cosmides, 2010). This is not to imply that the process is fully logical or even fully conscious; these assessments could be made in a more intuitive or heuristic and less than fully conscious manner. In summary, factors that affect *exploitation risk* and *relationship value* should be weighed most heavily and considered most important in making decisions to forgive and in considering the outcomes of such forgiveness.

This evolutionary approach to forgiveness can be used as a building block for future inquiry into the health consequences of forgiveness in different types of relationships. For example, relationship value may be greater in romantic relationships relative to friendships such that holding a grudge against a dating partner would be more costly to health. In addition, if individuals are inclined to forgive even if exploitation risk remains and/or the relationship holds little or no value to them, then forgiveness could be costly. Indeed, forgiving a perpetrator in the absence of amends (a signal that future exploitation risk is high) erodes self-respect and self-concept clarity (Luchies et al., 2010). Forgiving a perpetrator who has not signaled that the victim will be safe and valued in future interactions could influence health outcomes in a similar fashion. Future inquiry into health consequences of forgiveness could benefit from an investigation examining relationship value and exploitation risk and subsequent physical, emotional, and relationship health outcomes. For example, although forgiveness when value is low and exploitation is high may be costly to the individual in terms of mental health outcomes, it might contribute to relationship health.

Attachment Theory According to attachment theory, individuals seek protection and comfort from a primary attachment figure when feeling vulnerable or stressed. The attachment behavioral systems include proximity seeking, safe haven (source of safety when feeling threatened), and secure base (well of emotional support that serves as a launching pad for exploration). Individuals vary in the extent to which they have *avoidant* (beliefs that others tend to be unresponsive to needs or discomfort with dependency on others) and *anxious* (beliefs that others may reject them or that they are unworthy of love) orientations. Importantly, anxious and avoidant attachment are negatively associated with dispositional forgivingness (Burnette, Davis, Green, Worthington, & Bradfield, 2009). Anxious individuals tend to exaggerate the impact of transgressions and thus engage in greater angry rumination (Burnette, Taylor, Worthington, & Forsyth, 2007), and avoidant individuals tend to respond to transgressions with distancing and withdrawal and thus experience reduced empathy; both of these responses yield unforgiveness (Burnette et al., 2009). Among individuals whose blood pressure was monitored before and during an interview regarding a past betrayal (Lawler-Row et al., 2006), secure attachment was associated with greater forgiveness as well as reduced systolic blood pressure and greater blood pressure recovery. Recent work also highlights changes in cortisol production as a key mechanism linking attachment anxiety to reduced health in the aftermath of conflict (Jaremka et al., 2013). Securely attached individuals tend to more readily let go of negative emotions, leading to health benefits. However, insecurely attached individuals tend to be more vulnerable to stress, less likely to benefit from social support networks, and rely more heavily on external coping methods (e.g., alcohol, overeating) when they encounter stress (Lawler-Row, Hyatt-Edwards, Wuensch, & Karremans, 2011; Maunder & Hunter, 2001). Thus, forgiveness may be the "key mediator of the association between attachment and health" (Lawler-Row et al., 2011, p. 179).

Secure and caring relationships are critical to mental health, but emotional bonds take time to form; attachment is a process that unfolds relatively slowly over the course of months or years (Hazan & Zeifman, 1994). Across the lifespan, individuals' attachment needs are met by a series of primary attachment figures, from parents in childhood to friends in adolescence to romantic partners in adulthood. However, individuals can have multiple concurrent attachments and may seek out different individuals (e.g., friends and romantic partners) to serve various attachment-related needs like security and caregiving (Fraley & Davis, 1997). Unforgiveness of a romantic partner may have the greatest negative health impact for those who are insecurely attached. However, unforgiveness of friends, particularly long-term friends who are relatively unique (e.g., a best friend), may also have health consequences because the victim relies on that relationship to serve at least some attachment functions. Future research should investigate health consequences of forgiveness in friendships drawing on an attachment perspective.

Future Directions and Applications

In addition to the ideas proposed throughout the previous section, other potentially fruitful areas for future research involve expanding the focus of health outcomes beyond the victims of transgressions. For example, a conundrum exists when individuals have forgiven a romantic partner for a transgression, but a close partner of theirs (e.g., a friend or family member) has not. Research on *third-party forgiveness* suggests that third parties (close partners of the victim) are less forgiving than first parties (the victims themselves) because first parties are more likely to feel greater commitment to the perpetrator and make more benign attributions for the perpetrator's behavior (Green, Burnette, & Davis, 2008). This research suggests that forgiveness and unforgiveness could have significant effects beyond the dyad. An extension of this research could be to examine whether first parties (victims) of transgressions experience health benefits associated with their forgiveness, whereas third parties may experience health costs associated with their unforgiveness; such health costs most likely would be linked to the quality of their relationship to the victim (e.g., commitment, attachment, relationship value). Furthermore, it would be interesting to explore the extent to which health benefits from forgiveness for victims are attenuated in the face of third-party unforgiveness; it seems likely that individuals would experience tension or stress when their close friend or family member maintains vengeful feelings toward their romantic partner, and such stress could lead to poor health outcomes. These broader social network effects of forgiveness or unforgiveness may tend to be overlooked by practitioners and individuals themselves, but may be important to consider.

In another example of context beyond the dyad, past research has examined how aspects of individuals' work environments influence forgiveness; future research could explore in what ways such organizational variables are linked to health. For example, perceptions of procedural justice affect forgiveness, especially for victims with less power (Aquino, Tripp, & Bies, 2006). If individuals do not feel that the "system" is fair and their grievance has been taken seriously, festering feelings of anger, avoidance, and revenge could lead to deleterious health outcomes. More broadly, future work should explore health benefits of forgiveness in the workplace; coworker relationships are an important but understudied category of interpersonal relationships. Although a great deal of research has examined processes relating to conflict and forgiveness in workplace settings, very little research has measured health outcomes (Cox et al., 2012).

Another understudied area is that of the perpetrator. Research has demonstrated a range of health benefits (i.e., blood pressure reduction) of forgiveness for perpetrators as well as victims (Hannon, Finkel, Kumashiro, & Rusbult, 2012). Offering forgiveness to perpetrators communicates a victim's relationship commitment, facilitates prorelationship behaviors (Karremans & Van Lange, 2004), and leads perpetrators to experience greater feelings of trust, which increases relationship satisfaction (Wieselquist, 2009). Perpetrator outcomes generally are an understudied area. Any hypotheses advanced for victim health outcomes could be tested in parallel for perpetrators. Perpetrators may be motivated to make amends and seek forgiveness in order to repair their relationships, but they also could be motivated by potential physical and mental health benefits. Victims could be motivated to offer forgiveness not only to benefit their own health, but that of the perpetrator as well.

An important implication of this collective body of research is that physical, mental, and relationship health all are connected to forgiveness processes. Relationships among these domains of health may sometimes operate in parallel manner (increases in mental health could lead to increases in physical health), but may sometimes operate at odds with each other (increases in relationship health could lead to decreases in mental health if an unhealthy relationship is maintained due to forgiveness). For example, it is important for perpetrators to offer sincere amends for their transgressions to maximize mental health outcomes for victims (Luchies et al., 2010; Schumann, 2012). Recognition of these complex relationships could inform interventions designed to enhance forgiveness.

Conclusion

Forgiveness generally is associated with positive health benefits. Relationships theories provide useful tools for prediction, understanding underlying processes that enhance health benefits of forgiveness or magnify harm of unforgiveness. However, researchers need to examine multiple types of health to fully understand the links among them as well as the occasional tradeoffs. There are vast opportunities for future research to identify what constitutes "healthy" forgiveness and to expand forgiveness research into new areas. For example, health costs and benefits of unforgiveness and forgiveness likely exist for more than just the victim, but also for perpetrators and third parties. Researchers may have underestimated the importance of relationship quality of friendships and nonmarital relationships. Clinicians should be aware that unforgiveness can lead to poor health outcomes for victims and perpetrators even in nonmarital relationships.

References

Aquino, K., Tripp, T. M., & Bies, R. J. (2006). Getting even or moving on? Power, procedural justice, and types of offense as predictors of revenge, forgiveness, reconciliation, and avoidance in organizations. *Journal of Applied Psychology, 91*, 653–668.

Berry, J. W., & Worthington, E. L., Jr. (2001). Forgivingness, relationship quality, stress while imagining relationship events, and physical and mental health. *Journal of Counseling Psychology, 48*, 447–455.

Braithwaite, S. R., Selby, E. A., & Fincham, F. D. (2011). Forgiveness and relationship satisfaction: Mediating mechanisms. *Journal of Family Psychology, 25*, 551–559.

Burnette, J. L., Davis, D. E., Green, J. D., Worthington, E. L., Jr., & Bradfield, E. (2009). Insecure attachment and depressive symptoms: The mediating role of rumination, empathy, and forgiveness. *Personality and Individual Differences, 46*, 276–280.

Burnette, J. L., McCullough, M. E., Van Tongeren, D. R., & Davis, D. E. (2012). Forgiveness results from integrating information about relationship value and exploitation risk. *Personality and Social Psychology Bulletin, 38*, 345–356.

Burnette, J. L., Taylor, K. W., Worthington, E. L., Jr., & Forsyth, D. R. (2007). Attachment and trait forgiveness: The mediating role of angry rumination. *Personality and Individual Differences, 42*, 1585–1596.

Cox, S. S., Bennett, R. J., Tripp, T. M., & Aquino, K. (2012). An empirical test of forgiveness motives' effects on employees' health and well-being. *Journal of Occupational Health Psychology, 17*, 330–340.

Coyle, C. T., & Enright, R. D. (1997). Forgiveness intervention with postabortion men. *Journal of Consulting and Clinical Psychology, 65*, 1042–1046.

Demir, M. (2010). Close relationships and happiness among emerging adults. *Journal of Happiness Studies, 11*, 293–313.

Dienstbier, R. A. (1989). Arousal and physiological toughness: Implications for mental and physical health. *Psychological Review, 96*, 84–100.

Duchaine, B., Cosmides, L., & Tooby, J. (2001). Evolutionary psychology and the brain. *Current Opinion in Neurobiology, 11*, 225–230.

Finkel, E. J., Rusbult, C. E., Kumashiro, M., & Hannon, P. A. (2002). Dealing with betrayal in close relationships: Does commitment promote forgiveness? *Journal of Personality and Social Psychology, 82*, 956–974.

Fraley, R. C., & Davis, K. E. (1997). Attachment formation and transfer in young adults' close relationships and romantic relationships. *Personal Relationships, 4*, 131–144.

Green, J. D., Burnette, J., & Davis, J. L. (2008). Third-party forgiveness: (Not) forgiving your close other's betrayer. *Personality and Social Psychology Bulletin, 34*, 407–418.

Greenberg, L., Warwar, S., & Malcolm, W. (2010). Emotion-focused couples therapy and the facilitation of forgiveness. *Journal of Marital and Family Therapy, 36*, 28–42.

Hannon, P. A., Finkel, E. J., Kumashiro, M., & Rusbult, C. E. (2012). The soothing effects of forgiveness on victims' and perpetrators' blood pressure. *Personal Relationships, 19*, 279–289.

Hannon, P. A., Rusbult, C. E., Finkel, E. J., & Kamashiro, M. (2010). In the wake of betrayal: Amends, forgiveness, and the resolution of betrayal. *Personal Relationships, 17*, 253–278.

Hazan, C., & Zeifman, D. (1994). Sex and the psychological tether. In K. Bartholomew & D. Pearlman (Eds.), *Advances in personal relationships: Vol. 5. Attachment processes in adulthood* (pp. 151–178). London, UK: Jessica Kingsley.

Huang, S. T., & Enright, R. D. (2000). Forgiveness and anger-related emotions in Taiwan: Implication for therapy. *Psychotherapy, 37*, 71–79.

Jaremka, L.M., Glaser, R., Loving, T.J., Malarkey, W.B., Stowell, J.R, & Kiecolt-Glaser, J.K. (2013). Attachment anxiety is linked to alterations in cortisol production and cellular immunity. *Psychological Science, 24*(3), 272–279.

Karremans, J. C., & Van Lange, P. A. M. (2004). Back to caring after being hurt: The role of forgiveness. *European Journal of Social Psychology, 34*, 207–227.

Kluwer, E. S., & Karremans, J. (2009). Unforgiving motivations following infidelity: Should we make peace with our past. *Journal of Social Clinical Psychology, 28*, 1298–1325.

Lawler, K. A., Younger, J. W., Piferi, R. L., Billington, E., Jobe, R., Edmondson, K., et al. (2003). A change of heart: Cardiovascular correlates of forgiveness in response to interpersonal conflict. *Journal of Behavioral Medicine, 26*, 372–393.

Lawler, K. A., Younger, J. W., Piferi, R. L., Jobe, R., Edmondson, K., & Jones, W. H. (2005). The unique effects of forgiveness on health: An exploration of pathways. *Journal of Behavioral Medicine, 28*, 157–167.

Lawler-Row, K. A., Hyatt-Edwards, L., Wuensch, K. L., & Karremans, J. C. (2011). Forgiveness and health: The role of attachment. *Personal Relationships, 18*, 170–183.

Lawler-Row, K. A., Younger, J. W., Piferi, R. L., & Jones, W. H. (2006). The role of adult attachment style in forgiveness following an interpersonal offense. *Journal of Counseling and Development, 84*, 493–502.

Le, B., & Agnew, C. R. (2003). Commitment and its theorized determinants: A meta-analysis of the investment model. *Personal Relationships, 10*, 37–57.

Lehmiller, J. J. (2010). Differences in relationship investments between gay and heterosexual men. *Personal Relationships, 17*, 81–96.

Luchies, L. B., Finkel, E. J., McNulty, J. K., & Kumashiro, M. (2010). The doormat effect: When forgiving erodes self-respect and self-concept clarity. *Journal of Personality and Social Psychology, 98*, 734–749.

Maunder, R. G., & Hunter, J. J. (2001). Attachment and psychometric medicine: Developmental contrubutions to stress and disease. *Psychometric Medicine, 63*, 556–567.

McCullough, M. E., Fincham, F. D., & Tsang, J. (2003). Forgiveness, forbearance, and time: The temporal unfolding of transgression related interpersonal motivations. *Journal of Personality and Social Psychology, 84*, 540–557.

McCullough, M. E., Pargament, K. I., & Thoresen, C. E. (Eds.). (2000). *Forgiveness: Theory, research, and practice*. New York, NY: Guilford Press.

McCullough, M. E., Orsulak, P., Brandon, A., & Akers, L. (2007). Rumination, fear, and cortisol: An in vivo study of interpersonal transgressions. *Health Psychology, 26*, 126–132.

McEwen, B. S. (2004). Protection and damage from acute and chronic stress: Allostasis and allostatic overload and relevance to the pathophysiology of psychiatric disorders. *Annals of the New York Academy of Sciences, 1032*, 1–7.

Morse, C. R., & Metts, S. (2011). Situational and communicative predictors of forgiveness following a relational transgression. *Western Journal of Communication, 75*, 239–258.

Orcutt, H. K. (2006). The prospective relationship of interpersonal forgiveness and psychological distress symptoms in college women. *Journal of Counseling Psychology, 53*, 350–361.

Orcutt, H. K., Pickett, S. M., & Pope, E. B. (2008). The relationship of offense-specific forgiveness to posttraumatic stress disorder symptoms in college students. *Journal of Aggression, Maltreatment & Trauma, 16*, 72–91.

Petersen, M. B., Sell, A., Tooby, J., & Cosmides, L. (2010). To punish or repair? Evolutionary psychology and lay intuitions about modern criminal justice. *Evolution and Human Behavior, 33*, 682–695.

Riek, B. M., & Mania, E. W. (2012). The antecedents and consequences of interpersonal forgiveness: A meta-analytic review. *Personal Relationships, 19*, 304–325.

Rusbult, C. E. (1980). Commitment and satisfaction in romantic associations: A test of the investment model. *Journal of Experimental Social Psychology, 16*, 172–186.

Rye, M. S., & Pargament, K. I. (2002). Forgiveness and romantic relationships in college: Can it heal the wounded heart? *Journal of Clinical Psychology, 58*, 419–441.

Rye, M. S., Pargament, K. I., Pan, W., Yingling, D. W., Shogren, K. A., & Ito, M. (2005). Can group interventions facilitate forgiveness of an ex-spouse? A randomized clinical trial. *Journal of Consulting and Clinical Psychology, 73*, 880–892.

Schumann, K. (2012). Does love mean never having to say you're sorry? Associations between relationship satisfaction, perceived apology sincerity, and forgiveness. *Journal of Social and Personal Relationships, 29*, 997–1010.

Stoia-Caraballo, R., Rye, M. S., Pan, W., Kirschman, K. J. B., Lutz-Zois, C., & Lyons, A. M. (2008). Negative affect and anger rumination as mediators between forgiveness and sleep quality. *Journal of Behavioral Medicine, 31*, 478–488.

Strelan, P., & Covic, T. (2006). A review of forgiveness process models and a coping framework to guide future research. *Journal of Social and Clinical Psychology, 25*, 1059–1085.

Struthers, C. W., Dupius, R., & Eaton, J. (2005). Promoting forgiveness among co-workers following a workplace transgression: The effects of social motivation training. *Canadian Journal of Behavioural Science, 37*, 299–308.

Tsang, J., McCullough, M. E., & Fincham, F. D. (2006). The longitudinal association between forgiveness and relationship closeness and commitment. *Journal of Social and Clinical Psychology, 25*, 448–472.

Tse, W. S., & Yip, T. H. J. (2009). Relationship among dispositional forgiveness of others, interpersonal adjustment and psychological well-being: Implication for interpersonal theory of depression. *Personality and Individual Differences, 46*, 365–368.
Wieselquist, J. (2009). Interpersonal forgiveness, trust, and the investment model of commitment. *Journal of Social and Personal Relationships, 26*, 531–548.
Witvliet, C. V. O., Ludwig, T. E., & Laan Vander, K. L. (2001). Granting forgiveness or harboring grudges: Implications for emotion, physiology, and health. *Psychological Science, 12*, 117–123.
Worthington, E. L., Jr. (2003). *Forgiving and reconciling: Bridges to wholeness and hope*. Downers Grove, IL: Intervarsity Press.
Worthington, E. L., Jr. (2006). *Forgiveness and reconciliation: Theory and application*. New York, NY: Routledge/Taylor & Francis Group.
Worthington, E. L., Jr., Jennings, D. J. I. I., & DiBlasio, F. A. (2010). Interventions to promote forgiveness in couple and family context: Conceptualization, review, and analysis. *Journal of Psychology and Theology, 38*, 231–245.
Worthington, E. L., Jr., & Scherer, M. (2004). Forgiveness is an emotion-focused coping strategy that can reduce health risks and promote health resilience: Theory, review, and hypotheses. *Psychology and Health, 19*, 385–405.
Ysseldyk, R., Matheson, K., & Anisman, H. (2009). Forgiveness and the appraisal-coping process in response to relationship conflicts: Implications for depressive symptoms. *Stress: The International Journal on the Biology of Stress, 12*, 152–166.
Ysseldyk, R., & Wohl, M. J. A. (2012). I forgive therefore I'm committed: A longitudinal examination of commitment after a romantic relationship transgression. *Canadian Journal of Behavioral Science, 44*, 257–263.

Chapter 17
Forgiveness, Family Relationships and Health

Frank D. Fincham

Family relationships play an integral role in the psychological and physical health of family members, as well as the economic well-being of the family (see Beach & Whisman, 2012; Fincham & Beach, 2010). Paradoxically it is in family relationships that many of our important needs are met and yet some of our deepest hurts occur. These hurts can be occasioned by a violation of an implicit or explicit relationship norm, deceit, betrayal and so on. Although various options exist for dealing with such hurts (e.g., withdrawal, denial, condoning, reframing the transgressions), over the course of long-term relationships such as marriage they are unlikely to suffice. Little surprise, then, that the well known journalist/humorist, Robert Quillen (2008, p. 255), the Garrison Keillor of his day, wrote that "a happy marriage is the union of two good forgivers."

What are the consequences of forgiving versus not forgiving in family relationships? To the extent that failure to forgive results in destructive conflict and/or disruption of the family relationship, the results can be costly for those involved in the transgression as well as other family members. For example, the deleterious effect of marital discord on the psychological and physical health of spouses is well documented (e.g., Kiecolt-Glaser et al., 2005; Whisman, 2007), as is the panoply of effects it has on both child and adult offspring (e.g., Amato, 2010; Rhoades, 2008; Troxel & Mathews, 2004).

It is widely accepted that even though forgiveness (an intrapersonal process) should not be confused with relationship reconciliation (a dyadic process), it promotes prosocial motivational process that can lead to relationship repair and the

Preparation of this chapter was supported by a grant from the John Templeton Foundation.

F.D. Fincham (✉)
Florida State University, 120 Convocation Way, Tallahassee, FL 32306-1491, USA
e-mail: ffincham@fsu.edu

L.L. Toussaint et al. (eds.), *Forgiveness and Health*,
DOI 10.1007/978-94-017-9993-5_17

re-emergence of a healthy relationship. At a conceptual level then, it is apparent that forgiveness in family relationships can play a critical role in both the psychological and physical health of family members. The present chapter examines whether this is indeed the case.

Dimensions of Health

Psychological Health Even though there is a burgeoning literature on interventions to promote forgiveness in marital and family contexts (see Worthington & Jennings, 2010), most of these interventions are primarily psycho-educational and not specifically designed to deal with patient populations. Because certain conditions such as depression and marital discord tend to be co-morbid, it is quite possible that psychopathology may be present in distressed couples who seek such interventions. However, forgiveness intervention research and work on forgiveness in families more generally tends to focus on community samples and make use of dimensional measures of symptoms (e.g., anger, depression).

Physical Health There is growing evidence from large, national probability samples as well as smaller scale studies that forgiving a transgressor is associated with psychophysiological and psychoneuroimmunological processes, as well as self-reported measures of health (e.g., Lawler-Row, Karremans, Scott, Edlis-Matityahou, & Edwards, 2008; Worthington, Witvliet, Pietrini, & Miller, 2007). In fact, forgiveness is associated with cardiac risk in both community and patient populations (Friedberg, Sonia, & Srinivas, 2007; Toussaint & Cheadle, 2009). One study has even shown that conditional forgiveness, forgiveness that depends on the post transgression behavior of the transgressor, predicts mortality (Toussaint, Owen, & Cheadle, 2012). In sum, failure to forgive unconditionally poses health risks and appears to be life threatening.

In contrast to psychological health, relatively few studies on forgiveness and family relationships include indices of physical health and research on patient samples is conspicuous by its absence. In the absence of a body of research on diagnosed psychological or physical disorders in the literature on forgiveness and family relationships, caution should be used in generalizing observations made in this chapter to clinical populations.

Dimensions of Forgiveness in Family Relationships

Although the conceptualization and measurement of forgiveness are discussed elsewhere (see Chaps. 1 and 3), there are particular dimensions of forgiveness that require mention in the context of family relationships. Forgiveness has been most frequently characterized in terms of a motivational change in which resentment, anger, retaliatory impulses, and so forth are overcome. But is this decrease in unforgiveness sufficient in the context of ongoing family relationships? It is a logical error to infer the presence of the positive (e.g., health, forgiveness) from the absence of the negative (e.g., illness, unforgiveness). Therefore, it bears noting that equally fundamental to forgiveness is "an attitude of real goodwill towards the offender as a person" (Holmgren, 1993), and this is especially relevant to ongoing relationships, such as those that occur in a family. Although this benevolence dimension is not entirely absent from general research on forgiveness (e.g., TRIM-18; McCullough, Root, & Cohen, 2006), concerns about measuring forgiveness adequately in close relationships has led to development of relationship specific measures (e.g., The Marital Offence Forgiveness Scale; Paleari, Regalia, & Fincham, 2009). There is even some evidence to show that positive and negative dimensions of forgiveness have different correlates in family relationships. For example, unforgiveness but not forgiveness, was associated with spousal aggression (Fincham & Beach, 2002) and with partner reports of marital satisfaction (Paleari et al., 2009). Moreover, wives' forgiveness predicted husbands' reports of conflict resolution 12 months later whereas neither spouse's unforgiveness predicted later partner reports (Fincham, Beach & Davila, 2007).

Forgiveness can also be conceptualized at different levels of specificity: as a trait, as a tendency toward a specific relationship partner, and as an offense-specific response (see McCullough, Hoyt, & Rachal, 2000). Trait forgiveness, or forgivingness, occurs across relationships, offenses and situations whereas the tendency to forgive a particular relationship partner, sometimes referred to as dyadic forgiveness (Fincham, Hall, & Beach, 2006), is the tendency to forgive him or her across multiple offenses. Finally, offense-specific forgiveness is defined as a single act of forgiveness for a specific offense within a particular interpersonal context. Associations among these levels of forgiveness is modest at best (e.g., Allemand, Amberg, Zimprich, & Fincham, 20072007; Eaton, Struthers, & Santelli, 2007). In fact, Paleari et al. (2009) found that both positive and negative dimensions of forgiveness were more strongly related to relationship variables than to trait forgivingness, arguing that "relational characteristics may be more important in understanding forgiveness of interpersonal transgressions in close relationships than a global disposition to forgive" (Paleari et al., 2009, p. 205).

It can thus be argued that forgiveness in families most likely serves a purpose that is linked to the nature and functioning of the family relationship involved. For example, the operation of forgiveness should depend greatly on whether it occurs between two spouses, a parent and a child, two similarly aged siblings, parent and adult offspring and so on because each involves different roles and serves different psychological needs. For example, an evolutionary perspective suggests that avoidance engendered by unforgiveness should lead to less parental care in the parent–child relationship, causing unforgiving parents to have a decreased chance of gene replication (Trivers, 1985). This reproductive disadvantage alone suggests that forgiveness is different in the parent–child relationship from forgiveness in relationships between parents. Karremans and van Lange (2009) have similarly argued, and provided supportive data, for the view that forgiveness becomes part of the mental representation of a relationship, and it follows that forgiveness may be represented differently in different relationships. Attempts to examine forgiveness across different family relationships are limited but, as will be seen, they do support the above argument.

Theoretical/Conceptual Models of the Forgiveness-Health Connection in Families

Conceptual work on the forgiveness-health connection specifically in the context of families is lacking. This is hardly surprising given the relatively recent emergence of focused research on the forgiveness-health connection more generally. Indeed, after reviewing extant research relating to physical health, Harris and Thoresen (2005, p. 331) concluded, "we can reasonably hypothesize, yet not conclude, that chronic and intense unforgiveness are health risks." The need for conceptual development is particularly acute as evidenced in reviews of relevant literature (e.g., Worthington, Witvliet, Pietrini & Miller, 2007) where inferences made are sometimes quite tenuous and conclusions drawn often lack theoretical integration.

The above observations underline the importance of work by Witvliet and McCullough (2007) and McCullough, Root, Tabak, and Witvliet (2009) that examines potential pathways by which forgiveness may influence health. This work emphasizes the role of forgiveness in emotion regulation and the reduction of negative coping behaviors (e.g., substance use) that influence health. It may well be that the mechanism linking forgiveness and health is the stress response and physiological evidence documents a clear link between forgiveness and indices of stress (e.g., Lawler, Younger, Piferi, & Jones, 2006; McCullough et al., 2007; Witvliet, Ludwig & Van Der Laan, 2001). Lacking in these analyses, though, is consideration of how relationship functioning fits into the picture. Consider the two patterns of physiological arousal that have been associated with long-term health risk—sustained or chronic elevation of physiological processes and their acute reactivity to situational stressors such as partner transgressions. Poor quality relationships may make it harder to forgive the partner thereby facilitating chronic physiological arousal. In a similar vein, poor quality marital relationships are characterized by heightened reactivity to negative partner behavior (see Fincham, 2003). Indeed in low quality relationships merely imagining a typical interaction with the partner increases stress hormone levels (Berry & Worthington, 2001). In light of these observations, it is not surprising that poor marital quality is an important prognosticator of the occurrence of the metabolic syndrome, a cluster of risk factors for cardiovascular disease (Troxel, Matthews, Gallo, & Huller, 2005).

In short, a stress-and-coping framework wherein forgiveness ameliorates chronic (and possibly acute) stress responses to a transgression is likely to be helpful in understanding how forgiveness may impact health (see Worthington & Scherer, 2004). It is hypothesized that in such a framework the nature of the transgressor-victim relationship will be pivotal. Specifically, the nature of the relationship is hypothesized to moderate the link; there is likely to be a stronger relationship between unforgiveness and health in lower quality relationships than high quality ones. Whether the positive dimension of forgiveness will operate similarly is open to question. Fincham (2000) points out that the behaviors associated with the positive dimension of forgiveness do not have a unique topography and instead they simply comprise anything that reflects "an attitude of real goodwill." In contrast, unforgiveness is more readily identified as a cluster of negative emotions and motivations that include vengeance, resentment, bitterness, anger, fear, avoidance and rumination initiated by a transgression. It is little wonder, then, that it is unforgiveness that has typically been related to health outcomes.

Empirical Evidence of Forgiveness and Health in Families

As noted, forgiveness can be distinguished from unforgiveness, and both are viewed as important in ongoing relationships such as those found in families. It is posited that forgiveness and reduced unforgiveness may both be related to health outcomes indirectly by facilitating healthy relationships; however direct relationships to health outcomes may also exist. Each of these possibilities is now considered.

Is Forgiveness Associated with Relationship Properties Known to Increase Health Risk? Relationship quality is widely accepted as the final common pathway that leads couples and families to seek help. Not surprisingly, it has been a focus of research on forgiveness in family contexts. An association exists between both forgiveness and unforgiveness and marital quality (see Fincham, 2010; Fincham et al., 2006), with some indication of a more robust relationship for unforgiveness (Gordon, Hughes, Tomcizk, Dixon & Litzinge, 2009).[1] Longitudinal evidence suggests that marital quality predicts later forgiveness and that forgiveness also predicts later marital satisfaction (Fincham & Beach, 2007; Paleari et al., 2005). Turning to mechanisms that might account for the association, Fincham et al. (2004) suggested that unresolved transgressions may spill over into future conflicts and, in turn, impede their resolution, thereby putting the couple at risk for developing the negative cycle of interaction that characterizes distressed marriages. This would provide a mechanism that links forgiveness and relationship satisfaction and is further supported by the finding that forgiveness predicts behavioral responses to partner transgressions (Fincham, 2000). Indeed, unforgiveness predicts partner reported acts of psychological aggression in marriage whereas forgiveness predicts partner reports of constructive communication (Fincham & Beach, 2002). There is also some evidence that trust mediates the forgiveness-marital satisfaction association

[1]Many studies do not use separate measures of forgiveness and unforgiveness. Instead, they use a single unidimensional measure that comprises both types of items. For ease of presentation the word forgiveness is used in describing results from these studies.

in the case of both positive and negative forgiveness dimensions (Gordon et al., 2009). Finally, Schumann (2012) provides evidence to suggest that partners with higher relationship satisfaction are more forgiving as they tend to view apologies offered by the transgressor as more sincere.

Finkel, Rusbult, Kumashiro, and Hannon (2002) argue, however, that forgiveness in relationships is driven by the intent to persist in a relationship or commitment. They provide experimental data to support this view and there is no doubt a strong relationship between commitment and forgiveness (see Karremans & van Lange, 2008). However, Tsang, McCullough, and Fincham (2006) offered longitudinal evidence that forgiveness also promotes increases in commitment. Braithwaite, Selby, and Fincham (2011) specifically examined commitment and satisfaction together in examining the mechanism(s) linking forgiveness and relationship satisfaction. They found that conflict mediated the association between forgiveness and later relationship satisfaction independently of commitment and initial levels of relationship satisfaction. Their study also showed that behavioral regulation of relationship relevant behavior mediated the temporal association between forgiveness and relationship satisfaction.

In a similar vein, the quality of parent-child relationships was related to adolescent forgiving of parents, which, in turn, was associated with decreased parent-adolescent conflict (Paleari, Fincham, & Regalia, 2003). Maio, Thomas, Fincham, and Carnelley (2008) showed that forgiveness in families is specifically related to aspects of the relationship with the transgressor and not with other family members. However, they did show that higher forgiveness among family members correlated with a more positive experience of the family environment. Cross lagged analyses of longitudinal data also showed that child and mother forgiveness of the father predicted greater family expressiveness and less family conflict 12 months later; whereas child and father forgiveness of the mother predicted later family expressiveness and cohesiveness. Forgiveness of the child did not predict later family functioning. Importantly, these family level variables did not predict later forgiveness.

Hoyt, Fincham, McCullough, Maio, and Davila (2005) used the social relations model to examine variation within families in who tends to forgive (forgivingness) and who tends to be forgiven by others (forgivability). In doing so, they were able to partition variance into actor, partner, and relationship effects. The constellation of these effects varied across family relationships. However, relationship effects for both forgivingness and forgivability were consistently predicted by the degree of conflict present in the relationship. In a second study, they also found that trust significantly predicted the variance in forgivingness attributable to the relationship in the mother-father and mother-child relationships. Interestingly, relationship closeness was unrelated to variance in forgivingness and forgivability uniquely reflected in the relationship effects.

Finally, it has been found that in emerging adults forgiveness measures either fully or partially mediated associations between both parent–child relationship quality and interparental conflict and offspring psychological distress (Toussaint

& Jorgersen, 2008). Coop Gordon et al. (2009) also found effects involving interparental conflict in that husbands and wives'unforgiveness (but not forgiveness) predicted 11–16 year olds reports of interparental conflict properties.

It is possible to continue in this vein and document further aspects of relationships related to forgivingness (only Hoyt et al., 2005, studied forgivability). However, there is no need to do so, as it is readily apparent that forgivingness likely influences relationship health and vice versa. And relationships, especially in the family, can impact mental and physical health. We can thus conclude that forgiveness in family relationships is no doubt associated indirectly with health. This leaves us with the question of whether there is a direct relationship between forgiveness of family members and psychological and physical health.

Is There a Direct Association Between Forgiveness of Family Members and Health? In regard to the question just posed, a particular problem arises in relationship research, especially the marital research literature. This literature is strewn with studies in which constructs merely act as proxies for relationship quality, often giving rise to tautologies (see Fincham & Bradbury, 1987). As a result, Fincham et al. (2004) proposed the surplus value test whereby it is necessary to show that constructs do more than capture variance in commonly used measures of relationship quality. Absent such a requirement, forgiveness may simply function as a proxy index of relationship quality. They went on to show that forgiveness did pass this test in their studies. The importance of this test is emphasized by a finding obtained by Coop Gordon et al. (2009). They showed that both husband and wife unforgiveness strongly predicted the parenting alliance between spouses but that when marital satisfaction was added to the model the unforgiveness-parenting alliance became nonsignificant (i.e., unforgiveness was acting as a proxy for marital satisfaction in that particular link). However, forgiveness remained a significant predictor of parenting alliance in the full model. So in terms of predicting parenting alliance, unforgiveness did not pass the surplus value test but forgiveness did. Unfortunately, the surplus value test is not routinely applied in marital and family research.

A further problem in addressing our question stems from the fact that forgiveness research in family contexts rarely sets out to investigate issues of health per se. Nonetheless some data exist that are relevant to our question. As these data are often collected in the context of other endeavors, such as developing a new measure of forgiveness, they do not allow us to address the important question of whether forgiveness is related to health outcomes net of the characteristics of the relationship context in which it occurs. Most of the relevant data concern mental health but there are a few studies that examine indices relevant to physical health. Each is briefly reviewed.

More data exist on depressive symptoms and forgiveness in families than perhaps any other variable. There is a robust inverse relationship between depressive symptoms and forgiveness in marriage (e.g., Kachadourian, Fincham, & Davila, 2004). Paleari et al. (2009) showed that this association held for both unforgiveness and forgiveness and for both husbands and wives. A similar forgiveness-depression association was found with 12–16 year old children's forgiveness of a parent, but not, as might be expected, for parent forgiveness of the child (Maio et al., 2008). That may be because evolutionary considerations as well as social norms regarding forgiveness of children, should lead to parents forgiving children regardless of parents' depressive symptoms.

In many studies of forgiveness, trait level forgivingness is studied. However, the evidence reviewed thus far suggests that general trait forgivingness ignores the importance of relationship context for understanding forgiveness. This is true for also understanding any health correlate and is supported by data reported by Karremans, van Lange, Ouwerkerk, and Kluwer (2003, Study 4). They found that general forgiveness and partner forgiveness were only moderately correlated and that for both men and women spouse-specific forgiveness was more strongly correlated with a measure of life satisfaction than was general forgiveness. In a sample of emerging adults who self-identified as Christian, Toussaint and Jorgersen (2008) found that trait forgivingness as well as forgiveness of a wrong perpetrated by the mother and one by the father were negatively related to an overall measure of psychological distress. Although they did not test for differences involving dyadic forgiveness versus trait forgiveness, tests conducted for this chapter using the correlations they reported showed that they did not differ.

Finally, relevant evidence regarding psychological health is provided by a growing literature on forgiveness intervention studies (see Worthington & Jennings, 2010, for a review). In this literature, there is evidence to show that forgiveness interventions have led to decreased psychological symptoms and in some studies increased relationship satisfaction. Unfortunately, this literature includes numerous studies that use small sample sizes and are therefore underpowered. Nonetheless, consistency with the findings reviewed earlier is worthy of note.

Data regarding physical health is limited to three studies. Berry and Worthington (2001) found that a composite measure comprising forgiveness, unforgiveness and trait anger that they labeled 'forgiving personality' was related to cortisol reactivity to imagined interaction with the partner. However, this association was reduced to a nonsignificant level when relationship quality was considered (the surplus value test). Although forgiving personality was also related to a self-report measure of physical health (SF-36 Health Survey), their findings must be viewed with considerable caution as this study used an extreme groups design and there is no indication that correlations were computed within groups and then averaged in conducting the regression analyses reviewed here. Without computing correlations within extreme groups and then averaging them, the correlation found can be spurious and simply reflect the sampling of extreme groups. It is thus possible that the associations reported are an artifact of the design used. The remaining two studies examine the marital and parent–child relationships, respectively.

Hannon, Finkel, Kumashiro, and Rusbult (2012) examined whether conciliatory behavior—viewed as a proxy for forgiveness when displayed by the victim and amends when displayed by the perpetrator—during discussion of an unresolved marital transgression predicted blood pressure 40 min after the discussion. When examining dyadic data it is important to recognize that the data provided by each partner are not independent and therefore violate an important assumption of most statistical tests. As a result, specialized procedures have been developed that allow actor (intrapersonal) and partner (interpersonal) effects to be computed. Hannon et al. (2012) used one of these, the actor-partner interdependence model, to analyze their data. They found that victim, but not perpetrator, conciliatory behavior was inversely related to own and spouse's diastolic and systolic blood pressure. This finding remained when both relationship commitment and trait forgivingness were controlled and were altered only slightly when transgression severity and betrayal resolution were also controlled. Two observations are relevant in evaluating these findings. First, there is the question of whether the study measured something different from positive and negative interaction behavior (both types were used to assess conciliatory behavior) as there is a robust literature showing the link between such behaviors and health outcomes. Second, the absence of a baseline measure of blood pressure is problematic as are the nature of some of the tasks performed in the 40 min after the discussion (e.g., ego-depletion task). Notwithstanding such concerns, the results of the study are intriguing.

Turning to the parent-child relationship, Lawler-Row, Hyatt-Edwards, Wuench, and Karremans (2011) examined the relationships among attachment, forgiveness, and health. Premised, in part, on the view that insecure attachment is associated with stress and cardiovascular predictors of poorer health, these authors suggested that, "... focusing on the role of forgiveness in maintaining meaningful and satisfying relationships may prove to be a more fruitful explanatory concept than anger for understanding the link between forgiveness and health" (p. 171). They showed that forgiveness was inversely related to self-reported health problems and that forgiveness mediated the relation between insecure attachment and health. Moreover, both state forgiveness and trait forgivingness were related to heart rate and heart rate reactivity in response to and recovery from a stressor, a recalled hurt by one or both parents. Systolic blood pressure similarly showed reactivity to stress in that, for women but not men, a higher forgiveness group showed lower systolic blood pressure than a lower forgiveness group. An important concern in evaluating these findings is that they may be sample-specific given that groups were formed by a median split (which arbitrarily defines "high" versus "low").

Limitations of Existing Work on Forgiveness in the Family Context and Health
The modest size of the literature on forgiveness and families limits the conclusions that can be drawn about forgiveness of family members and health. Most notable is the paucity of research on health outcomes in a family context. Nonetheless, there is strong evidence that forgiveness in families is associated with important relationship characteristics. These characteristics (e.g., relationship quality, relationship conflict) have, in turn, been shown to predict both psychological and physical health outcomes. Consequently, we can infer that forgiveness is indirectly related to health via its impact on relationships. But we also know that relationship quality predicts later forgiveness and in this case, forgiveness might mediate the association between relationships and health. This said, it is still important to emphasize that we are

making inferences here, albeit reasonable ones, and that these inferences need to be the subject of research.

More direct evidence comes from examining direct relationships between forgiveness in family relationships and health. Here the evidence is somewhat scattered in that few studies set out specifically to examine this relationship. The very few studies that have done so represent a beginning but, as noted in describing them, each is subject to important limitations. These include use of correlational analyses in an extreme-groups design, use of median splits to form groups that may render results sample specific, and failure to control important variables that influence physiological functioning. For example, hemodynamic functioning follows a circadian rhythm, yet none of the studies control for time of day in data collection. Moreover, there is little evidence that forgiveness is related to health outcomes independently of the quality of the relationship between the family member who perpetrates the wrong and the family member victim.

Conclusions Notwithstanding the above limitations, several reasonable conclusions can be drawn. First, forgiveness of family members differs as a function of the relationship involved. In particular, forgiveness in parent–child relationships is quite different in that parent forgiveness of children has a strong evolutionary basis and is socially normative. Second, forgiveness impacts and is impacted by the quality of the relationship between the transgressor and victim, and it is well established that the quality of family relationships is associated with health outcomes. Thus, it seems that forgiveness, at a minimum, is indirectly related to health because of its impact on characteristics of the relationship. Third, there is a direct association between forgiveness of family members and psychological health, especially depressive symptoms. Fourth, research on forgiveness of family members and physical health is beginning, but it is too early to draw any conclusions in this regard. However, it seems likely that forgiveness of family members is related to physiological indices of stress.

Agenda for Future Research on Forgiveness in Families

It follows from the preceding observations that the first order of business for future research is to explicitly set out to investigate health outcomes of forgiveness in family relationships. In doing so, it is important for the field also to be cognizant of potential adverse effects of forgiveness. McNulty (2010), for example, has found that more forgiving spouses experienced stable or growing levels of psychological and physical aggression over the first 5 years of marriage, whereas less forgiving spouses experienced declines in partner transgression (see McNulty & Fincham, 2012, for further data and discussion). And, psychological and physical aggression are linked to poorer health.

Also central to this new endeavor is the need to expand the focus beyond that of the victim and to gather data on health outcomes for perpetrators. Causing harm to a family member has the potential to have a deleterious effect on the perpetrator and points to the potential role of self-forgiveness in family relationships. The importance of this topic is emphasized by a recent study that showed for both husbands and wives, transgressors were more satisfied with their marriages to the extent that they engaged in less self-unforgiveness and more self-forgiveness, whereas victimized partners were more satisfied with the relationship when the offending partner displayed less self-unforgiveness; more transgressor self-forgiveness was unrelated to their perceived relationship quality (Pelucci, Regalia, Paleari, & Fincham, 2013).

Consideration of both self-forgiveness and forgiveness of the other in family relationships highlights an important feature of family and, indeed, all ongoing relationships. In such relationships partners tend to be, simultaneously or alternatively, perpetrators and victims of transgressions. The imperfection of each partner necessarily gives rise to a history of hurts in a relationship.

This has several important implications for future research. First, and at the most fundamental level, is the need for clarity on what is forgiven. It is possible to consider forgiveness in regard to a hurtful relationship, as well as in regard to specific hurts. Forgiveness of a hurtful relationship is likely what was at issue in the finding that women at a domestic violence shelter who were more forgiving, reported being more likely to return to their abusive partners (Gordon, Burton, & Porter, 2004). It is hard to imagine anything but an inverse relationship between forgiveness and future health in such circumstances. Second, relationship partners are likely to develop a sense of how frequently they forgive their partner for transgressions and how frequently their partner forgives them. This can lead to feeling inequity, or imbalance (feeling underbenefited or overbenefited), when it comes to forgiveness. In the only study investigating the consequences of imbalance between giving and receiving forgiveness in marriage, it was found that among wives inequity in marital forgiveness predicted a decrease in personal and relational subjective well-being over a 6-month period (Paleari, Regalia, & Fincham, 2011). Finally, such findings make clear that the history of forgiveness in the family relationship studied is likely to be important for understanding the association between forgiveness and health in that relationship.

Perhaps the most obvious need for future research is to study patient populations—both those with acute physical disorders and those with intractable disorders. This is critical for providing a more complete understanding of the forgiveness-health association and opens up a number of new issues. For example, does unforgiveness and with it potential rumination lead to poorer treatment adherence, and under what conditions might it do so? Similarly, it is important to document how forgiveness and unforgiveness with a family member, especially one who assumes the role of care-giver impacts recovery from an illness and, where recovery is not possible (e.g., spinal cord injury), adaptation to the health condition. In these circumstances it is not only forgiveness by the patient but also by the care-giver that is likely to be important, especially when forgiveness is relevant to the burden imposed by the illness.

Implications for Health Enhancement, Medicine, Integrative Treatment

In considering the implications of forgiveness in families it behooves us to remember that forgiveness is a motivated behavior. And like all motivated behavior it can arise from good and bad motives. Thus forgiveness can be used strategically to manipulate others, to put them down and so on. Under such circumstances forgiveness can be quite harmful. However, if the outward expressions of forgiveness truly reflect internal motivations, it is safe to conclude that forgiveness plays an important salutary role in amicable family relationships and that this role promotes health both directly and indirectly by repairing the relationship. This is perhaps most poignantly captured by the philosopher Boleyn-Fitzgerald's (2002) observation that forgiveness is "arguably the most important virtue for controlling anger" (p. 483). Acute anger can impact health, especially when accompanied by physical violence, and the adverse impact of chronic anger on health is well known.

However, it is worth noting the qualifier "amicable" in the above statement. There is now evidence that the impact of expressing forgiveness can be moderated by context. As McNulty's (2008) work shows, expressing forgiveness in the context of on-going conflictual relationships predicts lower satisfaction in newlyweds over the first year of marriage and perhaps indirectly leads to poorer health. McFarland, Smith, Toussaint, and Thomas (2012) found that the relationship between forgiveness and health was negative for people who lived in more dilapidated or run-down conditions and positive for those who lived in more affluent conditions. They concluded that "...forgiveness was beneficial in some settings but had a deleterious impact in more noxious environments" (p. 66). Although the referent in their case was neighborhoods, the conclusion is equally applicable to relationships. Some relationships are simply not healthy and should be terminated. There is nothing inconsistent in simultaneously ending such relationships and engaging in forgiveness of the partner. Indeed, both ending the relationship and forgiving the partner is likely to yield the best health outcome.

Assuming forgiveness is prudent and safe, it may be the preferred option and one that promotes mental and physical health. In this case it is advantageous to recognize that forgiveness is a process that takes time. It is not achieved immediately, a circumstance that can lead to problems when the offending spouse takes a partner's statement of forgiveness ("I forgive you") literally rather than as a promissory note ("I am trying to forgive you"). Thus, when hurt feelings regarding a transgression arise after a statement of forgiveness, the offending partner may experience confusion or anger if he or she believes that the matter had been previously resolved. The temptation to equate forgiveness with a specific act at a specific point in time (usually now) is strong. Accordingly, both transgressor and victim need to be mindful of the temporal dimension of forgiveness and that resurfacing of feelings associated with the initial transgression at a later time is normal and does not negate the forgiveness process.

It remains to note again the growing literature on forgiveness interventions in family contexts (Worthington & Jennings, 2010). Given the difficulty of doing experimental work in this area, intervention studies have the potential to provide much needed information on mechanisms involved in forgiveness. To date, however, this potential remains largely untapped because the dismantling of these multicomponent interventions to determine the active ingredients for changing forgiveness is notably absent. To realize more fully their potential to advance understanding of forgiveness in family relationships and health, intervention studies, like more general research, also need to include assessments of both relationship characteristics relevant to health as well as measures of psychological and physical health.

To conclude, forgiveness in the family context holds considerable potential for understanding, and ultimately improving, both mental and physical health. Whether this potential is realized will depend on the emergence of methodologically sound, programmatic work linking forgiving in family relationships and health. The observations offered in this chapter represent an attempt to shape a future in which the above mentioned potential is realized.

References

Allemand, M., Amberg, I., Zimprich, D., & Fincham, F.D. (2007). The role of trait forgiveness and relationship satisfaction in episodic forgiveness. *Journal of Social and Clinical Psychology, 26*, 199–217.

Amato, P. (2010). Research on divorce: Continuing trends and new developments. *Journal of Marriage and Family, 72*, 650–666.

Beach, S. R. H., & Whisman, M. (2012). Relationship distress: Impact on mental illness, physical health, children, and family economics. In S. R. H. Beach, R. Heyman, A. Smith Slep, & H. Foran (Eds.), *Family problems and family violence* (pp. 91–100). New York, NY: Springer.

Berry, J. W., & Worthington, E. L. (2001). Forgivingness, relationship quality, stress while imagining relationship events, and physical and mental health. *Journal of Counseling Psychology, 4*, 447–455.

Boleyn-Fitzgerald, P. (2002). What should "forgiveness" mean? *The Journal of Values Inquiry, 36*, 483–498.

Braithwaite, S., Selby, E., & Fincham, F. D. (2011). Forgiveness and relationship satisfaction: Mediating mechanisms. *Journal of Family Psychology, 25*, 551–559.

Eaton, J., Struthers, C. W., & Santelli, A. G. (2006). Dispositional and state forgiveness: The role of self-esteem, need for structure, and narcissism. *Personality and Individual Differences, 41*, 371–380.

Fincham, F. D. (2000). The kiss of the porcupines: From attributing responsibility to forgiving. *Personal Relationships, 7*, 1–23.

Fincham, F. D. (2003). Marital conflict: Correlates, structure and context. *Current Directions in Psychological Science, 12*, 23–27.

Fincham, F. D. (2010). Forgiveness: Integral to a science of close relationships? In M. Mikulincer & P. Shaver (Eds.), *Prosocial motives, emotions, and behavior: The better angels of our nature* (pp. 347–365). Washington, D.C: American Psychological Association.

Fincham, F. D., & Beach, S. R. H. (2002). Forgiveness in marriage: Implications for psychological aggression and constructive communication. *Personal Relationships, 9*, 239–251.

Fincham, F. D., & Beach, S. R. H. (2007). Forgiveness and marital quality: Precursor or consequence in well-established relationships. *Journal of Positive Psychology, 2*, 260–268.

Fincham, F. D., & Beach, S. R. H. (2010). Marriage in the new millennium: A decade in review. *Journal of Marriage and Family, 72*, 630–649.

Fincham, F. D., Beach, S. R. H., & Davila, J. (2004). Forgiveness and conflict resolution in marriage. *Journal of Family Psychology, 18*, 72–81.

Fincham, F. D., Beach, S. R. H., & Davila, J. (2007). Longitudinal relations between forgiveness and conflict resolution in marriage. *Journal of Family Psychology, 21*, 542–545.

Fincham, F. D., & Bradbury, T. N. (1987). The assessment of marital quality: A reevaluation. *Journal of Marriage and the Family, 49*, 797–809.

Fincham, F. D., Hall, J., & Beach, S. R. H. (2006). Forgiveness in marriage: Current status and future directions. *Family Relations, 55*, 415–427.

Finkel, E. J., Rusbult, C. E., Kumashiro, M., & Hannon, P. A. (2002). Dealing with betrayal in close relationships: Does commitment promote forgiveness? *Journal of Personality and Social Psychology, 82*, 956–974.

Friedberg, J. P., Sonia, S., & Srinivas, V. S. (2007). Relationship between forgiveness and psychological and physiological indices in cardiac patients. *International Journal of Behavioral Medicine, 16*, 205–211.

Gordon, K. C., Burton, S., & Porter, L. (2004). Predicting the intentions of women in domestic violence shelters to return to partners: Does forgiveness play a role? *Journal of Family Psychology, 18*, 331–338.

Gordon, K. C., Hughes, F. M., Tomcik, N. D., Dixon, L. J., & Litzinger, S. C. (2009). Widening spheres of impact: The role of forgiveness in marital and family functioning. *Journal of Family Psychology, 23*, 1–13.

Hannon, P. A., Finkel, E. J., Kumashiro, M., & Rusbult, C. E. (2012). The soothing effects of forgiveness on victims' and perpetrators' blood pressure. *Personal Relationships, 19*, 279–289.

Harris, A. H. S., & Thoresen, C. E. (2005). Forgiveness, unforgiveness, health and disease. In E. L. Worthington Jr. (Ed.), *Handbook of forgiveness* (pp. 321–334). New York, NY: Brunner-Routledge.

Holmgren, M. R. (1993). Forgiveness and the intrinsic value of persons. *American Philosophical Quarterly, 30*, 342–352.

Hoyt, W. T., Fincham, F. D., McCullough, M. E., Maio, G., & Davila, J. (2005). Responses to interpersonal transgressions in families: Forgivingness, forgivability, and relationship-specific effects. *Journal of Personality and Social Psychology, 89*, 375–394.

Kachadourian, L. K., Fincham, F. D., & Davila, J. (2004). The tendency to forgive in dating and married couples: Association with attachment and relationship satisfaction. *Personal Relationships, 11*, 373–393.

Karremans, J. C., & van Lange, P. A. M. (2008). Forgiveness in personal relationships: Its malleability and powerful consequences. *European Review of Social Psychology, 19*, 202–241.

Karremans, J.C. & van Lange, P. A. (2009). The malleability of forgiveness. In M. Mikulincer & P.R. Shaver (Eds.), *Prosocial motives, emotions, and behavior* (pp. 285–302). Washington, DC: American Psychological Association.

Karremans, J. C., van Lange, P. A. M., Ouwerkerk, J. W., & Kluwer, E. S. (2003). When forgiveness enhances psychological well-being: The influence of interpersonal commitment. *Journal of Personality and Social Psychology, 84*, 1011–1026.

Kiecolt-Glaser, J. K., Loving, T. J., Stowell, J. R., Malarkey, W. B., Lemeshow, S., Dickinson, S. L., & Glaser, R. (2005). Hostile marital interactions, proinflammatory cytokine production, and wound healing. *Archives of General Psychiatry, 62*, 1377–1384.

Lawler-Row, K. A., Hyatt-Edwards, L., Wuench, K. L., & Karremans, J. C. (2011). Forgiveness and health: The role of attachment. *Personal Relationships, 18*, 170–183.

Lawler-Row, K. A., Karremans, J. C., Scott, C., Edlis-Matityahou, M., & Edwards, L. (2008). Forgiveness, physiological reactivity and health: The role of anger. *International Journal of Psychophysiology, 68*, 51–58.

Lawler-Row, K. A., Younger, J., Piferi, R. L., & Jones, W. H. (2006). The role of adult attachment style in forgiveness following an interpersonal offense. *Journal of Counseling and Development, 84,* 493–502

Maio, G. R., Thomas, G., Fincham, F. D., & Carnelley, K. (2008). Unraveling the role of forgiveness in family relationships. *Journal of Personality and Social Psychology, 94,* 307–319.

McCullough, M. E., Orsulak, P., Brandon, A., & Akers, L. (2007). Rumination, fear, and cortisol: An in vivo study of interpersonal transgressions. *Health Psychology, 26,* 126–132.

Mc Nulty, J. K., & Fincham, F. D. (2012). Beyond positive psychology? Toward a contextual view of psychological processes and well-being. *American Psychologist, 67,* 101–110.

McCullough, M. E., Hoyt, W. T., & Rachal, K. C. (2000). What we know (and need to know) about assessing forgiveness constructs. In M. McCullough, K. I. Pargament, & C. E. Thoresen (Eds.), *Forgiveness: Theory, research and practice* (pp. 65–90). New York, NY: Guilford.

McCullough, M. E., Root, L. M., & Cohen, A. D. (2006). Writing about the benefits of an interpersonal transgression facilitates forgiveness. *Journal of Consulting and Clinical Psychology, 74,* 887–897.

McCullough, M. E., Root, L. M., Tabak, B., & Witvliet, C. V. O. (2009). Forgiveness. In S. J. Lopez (Ed.), *Handbook of positive psychology* (2nd ed., pp. 427–435). New York, NY: Oxford.

McFarland, M. J., Smith, C. A., Toussaint, L., & Thomas, P. A. (2012). Forgiveness of others and health: Do race and neighborhood matter? *Journals of Gerontology. Series B, Psychological Sciences and Social Sciences, 67,* 66–75.

McNulty, J. K. (2008). Forgiveness in marriage: Putting the benefits into context. *Journal of Family Psychology, 22,* 171–175.

McNulty, J. K. (2010). Forgiveness increases the likelihood of subsequent partner transgressions in marriage. *Journal of Family Psychology, 24,* 787–790.

Paleari, F. G., Regalia, C., & Fincham, F. D. (2003). Adolescents' willingness to forgive parents: An empirical model. *Parenting: Science and Practice, 3,* 155–174.

Paleari, G., Regalia, C., & Fincham, F. D. (2005). Marital quality, forgiveness, empathy, and rumination: A longitudinal analysis. *Personality and Social Psychology Bulletin, 31,* 368–378.

Paleari, F. G., Regalia, C., & Fincham, F. D. (2009). Measuring offence-specific forgiveness in marriage: The Marital Offence-Specific Forgiveness Scale (MOFS). *Psychological Assessment, 21,* 194–209.

Paleari, F. G, Regalia, C., & Fincham, F. D. (2011). Inequity in forgiveness: Implications for personal and relational well-being. *Journal of Social and Clinical Psychology, 30,* 297–324.

Pelucci, S., Regalia, C., Paleari, F. G. & Fincham, F. D. (2013). Self-forgiveness in romantic relationships: It matters to both of us. *Journal of Family Psychology, 27,* 541–549.

Quillen, R. (2008). In J. H. Moore (Ed.), *The voice of small town America: The selected writings of Robert Quillen, 1920–1948.* Columbia, SC: University of South Carolina Press.

Rhoades, K. A. (2008). Children's responses to interparental conflict: A meta-analysis of their associations with child adjustment. *Child Development, 79,* 1942–1956.

Schumann, K. (2012). Does love mean never having to say you're sorry? Associations between relationship satisfaction, perceived apology sincerity, and forgiveness. *Journal of Social and Personal Relationships, 29,* 997–1010

Toussaint, L., & Cheadle, A. C. D. (2009). Unforgiveness and the broken heart: Unforgiving tendencies, problems due to unforgiveness, and 12-month prevalence of cardiovascular health conditions. In M. T. Evans & E. D. Walker (Eds.), *Religion and psychology.* New York, NY: Nova.

Toussaint, L., & Jorgersen, K. M. (2008). Inter-parental conflict, parent-child relationship quality, and adjustment in Christian adolescents: Forgiveness as a mediating variable. *Journal of Psychology and Christianity, 27,* 337–346.

Toussaint, L. L., Owen, A. D., & Cheadle, A. C. D. (2012). Forgive to live: Forgiveness, health, and longevity. *Journal of Behavioral Medicine, 35,* 375–386.

Trivers, R. (1985). *Social evolution.* Menlo Park, CA: Benjamin/Cummings.

Troxel, W. M., & Matthews, K. A. (2004). What are the costs of marital conflict and dissolution to children's physical health? *Clinical Child and Family Psychology Review, 7*, 29–57.

Troxel, W. M., Matthews, K. A., Gallo, L. C., & Huller, L. H. (2005). Marital quality and occurrence of the metabolic syndrome in women. *Archives of Internal Medicine, 165*, 1022–1027.

Tsang, J. A., McCullough, M. E., & Fincham, F. D. (2006). Forgiveness and the psychological dimension of reconciliation: A longitudinal analysis. *Journal of Social and Clinical Psychology, 25*, 404–442.

Whisman, M. A. (2007). Marital distress and *DSM-IV* psychiatric disorders in a population-based national survey. *Journal of Abnormal Psychology, 116*, 638–643.

Witvliet, C. V. O., Ludwig, T. E., & Vander Laan, K. L. (2001). Granting forgiveness or harboring grudges: Implications for emotion, physiology, and health. *Psychological Science, 121*, 117–123.

Witvliet, C. V. O., & McCullough, M. E. (2007). Forgiveness and health: A review and theoretical exploration of emotion pathways. In S. G. Post (Ed.), *The science of altruism and health* (pp. 259–276). New York, NY: Oxford Press.

Worthington, E. L., Jr., & Jennings, D. J. (2010). Interventions to promote forgiveness in couple and family context: Conceptualization, review, and analysis. *Journal of Psychology and Theology, 38*, 231–245.

Worthington, E. L., Jr., & Scherer, M. (2004). Forgiveness as an emotion focused coping strategy that can reduce health risks and promote health resilience: Theory, review and hypotheses. *Psychology and Health, 19*, 385–405.

Worthington, E. L., Jr., Witvliet, C. V. O., Pietrini, P., & Miller, A. J. (2007). Forgiveness, health and wellbeing: A review of evidence for emotional versus decisional forgiveness, dispositional forgivingness, and reduced unforgiveness. *Journal of Behavioral Medicine, 30*, 291–302.

Chapter 18
Forgiveness Interventions to Promote Physical Health

Barbara Elliott

Forgiveness and unforgiveness are linked with how we live our lives, our relationships with others, and our health experiences. The connections between forgiveness, unforgiveness, mental health diagnoses, and relational pathologies are well described (Harris & Thoresen, 2005). These concepts encompass the mental health response and consequences of dealing with a perceived offense. For those who think beyond the mind and consider psychophysiology, human coping mechanisms, and other mind-body connections, additional questions emerge regarding the physical experiences of forgiveness and unforgiveness.

Forgiveness and unforgiveness have been linked to short-term physiological responses (Witvliet, Ludwig, & Vander Laan, 2001; Worthington, Witvliet, Pietrini, & Miller, 2007), providing the basis to hypothesize, if not conclude, that chronic and continuing unforgiveness may present a risk to human physical health (Worthington et al., 2007), and/or that forgiveness interventions may have a role to play in reducing these physical experiences (Worthington & Scherer, 2004). More recently, observations about parallels between the physical impact of chronic or longstanding unforgiveness and experiences of chronic illnesses open the possibilities that forgiveness interventions may also have important personal and public health relevance and impact (Elliott, 2011).

The purpose of this chapter is to (a) review how unforgiveness and forgiveness are experienced physically and what impact forgiveness interventions have on human physiology and health conditions; (b) propose a model describing these relationships; and (c) identify a research agenda to move this scholarship forward.

B. Elliott (✉)
Department of Family Medicine and Community Health, University of Minnesota, 1035 University Drive, Duluth, MN 55812, USA
e-mail: belliott@d.umn.edu

L.L. Toussaint et al. (eds.), *Forgiveness and Health*,
DOI 10.1007/978-94-017-9993-5_18

Definitions

Health In 1948 the World Health Organization defined health using a definition that has not been changed in more than 60 years: "Health is a state of complete physical, mental and social well-being and not merely the absence of disease or infirmity" (World Health Association, 1948). This definition clearly includes mental, relational, and physical health experiences, and notes that variations or disruptions in this desired experience and well-being can be understood as un-health or labeled as illness, disease, or pathology.

Current Western scholarship is endorsing the bio-psycho-social-spiritual (BPSS) model (Engel, 1977; Parse, 1981) to better explain the complexity of human health experience. The BPSS model defines human health and well being as the result of multiple life dimensions.

Unforgiveness and Forgiveness It is important to note specific dimensions of forgiveness that are particularly relevant to this discussion of unforgiveness, forgiveness and physical health. First, for purposes of this discussion, *unforgiveness* is recognized as a state of mind-body experience that develops when people perceive themselves to have been victimized and continue to attribute power and control over their well being to an offender for the action. Unforgiveness can become a chronic state of being, continuing over time and engaging the body's stress response (Elliott, 2011; Harris & Thoresen, 2005; Lavelock, Griffin, & Worthington, 2013; Sapolsky, 2005; Worthington et al., 2007).

Forgiveness has been conceptualized both as a coping mechanism and as a description of the state of mind-body experience when the forgiveness coping mechanism has been engaged. This experience can be based in either spiritual or secular processes, and forgiveness is used to cope with the BPSS stresses of living with unforgiveness. Forgiveness can be focused to neutralize an offense perceived as committed by others (*forgiveness of others*), or it can be employed to forgive ones-self (*self-forgiveness*) for perceived burdens resulting from one's own behaviors. *Decisional forgiveness* references the use of this coping mechanism at a cognitive level, where a decision is made to change one's behavior regarding the offender. Alternately, forgiveness as a coping mechanism can be engaged more broadly, involving cognitive, emotional and motivational levels. This coping process is termed *emotional forgiveness*, and results in the elimination of the attributed power and control. Emotional forgiveness is documented to be more powerful physiologically compared to decisional forgiveness (Worthington et al., 2007) and has been described as an emotional and spiritual transformation (Lawler et al., 2005). When people accomplish emotional forgiveness, the literature describes them as having achieved the mind-body state of forgiveness. Throughout this writing, when the term forgiveness is used, it will reference the state of well being achieved through emotional forgiveness, unless specified differently.

It is also important to note the variety of approaches that can be engaged to teach how to use the forgiveness coping mechanism, which can lead to the state of forgiveness and its related physiological changes. Effective forgiveness education and counseling can be spiritually based (Harris, Thoresen, McCullough, & Larson, 1999; Lavelock et al., 2013; Post & Wade, 2009) or educationally designed (Toussaint, Owen, & Cheadle, 2012); in addition forgiveness training can be accomplished at the bedside by nursing personnel (Recine, Wener, & Recine, 2009), others in community educational programs (Toussaint et al., 2012), and still others through one-on-one sessions with counselors who may be spiritually based (Lavelock et al., 2013). In any case, if the coping mechanism of forgiveness is to become recognized as an effective intervention for physical conditions, from what we know to date, each of these methods can be engaged successfully (Wade, Hoyt, Meyer, & Worthington, 2014).

The Physiology of the Stress Response To survive, the human body protects itself with its response to the stressors it encounters. Stressors are perceived through the senses, and the brain coordinates the physiologic responses through the nervous, endocrine and immune systems, with brief as well as long-term impacts on the body. In most settings these responses are part of maintaining normal physiologic functioning of the human organism (e.g., *homeostasis*) in its environments; when the stressors are long-standing, the continuing responses create a physiologic *allostasis* Thoresen, Harris, & Luskin, 2001, with the chronic physiologic burden, termed the *allostatic load* (Sapolsky, 2005).

With the perception of a stressor, the brain becomes both the generator and recipient of the chemical responses. The endocrine system is engaged and activates the HPA (hypothalamic-pituitary-adrenal) while the autonomic nervous system engages the SAM (Sympathetic-Adrenal Medullary) system. Among the first and most powerful of these chemicals are the corticosteroids and catecholamines that impact heart and respiration rates, blood glucose levels, constriction of blood vessels, gastro-intestinal (GI) track functioning, heightened brain responses (perception, physical withdrawal, depression, memory, etc.), physical shaking, and (within the immune system) T- helper and T- suppression cells. If the heightened stress response becomes chronic because the perceived stress is ongoing, the body adjusts to this allostatic load, which also impacts the brain's neuroplasticity and structural integrity. These biomarkers and brain findings are the primary physiologic indicators of the stress response. (Cohen, Janicki-Deverts, & Miller, 2007; Dickerson & Kemeny, 2004; Ganzel, Morris & Wethinton, 2010; Kemeny, 2003).

Mechanisms Connecting Stress and Health

Scientific theories suggest how the experiences of chronic stress and specific health outcomes are connected (Shonkoff, Boyce, & McEwen, 2009), and recent experimental work describes the biological pathways that are implicated with these theories (de Kloet, Joels, & Holsboer, 2005; Miller, Cohen, & Ritchey, 2002). Theory suggests that the allostatic load becomes toxic as it accumulates over time, and the body's endocrine, immune and/or cardiac systems are permanently changed to adjust to the biochemical burden. These ideas are complemented with the observation that when a stress burden occurs at a particularly sensitive developmental period, it becomes incorporated in the person's brain and physiology.

A variety of studies in the medical literature support these theories by describing how the chronic stress experience impacts a person's health. People with a history of maltreatment have been documented to live with an up-regulation of their immune system's inflammatory response, compared to those with no history of maltreatment (Danese, Pariante, Caspi, Taylor, & Poulton, 2007). Another study has documented that the stress management systems (e.g., stress hormones, heart rate, blood pressure, flight/fear readiness) that are controlled by the brains in those with history of chronic stress are dysregulated, compared to non-exposed adults (McEwen, 1998, 2000). The chronic stress of this experience is recognized to result in physiologic "weathering" (Geronimus, 1992); this experience is biologically exhausting and results in shortened life spans (Geronimus, Hicken, Keene, & Bound, 2006).

Complementing these studies is the developing brain imaging research that has also been focusing on the brain impacts of chronic stressors. Brain imaging has investigated how experiences change the brain at developmentally sensitive times, and which parts of the brain are impacted by particular circumstances. These neuroimaging studies have revealed changes in both brain anatomy and brain activity, and attribute the changes to the chronic stress (Shonkoff et al., 2009).

Modeling the Stress-Forgiveness-Physical Health Connection

As noted above, the bio-psycho-social-spiritual (BPSS) model of understanding human health explains that health is experienced as the result of these multiple dimensions, creating a level of perceived well being. The reality of this complex structure-and-function connection is displayed by brain imaging studies. These studies reveal that the parts of the brain that are engaged with psychological-social-spiritual experiences of forgiveness (especially in the left frontal cortex) are also actively engaged with the body's physical responses to the environment (Farrow et al., 2001; Farrow & Woodruff, 2005; Newberg & deMarici, 2001).

The most widely accepted theoretical explanation connecting these brain-imaging results and a person's physical response to experiencing forgiveness is the stress-and-coping model. This theoretical approach was first presented in 2004 (Worthington & Scherer, 2004) and discussed more fully in 2006 (Strelan & Covic, 2006; Worthington, 2006); it has been recently expanded by Lavelock and her colleagues (2013). In the past the stress-and-coping understanding of forgiveness was used to explain the personal and relational consequences resulting from offensive experiences. Lavelock's recent work reviews the literature examining

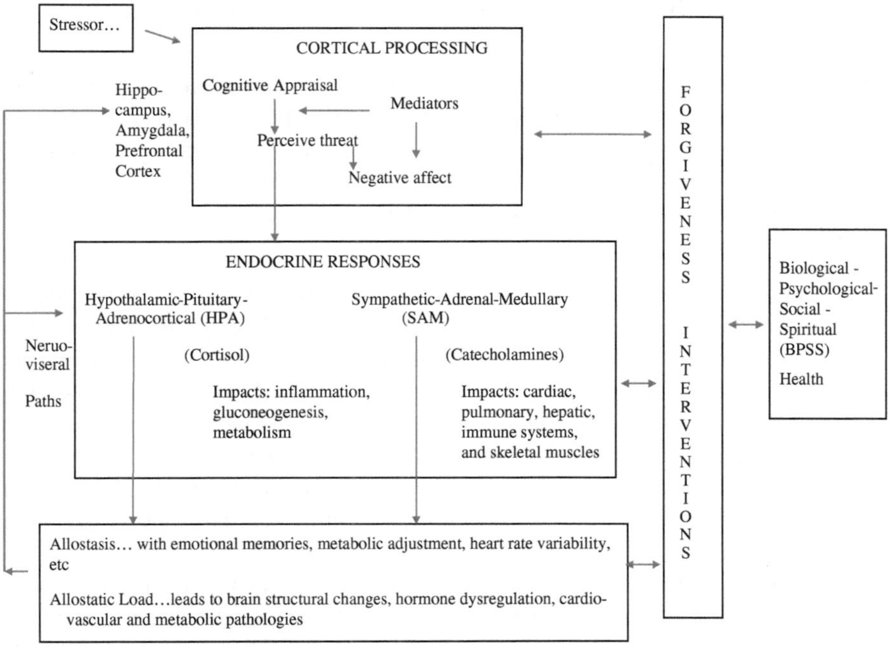

Fig. 18.1 Stress, forgiveness, and bio-psycho-social-spiritual health

the theoretical role of forgiveness in offenses that have resulted in physical consequences. The Lavelock diagram of the stress response model further develops earlier efforts with inclusion of Lazarus' work (Lazarus, 1999), describing how the mind engages the (various) forgiveness coping responses to effectively mitigate the stress experience with its resulting outcomes, including physical consequences.

The stress-and-coping model proposed in Fig. 18.1 builds on both the work in the medical sciences described above and Lavelock's recent work. Figure 18.1, presented here, postulates that when a person perceives an offense, the experience engages the psychological, social, and spiritual as well as physiologic stress responses, and forgiveness is considered one of the available coping options in this process. Figure 18.1 proposes that people perceive threats, experience those (chronic) stressors, can employ forgiveness as a coping strategy, and then experience that full response within their biological, psychological, social and/or spiritual health experiences.

It is interesting to note that recent quantitative assessments of the role of forgiveness in the health research also support this model. These studies have used structural equation modeling and path analysis to document that the coping mechanism of forgiveness functions in a mediating way with hostility in health (Lutjen, Silton, & Flannelly, 2012) and with anger and health (Lawler-Row, Karremans, Scott, Edlis-Matityahou, & Edwards, 2008).

Empirical Evidence of Forgiveness Interventions and Health

The Physiologic Impact of Forgiveness Interventions and Identified Mediators To date, most of the research regarding the physiology of forgiveness and its impact on bodily functioning has documented particular physiologic responses in settings of forgiveness and unforgiveness. Returning to Fig. 18.1, the findings in this area of scholarship describe changes represented to the left of the Forgiveness Interventions portion in the model.

Unforgiveness is experienced as negative emotions resulting in a cascade of biological and brain responses that create allostatic load. Findings about the body's hormone response to unforgiveness reveal that unforgiveness is reflected in specific cortisol levels, adrenaline production and cytokine balance (Worthington, Witvliet, Lerner, & Scherer, 2005), with patterns that parallel those reported in people living with high stress. These hormone patterns are known to compromise the immune system (Berry & Worthington, 2001; Seybold, Hill, Neumann, & Chi, 2001) with the long-term consequence of leading to several identified chronic illnesses (Danese et al., 2007).

The body's response to stress has also been investigated in people who have accomplished forgiveness, compared to those of others who have continuing unforgiveness. Forgiveness reportedly results in beneficial physiologic changes, including lower heart rate, increased rate of cardiovascular recovery (including heart rate variability or HRV), lower cholesterol ratios, reduced resting blood pressure, less EMG tension, and reduced skin conductance (Friedberg, Suchday, & Srinivas, 2009; Lawler et al., (2003); Witvliet et al., 2001, 2007). Each of these physiologic markers is documented to normalize with forgiveness.

It is important to note that the research efforts have been investigating the relationships between forgiveness and physiologic markers of health are now also incorporating mediating variables in their analyses. This increasing sophistication also refines the theoretical models about stress, forgiveness, and health, and adds to our understanding of how forgiveness is experienced as part of a person's well being. The possibility of accomplishing forgiveness seems to be variably available to people, depending on their mental health, personality traits, and social experiences. Some people have personality characteristics (or make attributions about others' characteristics) that impair their ability to forgive (Tabak & McCullough, 2011). Others are less able to forgive because of their social circumstances, including their race, neighborhood, faith or other social experiences (Lavelock et al., 2013; McFarland, Smith, Toussaint, & Thomas, 2011). Still others need to "grow into" their ability to forgive: older people and those nearing the end of their lives seem more adept at forgiving (Girard & Mullet, 1997; Toussaint, Williams, Musick, & Everson, 2001; Worthington et al., 2007; also see Chap. 14 of this volume).

Interestingly, it seems that the ability to forgive can be cultivated among those with a predisposition to forgive also termed "forgivingness" (Harris et al., 2006; Wade & Worthington, 2005; Worthington et al., 2007); this is important information for understanding and creating educational and therapeutic approaches to accomplishing forgiveness. And it is this observation that moves us again into the physical sphere: there may, at least in part, be a genetic predisposition that allows this experience. This of course, will need future investigations (for preliminary research in this area see Chap. 5 of this volume).

Forgiveness Interventions' Impact on Health Status and Health Conditions Reviews of the relationships between forgiveness, unforgiveness, health and disease were summarized in Harris and Thoresen's (2005) review, and hypotheses were proposed to explain how physiologic changes might be expected with forgiveness interventions (Worthington & Scherer, 2004), anticipating broader health benefits that might accompany this transformation (Lawler et al., 2005). Current reports are now describing research efforts that actually move to the right of the Forgiveness Interventions portion of Fig. 18.1. Most of the studies report correlational relationships between forgiveness interventions and experienced physical health. To date, only a few studies have completed clinical trials that document the impact of forgiveness intervention on physical health outcomes.

Correlational Investigations Correlational investigations have reported positive relationships between forgiveness and a variety of health outcomes, including the ultimate outcome of mortality. Toussaint's recent study documented that people who experience forgiveness also enjoy longer life spans, thus linking forgiveness and health at a population-level (Toussaint et al., 2012). Overall, in a community sample, forgiveness has been associated with indices of good health (Seybold et al., 2001).

At an individual level, studies have reported positive associations between forgiveness and health outcomes in segments of the population. Among people living with cardiac problems, studies have reported that people living with higher forgiveness also experience reduced cholesterol levels (Friedberg, Suchday, & Srinivas, 2009), a higher heart rate variability (Lawler-Row et al., 2008), and reduced prevalence of heart events over 12 months (Toussaint & Cheadle, 2009). In addition, in people living with HIV forgiveness has been associated with improved quality of life (Martin, Vosvick, & Riggs, 2012), and enhanced immune system functioning (Owen, Hayward, & Toussaint, 2011).

Positive correlational findings specifying the relationships of self forgiveness and health outcomes add to these findings. These studies report: (a) improvements in health status, improved quality of life (SF-12) scores, and reduced pain experience among people in physical therapy (Svalina & Webb, 2012); (b) improvements in reported health outcomes and satisfaction with life among people living with Spinal Cord injuries (Webb, Toussaint, Kalpakjian, & Tate, 2010); and (c) improvements in quality of life scores among women living with breast cancer (Romero, Friedman, Kalidas, Ellidge, Chang, & Liscum, 2006); and (d) improvements in perceived physical health (Wilson, Milosovic, Carroll, Hart, & Hibbard, 2008).

For people who experience health conditions that are identified with both mental health and physical health diagnoses, correlational studies have also suggested the role of forgiveness is important in achieving health: (a) among college students with suicidal behaviors, forgiveness (of others and of self) are associated with fewer suicidal behaviors (Hirsch, Webb, & Jeglic, 2011); (b) for people living with eating disorders, increased self forgiveness is related to fewer symptoms (Watson et al., 2012); and (c) non-suicidal self-injuries increase when there is a lack of self forgiveness reported by participants (Westers, Rehfuss, Olson, & Biron, 2012).

Intervention Studies Recently, these correlation studies have been extended into intervention studies. The impact of forgiveness interventions in the cardiac health of people with coronary artery disease has been investigated. Waltman's study demonstrated that participants experienced positive cardiac health outcomes following a forgiveness intervention training: they experienced significantly fewer cardiac perfusion defects, compared to their pre-test levels and compared to the control group (Waltman, Russell, Coyle, Enright, Hoter, & Swoboda, 2009).

Research that investigated the development of a forgiveness education intervention was tested with people living with fibromyalgia. The exploratory trial with this intervention noted that the forgiveness intervention was followed by an improvement in the report of pain among those living with this condition (Toussaint et al., 2013).

Research has also documented that perceived health status is improved with forgiveness interventions in aging adults (Ingersoll-Dayton, Campbell & Ha, 2009), and forgiveness interventions also strengthen participants' willingness to continue in physical rehabilitation exercises (Lavelock et al., 2013).

In other studies with people who experience health conditions that are identified with both mental and physical health diagnoses, interventions toward self-forgiveness have also been shown to improve participants' perception of and experiences of health: (a) drinkers experience an increased efficacy in their refusal of drinking (Scherer, Worthington, Hook, & Campana, 2011); and (b) there is a reduction in vulnerability to drug use over 4 weeks (Wei-Fen Lin, 2010).

Implications for Health and Medicine

In addition to the studies discussed above, a variety of chronic physical health conditions, including obesity, chronic obstructive pulmonary disease (COPD), and cirrhosis, have been identified as health conditions with social and interpersonal etiologies that seem to impact the body through the consequences of living with the allostatic load related to adverse early life experiences. The seminal project in this research, the ACES study, documented that early experiences with one or more types of adversity result in shortened life spans due to chronic illnesses, mental health challenges, and social dysfunction (Edwards, Holden, Felitti, & Anda, 2003; Felitti, 1998), paralleling the scholarship reviewed above. These studies and many that have followed it (including Caspi, Harrington, Moffitt, Milne, & Poulton, 2006; Dong et al., 2004; Hills et al., 2004; Horwitz, Widom, McLaughlin, & White, 2001; Shilling, Aseltine, Gore, 2007) have consistently detailed relationships between early adverse experiences and later health outcomes.

The consistency of this scholarship within the medical and epidemiologic literatures further supports the observations in the stress-and-forgiveness literature that there are chronic physical (and psychological, social, and spiritual) health consequences of living with allostatic load.

Reports regarding the effectiveness of forgiveness interventions with people who live with chronic psychological, social and spiritual suffering have been described here. Integrating these findings using the model proposed in Fig. 18.1 suggests the mechanism by which forgiveness allows longer life spans through mitigation of the stress response to an allostatic load, resulting in improved physical (and psychological, social and spiritual) health.

Current work is investigating the link between allostatic load and health outcomes, documenting the biological pathways that create the dysfunctions (Miller, Chen, & Parker, 2011). To date, the studies investigating the link between forgiveness and health outcomes have not explored how the forgiveness interventions improve specific stress-related physical bio-markers or how they impact functioning more generally. These studies hold enormous potential for human health. In light of the early findings as described above, that people with cardiovascular disease who experience forgiveness have improved cardiac prognoses (Friedberg et al., 2009; Toussaint & Cheadle, 2009), we can hypothesize that the treatment and prevention of other identified stress-related chronic health conditions (e.g., addictions, obesity, COPD and cirrhosis) may also be improved with this intervention. These studies hold life-changing health consequences for the large numbers of people who live with these conditions.

Future Research Directions

Future research projects are needed to learn the extent to which and how forgiveness interventions impact human health and well-being. Sophisticated and controlled research projects are needed to further evaluate these emerging insights, especially projects that use longitudinal designs. Longitudinal methodologies can examine how the experience with forgiveness changes the experience of human health over time. Longitudinal projects are also needed to identify insights that will build on the model presented in this chapter. These projects will need to focus on the (a) the neurologic, endocrine and immunological markers in this psycho-physiologic relationship; b) the relationships between forgiveness and health at various points in the life course; and (c) the impact of social relationships and social support in the forgiveness-health process.

Future studies will also need to identify appropriate populations for this research. This process will involve identifying people who are living in settings that offer natural experiments involving forgiveness and chronic stress (e.g., Amish groups for whom forgiveness is both a spiritual and cultural norm); populations with certain life experiences that are lived as chronic stressors (e.g., victims of child abuse); or groups who live with certain stress-impacted health conditions (e.g., obesity, diabetes, COPD). The examples listed here are settings for potential studies, since each of these potential study populations lives with a type of chronic stress that is recognized to impact human health. These groups are suggested because their experiences would expand what is known regarding their health and physiologic responses when: (a) forgiveness is experienced despite chronic stressors; (b) past victimization is known to generate continuing allostatic load with physiologic consequences; or (c) physical (health) consequences are being impacted—and perhaps caused by—the chronic stress of the allostatic load. Of course, multiple additional groups offer additional settings to measure the physiologic markers and health circumstances in groups with and without forgiveness interventions.

Another important dimension of this needed future research is the assurance that effective forgiveness interventions are consistently delivered and achieved—otherwise the findings regarding the physical (and psychologic-social-spiritual) health changes for those experiencing the intervention will not be valid or consistent. There are models for this intervention, both secularly (Recine, Wener, & Recine, 2009; Toussaint et al., 2013; Wade et al., 2014) and religiously (Harris et al., 1999; Lavelock et al., 2013; Post & Wade, 2009) motivated—and both have been shown to be effective. Clearly, these future projects will involve multiple disciplines working together to observe the relationship between forgiveness and personal health experiences (Webb, Toussaint, & Conway-Williams 2012). These collaborative projects will need to include skilled facilitators for the interventions and other scientists to assure documentation of the observations and measurements of the physiologic and health consequences.

The collaborations in this future research will also need to include consistent focus on the participants' personal and social health, as well as other characteristics in these forgiveness studies. Current research models identify the "mediators", referencing those personal and social characteristics that impact how people perceive and respond to stress. Identifying and describing these mediators can offer important insights regarding who can access and physiologically benefit from a forgiveness intervention, with its genetic implications.

As these collaborations evolve, their findings will be reported and that will suggest the following generation of research questions. It is possible that additional theories, other than the stress-forgiveness-BPSS health model proposed here, will emerge to offer explanations of this forgiveness-health impact as well—and scholars will need to be open to interpreting research results in light of this potential paradigm shift.

Limitations

It is important to acknowledge a few cautions as we prepare for these next steps. Consistency in the delivery of the forgiveness intervention is essential, as noted above. Related to that is the importance of assuring the therapeutic skill (and motivation) of the person facilitating that intervention to avoid further victimizing a person participating as a subject in the research process. Also, future research must be exceedingly clear, as discussed in Chap. 2 of this volume, about the use of common definitions, concepts, and measurements of the variables of interest, whether they are psychological, social, spiritual or physical. This clarity is essential in order to move the field forward.

Funding has not been commonly available for studies that extend the traditional approaches to understanding disease and illness. Nonetheless, the findings presented here indicate that this approach has personal and public health benefit.

Conclusion

The review and analysis presented here suggest future collaborative research in clinical and research settings to assess the extent to which forgiveness therapies can address and heal the burdensome consequences of stress-related health experiences. It is exciting to recognize that these interventions may have an enormous personal and public health impact in treatment of the health consequences of chronic stress experiences.

References

Berry, J. W., & Worthington, E. L., Jr. (2001). Forgiveness, relationship quality, stress while imagining relationship events, and physical and mental health. *Journal of Counseling Psychology, 48*, 447–455.

Caspi, A., Harrington, H., Moffitt, T. E., Milne, B. J., & Poulton, R. (2006). Socially isolated children 20 years later: Risk of cardiovascular disease. *Archives of Pediatric and Adolescent Medicine, 160*(8), 805–811.

Cohen, S., Janicki-Deverts, D., & Miller, G. E. (2007). Psychological stress and disease. *Journal of the American Medical Association, 298*(14), 1685–1687.

Danese, A., Pariante, C. M., Caspi, A., Taylor, A., & Poulton, R. (2007). Childhood maltreatment predicts adult inflammation in a life-course study. *Proceedings of the National Academy of Science of the United States of America, 104*(4), 1319–1324.

De Kloet, E. R., Joels, M., & Holsboer, F. (2005). Stress and the brain: From adaptation to disease. *Nature Reviews/Neuroscience, 6*, 463–465.

Dickerson, S. S., & Kemeny, M. E. (2004). Acute stressors and cortisol responses: A theoretical integration and synthesis of laboratory research. *Psychological Bulletin, 130*(3), 355–391.

Dong, M., Giles, W. H., Felitti, V. J., Dube, S. R., Williams, J. E., Chapman, D. P., & Andra, R. F. (2004). Insights into causal pathways for ischemic heart disease: Adverse childhood experiences study. *Circulation, 110*(13), 1761–1766.

Edwards, V. J., Holden, G. W., Felitti, V. J., & Anda, R. F. (2003). Relationship between multiple forms of childhood maltreatment and adult mental health in community respondents: Results from the adverse childhood experiences study. *American Journal of Psychiatry, 160*(8), 1453–1460.

Elliott, B. A. (2011). Forgiveness therapy: A clinical intervention for chronic disease. *Journal of Religion and Health, 50*(2), 240–247.

Engel, G. L. (1977). The need for a new medical model: A challenge for biomedicine. *Science, 196*(4286), 129–136.

Farrow, T. F. D., & Woodruff, P. W. R. (2005). Neuroimaging of forgivability. In E. L. Worthington Jr. (Ed.), *Handbook of forgiveness* (pp. 259–272). New York, NY: Brunner-Rutledge.
Farrow, T. F. D., Zheng, Y., Wilkinson, I. D., Spence, S. A., Deakin, J. F. W., Tarrier, N., et al. (2001). Investigating the functional anatomy of empathy and forgiveness. *Neuroreport, 12*(11), 2433–2438.
Felitti, V. (1998). Relationship of childhood abuse and household dysfunction to many of the leading causes of death in adults: The adverse childhood experiences (ACES) study. *American Journal of Preventive Medicine, 14*(4), 245–258.
Friedberg, J. P., Suchday, S., & Srinivas, V. S. (2009). Relationship between forgiveness and psychological and physiological indices in cardiac patients. *International Journal of Behavioral Medicine, 16*(3), 205–211.
Ganzel, B. L., Morris, P. A., & Wetherington, E. (2010). Allostasis and the human brain: Integrating models of stress from the social and life sciences. *Psychological Review, 117*(1), 134–174.
Geronimus, A. T. (1992). The weather hypothesis and the health of African-American women and infants: Evidence and speculations. *Ethnicity and Disease, 2*(3), 207–221.
Geronimus, A. T., Hicken, M., Keene, D., & Bound, J. (2006). 'Weathering' and age patterns of allostatic load scores among blacks and whites in the United States. *American Journal of Public Health, 96*(5), 826–833.
Girard, M., & Mullet, E. (1997). Forgiveness in adolescents, young, middle-aged, and older adults. *Journal of Adult Development, 4*, 209–220.
Harris, A. H. S., Luskin, F., Norman, S. B., Standard, S., Bruning, J., Evans, S., et al. (2006). Effects of a group forgiveness intervention on forgiveness, perceived stress, and trait-anger. *Journal of Clinical Psychology, 62*(6), 715–733.
Harris, A. H. S., & Thoresen, C. E. (2005). Forgiveness, unforgiveness, health and disease. In E. L. Worthington Jr. (Ed.), *Handbook of forgiveness* (pp. 321–334). New York, NY: Brunner-Routledge.
Harris, A. H. S., Thoresen, C. E., McCullough, M. E., & Larson, D. B. (1999). Spiritually and religiously oriented health interventions. *Journal of Health Psychology, 4*(3), 413–433.
Hills, S. D., Anda, R. F., Dube, S. R., Felitti, V. J., Marchbanks, P. A., & Marks, J. S. (2004). The association between adverse childhood experiences and adolescent pregnancy, long-term psychosocial consequences and fetal death. *Pediatrics, 113*(2), 320–327.
Hirsch, J. K., Webb, J. R., & Jeglic, E. L. (2011). Forgiveness, depression, and suicidal behavior among a diverse sample of college students. *Journal of Clinical Psychology, 67*, 1–11.
Horwitz, A. V., Widom, C. S., McLaughlin, J., & White, H. R. (2001). The impact of childhood abuse and neglect on adult mental health: A prospective study. *Journal of Health and Social Behavior, 42*(2), 184–201.
Ingersoll-Dayton, B., Campbell, R., & Ha, J. (2009). Enhancing forgiveness: A group intervention for the elderly. *Journal of Gerontological Social Work, 52*(1), 2–16.
Kemeny, M. E. (2003). The psychobiology of stress. *Current Directions in Psychological Science, 12*, 124–129.
Lavelock, C. R., Griffin, B. J., & Worthington, T. L. (2013). Forgiveness, religiousness, spirituality and health in people with physical challenges: A review and a model. In R. L. Piedmont & A. Village (Eds.), *Research in the social scientific study of religion* (Vol. 24, pp. 53–92). Boston, MA: Brill.
Lawler, K. A., Younger, J. W., Piferi, R. L., Billington, E., Jobe, R., Edmondson, K. E., & Jones, W. H. (2003). A change of heart: Cardiovascular correlates of forgiveness in response to interpersonal conflict. *Journal of Behavioral Medicine, 26*, 373–393.
Lawler, K. A., Younger, J. W., Piferi, R. L., Jobe, R. L., Edmondson, K. A., & Jones, W. H. (2005). The unique effects of forgiveness on health: An exploration of pathways. *Journal of Behavioral Medicine, 28*(2), 157–167.
Lawler-Row, K. A., Karremans, J. C., Scott, C., Edlis-Matityahou, M., & Edwards, L. (2008). Forgiveness, physiological reactivity and health: The role of anger. *International Journal of Psychophysiology, 68*, 51–58.

Lazarus, R. S. (1999). *Stress and emotion: A new synthesis*. New York, NY: Springer.
Lin, W.-F. (2010). The treatment of substance abuse disorders by the psychological forgiveness. *Bulletin of Educational Psychology, 41*(4), 859–884.
Lutjen, L. J., Silton, N. R., & Flannelly, K. J. (2012). Religion, forgiveness, hostility and health: A structural equation analysis. *Journal of Religion and Health, 51*(2), 468–478.
Martin, L. A., Vosvick, M., & Riggs, S. A. (2012). Attachment, forgiveness, and physical health quality of life in HIV+ adults. *AIDS Care, 24*(11), 1333–1340.
McEwen, B. S. (1998). Protective and damaging effects of stress mediators. *New England Journal of Medicine, 338*(3), 171–179.
McEwen, B. S. (2000). The neurobiology of stress: From serendipity to clinical relevance. *Brain Research, 886*(1–2), 172–189.
McFarland, M. J., Smith, C. A., Toussaint, L., & Thomas, P. A. (2011). Forgiveness of others and health: Do race and neighborhood matter? *The Journals of Gerontology Series B: Psychological Sciences and Social Sciences, 67*(1), 66–75.
Miller, G. E., Chen, E., & Parker, K. J. (2011). Psychological stress in childhood and susceptibility to the chronic diseases of aging: Moving towards a model of behavioral and biological mechanisms. *Psychological Bulletin, 137*(6), 959–997.
Miller, G. E., Cohen, S., & Ritchey, A. K. (2002). Chronic psychological stress and the regulation of pro-inflammatory cytokines: A glucocorticoid-resistance model. *Health Psychology, 21*(6), 531–541.
Newberg, A. B., & deMarici, V. (2001). The neurophysiological correlates of forgiveness. In M. E. McCullough, K. I. Pargament, & C. E. Thoresen (Eds.), *Forgiveness: Theory, research and practice* (pp. 91–110). New York, NY: Guilford Press.
Owen, A. D., Hayward, R. D., & Toussaint, L. L. (2011, April). *Forgiveness and immune functioning in people living with HIV-AIDS*. Paper presented at the Society of Behavioral Medicine, Washington, DC.
Parse, R. R. (1981). *Man-living-health: A theory of nursing*. New York, NY: Wiley.
Post, B. C., & Wade, N. G. (2009). Religion and spirituality in psychotherapy: A practice-friendly review of research. *Journal of Clinical Psychology: In Session, 65*(2), 131–146.
Recine, A. C., Wener, J. S., & Recine, L. (2009). Health promotion through forgiveness intervention. *Journal of Holistic Nursing, 27*(2), 115–123.
Romero, C., Friedman, L. C., Kalidas, M., Ellidge, R., Chang, J., & Liscum, K. R. (2006). Self-forgiveness, spirituality and psychological adjustment in women with breast cancer. *Journal of Behavioral Medicine, 29*(1), 29–36.
Sapolsky, R. M. (2005). The physiology and pathophysiology of unhappiness. In E. L. Worthington Jr. (Ed.), *Handbook of forgiveness* (pp. 273–304). New York, NY: Brunner-Rutledge.
Scherer, M., Worthington, E. L., Jr., Hook, J. N., & Campana, K. L. (2011). Forgiveness and the bottle: Promoting self-forgiveness in individuals who abuse alcohol. *Journal of Addictive Diseases, 30*(4), 382–395.
Seybold, K. S., Hill, P. C., Neumann, J. K., & Chi, D. S. (2001). Physiological and psychological correlates of forgiveness. *Journal of Psychology and Christianity, 20*, 250–259.
Shilling, E. A., Aseltine, R. H., Jr., & Gore, S. (2007). Adverse childhood experiences and mental health in young adults: A longitudinal survey. *BMC Public Health, 7*, 30.
Shonkoff, J. P., Boyce, W. T., & McEwen, B. S. (2009). Neuroscience, molecular biology, and the childhood roots of health disparities: Building a new framework for health promotion and disease prevention. *Journal of the American Medical Association, 301*(21), 2252–2259.
Strelan, P. G., & Covic, T. (2006). A review of forgiveness process models and a coping framework to guide future research. *Journal of Social and Clinical Psychology, 10*, 1059–1085.
Svalina, S. S., & Webb, J. R. (2012). Forgiveness and health among people in outpatient physical therapy. *Disability & Rehabilitation, 34*(5), 383–392.
Tabak, B. A., & McCullough, M. E. (2011). Perceived transgressor agreeableness decreases cortisol response and increases forgiveness following recent interpersonal transgressions. *Biological Psychology, 87*, 386–392.

Thoresen, C. E., Harris, A. H. S., & Luskin, F. (2001). Forgiveness and health: An unanswered question. In M. E. McCullough & K. I. Pargament (Eds.), *Forgiveness: Theory, research, and practice* (pp. 254–280). New York, NY: Guilford Press.

Toussaint, L. L., & Cheadle, A. (2009). Unforgiveness and the broken heart: Unforgiving tendencies, problems due to unforgiveness, and 12-month prevalence of cardiovascular health conditions. In M. T. Evans & E. D. Walker (Eds.), *Religion and psychology* (pp. 97–135). New York, NY: Nova Science.

Toussaint, L. L., Williams, D. R., Musick, M. A., & Everson, S. A. (2001). Forgiveness and health: Age differences in a U.S. probability sample. *Journal of Adult Development, 8*, 249–257.

Toussaint, L., Owen, A. D., & Cheadle, A. (2012). Forgive to live: Forgiveness, health and longevity. *Journal of Behavioral Medicine, 35*, 375–386.

Toussaint, L., Vincent, A., Whipple, M., Finnie, D., Hathaway, J., McAllister, S., & Vickers, K. S. (2013). A psycho-educational forgiveness program for fibromyalgia patients: Development and preliminary evaluation (in press).

Toussaint, L., Vincent, A., Whipple, M., McAllister, S., Finnie, D., Hathaway, J., Oh, T. H., Fleming, K. C., & Vickers Douglas, K. S. (2014). Forgiveness education in fibromyalgia: A qualitative inquiry. *Pain Studies and Treatment, 2*(1), 11–16. http://dx.doi.org/10.4236/pst.2014.21003

Wade, N. G., & Worthington, E. L., Jr. (2005). In search of a common core: A content analysis of interventions to promote forgiveness. *Psycho-Therapy, 42*, 160–177.

Wade, N. G., Hoyt, W. T., Kidwell, J. E. M., & Worthington, E. L. (2014). Efficacy of psychotherapeutic interventions to promote forgiveness: A meta-analysis. *Journal of Consulting and Clinical Psychology, 82*, 154–170.

Waltman, M. A., Russell, D. C., Coyle, C. T., Enright, R. D., Holter, A. C., & Swoboda, C. (2009). The effects of a forgiveness intervention on patients with coronary artery disease. *Psychology and Health, 24*, 11–27.

Watson, M. J., Lydecker, J. A., Jobe, R. L., Enright, R. D., Gartner, A., Mazzeo, S. E., & Worthington, E. L., Jr. (2012). Self-forgiveness in anorexia nervosa and bulimia nervosa. *Eating Disorders: The Journal of Treatment & Prevention, 10*(1), 31–41.

Webb, J. R., Toussaint, L. L., Kalpakjian, C. Z., & Tate, D. G. (2010). Forgiveness and health related outcomes among people with spinal cord injury. *Disability and Rehabilitation, 32*(5), 360–366.

Webb, J. R., Toussaint, L., & Conway-Williams, E. (2012). Forgiveness and health: Psycho-spiritual integration and the promotion of better healthcare. *Journal of Health Care Chaplaincy, 18*, 57–73.

Westers, N. J., Rehfuss, M., Olson, L., & Biron, D. (2012). The role of forgiveness in adolescents who engage in nonsuicidal self-injury. *The Journal of Nervous and Mental Disease, 200*(6), 535–541.

Wilson, T., Milosovic, A., Carroll, M., Hart, K., & Hibbard, S. (2008). Physical health status in relation to self-forgiveness and other-forgiveness in health college students. *Journal of Health Psychology, 13*(6), 798–803.

Witvliet, C. V. O., Ludwig, T. E., & Vander Laan, K. L. (2001). Granting forgiveness or harboring grudges: Implications for emotion, physiology, and health. *Psychological Science, 12*(2), 117–123.

Witvliet, C. V. O., Worthington, E. L., Jr., Root, L. M., Sato, A. F., Ludwig, T. E., & Exline, J. J. (2007). Retributive justice, restorative justice, and forgiveness: An experimental psychophysiology analysis. *Journal of Experimental Social Psychology, 44*, 10–25.

World Health Association. (1948). Preamble to the constitution of the World Health Organization. In *International health conference* (Official records of the World Health Organization, no. 2, p. 100). New York, NY: World Health Association.

Worthington, E. L., Jr. (2006). *Forgiveness and reconciliation: Theory and application*. New York, NY: Routledge.

Worthington, E. L., Jr., & Scherer, M. (2004). Forgiveness is an emotion-focused coping strategy that can reduce health risks and promote health resilience: Theory, review, and hypotheses. *Psychology and Health, 19*(3), 385–405.

Worthington, E. L., Jr., Witvliet, C. V. O., Lerner, A. J., & Scherer, M. (2005). Forgiveness in health research and medical practice. *Psychology and Health, 1*(3), 169–176.

Worthington, E. L., Jr., Witvliet, C. V. O., Pietrini, P., & Miller, A. J. (2007). Forgiveness, health, and well-being: A review of evidence for emotional versus decisional forgiveness, dispositional forgivingness, and reduced unforgiveness. *Journal of Behavioral Medicine, 30*, 291–302.

Part V
Conclusion

Chapter 19
Concluding Thoughts: Summary and Integration, Models, and Research Agendas

Loren L. Toussaint, Everett L. Worthington, Jr., and David R. Williams

We began this book with the goal of understanding a relatively simple question. Is forgiveness related to health? In reading to this point, you have probably come to understand that the answer to that question is not so straightforward. On one hand, evidence supports the conclusion that forgiveness is related to health. For instance, Lavelock, Snipes, Griffin, Worthington, Davis, Hook, Benotsch, & Ritter (Chap. 3) reviewed 95 studies of forgiveness and health between 2003 and 2014. However, the evidence base is not a deep one. On some issues, we simply lack sufficient research to draw firm conclusions. In one case, Leach and Parazak (Chap. 15) state that, "Little research has been accomplished integrating international forgiveness research with health." In fact, the most consistent refrain heard from all research teams is the call for more research on forgiveness and health.

If we have enough research to conclude, albeit tentatively, that forgiveness is related to health, but if we need still more evidence to decipher the exact nature of the connection, then an important consideration is the research agenda that investigators might pursue. Thankfully, the expert writing teams that have contributed to this book have taken this as one of their charges. They have identified detailed agendas for future research in each of their respective areas. In addition, they have provided explicit conceptualizations of forgiveness and health that will

L.L. Toussaint (✉)
Department of Psychology, Luther College, College Dr. 700, 52101 Decorah, IA, USA
e-mail: tauslo01@luther.edu

E.L. Worthington, Jr.
Department of Psychology, Virginia Commonwealth University, Richmond, VA, USA
e-mail: eworth@vcu.edu

D.R. Williams
Harvard T.H. Chan School of Public Health, Huntington Ave. 677, 02115-6096 Boston, MA, USA
e-mail: DWILLIAM@hsph.harvard.edu

L.L. Toussaint et al. (eds.), *Forgiveness and Health*,
DOI 10.1007/978-94-017-9993-5_19

undoubtedly prove useful in moving this area forward. Furthermore, they have discussed useful theoretical and conceptual models that offer heuristic value. What follows is our attempt to consolidate some of the learning that can be gained reading through the chapters. We seek to crystalize the key themes and identify a few especially interesting and unique questions that arise in each of these areas. We begin by reviewing conceptualizations of forgiveness and health. Next, we highlight some of the most useful models that might move this area forward. Last, we review the most consistently mentioned limitations and directions for future work.

The basis of our concluding thoughts is a comprehensive 50-page table that examines the key contributions of each chapter. This table provides a side-by-side comparison of each chapter's contributions on each of the following issues: (1) forgiveness definition, (2) health definition, (3) conceptual models, (4) conceptual figures and tables, (5) empirical evidence, (6) limitations, (7) conclusions, (8) research agenda, and (9) implications. If not for its size, we would have included the table in the chapter. Instead, we encourage interested readers to request the table from Dr. Toussaint.

Definitions

Forgiveness Experts across all areas agree that forgiveness is multifaceted. The forgiveness literature was once dominated by an almost singular focus on forgiving others (Hall & Fincham, 2005), but it has recently grown to encompass several additional dimensions. Contributors to this book have commonly discussed forgiving others, forgiving oneself, and feeling forgiven by God. Forgiving others is usually done when one has experienced an injustice or hurt at their hands. Forgiving oneself or feeling forgiven (or not) by God usually occurs when one is the offender or perpetrator or when one condemns himself or herself for failings or unmet expectations. In considering the multiple dimensions of forgiveness, care has been taken to clearly distinguish these constructs along theoretical and theological lines. It is all too tempting to discuss forgiveness of self and others and feeling forgiven by God all in the same breath and to treat them as slightly different shades of grey. Over half of the chapters in this book explicitly define forgiveness as multidimensional. When they do, they take care to delineate these dimensions.

We hope to encourage the practice of carefully explicating the dimensional structure of forgiveness. We urge investigators to continue to seek ways to understand each aspect of forgiving from theological, theoretical, and empirical standpoints that reveal more about how these experiences are similar and different. Toward that end, Tucker, Bitman, Wade, and Cornish (Chap. 1) offer five key questions to ask when attempting to define forgiveness: (a) Are there implicit or explicit theological, moral, or lay perspectives? (b) Is there a distinction between decisional and emotional forgiveness? (c) Is there a distinction between reducing unforgiveness and forgiving? (d) What is the endpoint of forgiveness in terms of required changes in cognition, emotions, motivations, behaviors and their combinations? (e) Is there a distinction between state forgiveness and trait forgivingness? Tucker et al. provide a guiding framework from which to continue to explore and refine the meaning of forgiveness.

In 2005 in the concluding chapter of the *Handbook of Forgiveness*, Worthington (2005) suggested that there was good consensus across experts in the field on what forgiveness was *not* and that there was also good consensus on what forgiveness *is* if one accepts that forgiveness has multiple aspects. The emphasis at the time was almost singularly on forgiving others. A similar consensus exists for the pluralistic definition of forgiveness today that encompasses a much wider scope of aspects of forgiveness that go beyond simply forgiving others. For instance, consensus seems to be growing on the definition of self-forgiveness as including release from shame, guilt, and self-loathing—in short, self-condemnation—and the promotion of self-acceptance and benevolence toward the self (Fisher & Exline, 2010; Hall & Fincham, 2005; Worthington, 2013). Likewise, good conceptual work has been done on the construct of feeling forgiven by God (Exline, 2008; Krause & Ingersoll-Dayton, 2001). However, other dimensions—such as feeling forgiven by others, seeking forgiveness, and forgiving God (or constructively dealing with anger at God) have received less consistent attention. This is particularly true when considering how these dimensions may relate to health.

In sum, the understanding of forgiveness as a construct with multiple dimensions is common. As such, it is crucial that explicit and thorough definitions of each of the dimensions continue to be developed and refined for continued progress to be made in understanding how aspects of experiences of forgiveness are connected to health.

Health Like with forgiveness, investigators have also conceptualized health as multidimensional. Some investigators have assumed this multidimensionality and reviewed research from multiple health domains. Others have explicitly defined health as encompassing physical, mental, and social domains. The definition of health offered by the World Health Organization (1948) (which views it as a state of total mental, physical and social well-being and not simply the absence of illness) supports these views. The work being done by these research teams in the area of forgiveness and health then seems consistent with mainstream views on health. Unfortunately, it is all too easy to understand this definition of health in a way that portrays these outcomes as simply static, parallel, interrelated *outcomes*. Davis, Green, Reid, Moloney, and Burnette (Chap. 16) remind us that physical, mental, and social aspects of health can have reciprocal causal influences on one another and remembering this is important. As just one example, they suggest that forgiveness may have an important connection to mental and physical health through the mechanism of social health. Social relationships have long been known to predict health and mortality (e.g., Reblin & Uchino, 2008). Better understanding the bidirectional causation between social, mental, and physical health and how forgiveness influences each is certain to bring better understanding about the forgiveness and health connection. Future research should also give more explicit attention to identifying and testing the potential contribution of forgiveness along the entire continuum of disease. Psychosocial factors such as forgiveness could play a role in the prevention of illness, disease onset, the effect of treatment, the severity and progression of disease and the nature of the illness experience and quality of life.

Models

Stress-and-Coping Model of Forgiveness We mention above that a consistent refrain from investigators is that more research needs to be done in the area of forgiveness and health. Perhaps an equally common point made by the various authors was the utility of the stress-and-coping model of forgiveness in guiding this research (Worthington, 2006). Almost every chapter makes some reference to this model. Almost all authors treat it as almost axiomatic that forgiveness can be—and usually is—related to health through the amount and type of stress and also through how people cope with that stress. Worthington and Scherer (2004) lay out four theoretical propositions of the stress and coping model of forgiveness including: (1) unforgiveness is stressful; (2) forgiveness is just one of many ways of coping with unforgiveness; (3) forgiveness reduces the stress of unforgiveness; and (4) coping through forgiveness is related to health. Much of the research reviewed in this book attests to the validity of proposition 4, but often the extent to which the study design and measures actually examine forgiveness as a *coping style or mechanism* could be called into question. It might be more accurate to say that forgiving states and traits are related to health, just like states such as anger, hope, and anxiety are related to health. But just as anger, hope, and anxiety can be coping responses to certain experiences, they are not inherently coping variables. Similarly, it might turn out that neither state forgiveness, and certainly not the disposition of trait forgivingness, are inherently coping variables. Therefore, as useful as the stress and coping model appears to be, there are some critical gaps in our understanding of it at present.

To fill in the gaps in our understanding of forgiveness as an emotion-focused coping mechanism with implications for stress and health more research needs to examine all four of the propositions set forth by Worthington and Scherer (2004). Some research has already established that unforgiveness is linked to health, but proposition 1 states that unforgiveness is *stressful* and this needs further scrutiny. What types of stress are experienced as a result of unforgiveness? Does unforgiveness elicit stress that is acute or chronic, interpersonal or intrapersonal, or traumatic or minor annoyances? Exactly how is unforgiveness stressful? Does unforgiveness change thoughts, motivations, or nervous system functioning in a way that promotes stress responding?

Regarding proposition 2, some research has examined the coping profile of more forgiving versus less forgiving individuals and shown differences in types of coping utilized (Ysseldyk & Matheson, 2008). More forgiving individuals, as compared to less forgiving individuals, use more problem-focused coping and cognitive restructuring and less rumination, wishful thinking, and emotional expression. But little is known about whether forgiveness offers any unique advantage in resolving unforgiveness issues or whether it simply acts as a proxy variable for healthier coping profiles. That is, does forgiveness offer real health benefits or does it merely signal that someone is more likely to use adaptive coping mechanisms?

Finally, Worthington and Scherer (2004) argue that forgiveness can be seen as an emotion-focused coping mechanism, but several different coping rubrics exist including active-passive, adaptive-maladaptive, cognitive-behavioral, etc. and additional work could be done to determine more definitively where forgiveness aligns itself in the coping hierarchy. Even more, decisional forgiveness might lead to very different effects than does emotional forgiveness. For example, decisions about intentions about how to behave toward an offender might have effects other than simply reducing stress. They might induce caretakers to provide better healthcare, for example.

Proposition 3 requires that both unforgiveness and forgiveness are measured in the same study and that forgiveness can be shown to reduce the stress of unforgiveness. Few, if any, studies examine these constructs simultaneously. Furthermore, it is critical to show more than an inverse correlation between unforgiveness and forgiveness to provide support for proposition 3. Rather, good support for this proposition requires data that show unforgiveness causes stress and that forgiveness either mediates or moderates the effect.

It is tempting, when most of a field seems to conceptualize a phenomenon in some singular way, to ask the skeptical question. Is it really all that well established that health is related to forgiveness because unforgiveness is stressful or forgiveness is a coping method? Might there be other mechanisms to which we have thus far been blinded? For example, forgiveness of self and others is related to alcohol and drug abuse and thus to health. But do most people engage in alcohol and drug abuse because they are stressed? Do they cope better with it when they are not stressed? Or are more physical, social, and motivational reasons the primary drivers?

Several research teams invoke the stress-and-coping model of forgiveness (Worthington, 2006) to help organize their reviews and to support their own conceptual modeling efforts. In this way, the stress-and-coping model of forgiveness is useful; it offers a convenient conceptual framework from which to work. It also possesses good heuristic value and continues to challenge investigators to connect forgiveness to health in novel ways. However, while the stress-and-coping theory of forgiveness offers a meta-structure in which to develop this work, the empirical support for this model is still only in its infancy and future research should aim to test the propositions and seek to investigate their validity.

Other Useful Models While the stress-and-coping model of forgiveness is the most widely cited model for connecting forgiveness and health, many of the expert teams have provided more specialized conceptual models for each of their respective areas. Lavelock, Snipes, Griffin, Worthington, Davis, Hook, Benotsch, and Ritter (Chap. 3) devoted an entire chapter to providing a conceptual foundation for the study of forgiveness and health and offered a comprehensive model. Given the aim of their chapter, it is not surprising that their model is very broad and delineates the major causal architecture of the connections between forgiveness and health.

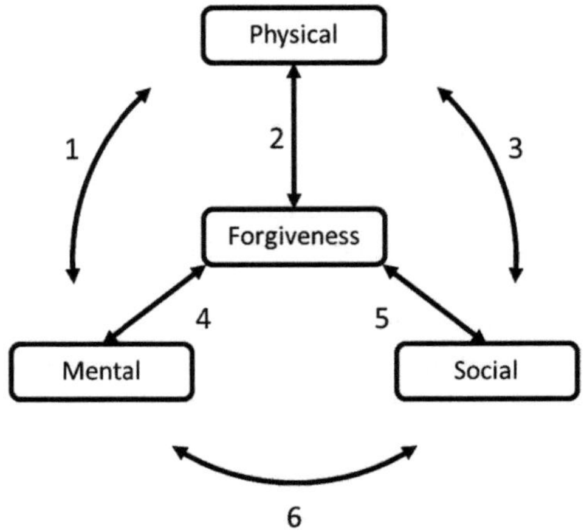

Fig. 19.1 Reciprocal causation model of intersections between forgiveness and multiple dimensions of health

Specifically, the model outlines the causal antecedents of forgiveness, a set of sequential mediators (i.e., psychosocial variables in the first step, mental health and well-being and physiological risk variables in the second step), and finally physical health outcomes.

As one additional panoramic view of the forgiveness and health connection, we offer a reciprocal causation model of intersections between forgiveness and multiple dimensions of health (see Fig. 19.1). This expands on the notion that Davis, Green, Reid, Moloney, and Burnette developed in Chap. 16—that forgiveness may act though social health to influence mental and physical health—and builds off the notion of transaction (Lazarus, 1966; Folkman, 1984) whereby we posit forgiveness-health transactions that occur at multiple levels. Simply put, this model explicitly expands the focus to highlight all possible directions of causation and all possible points of intersection between forgiveness and health. For instance, Davis et al. suggest that the effects of forgiveness on mental (path 4) and physical (path 2) health may be mediated through social health (path 5 then through paths 6 and 3). However, because of reciprocal causation, it could be equally likely that forgiveness could act on mental health (path 4) and physical health (path 2) and that these effects could in turn affect social health (through paths 6 and 3). Although the model offers only general labels, the constructs of physical, mental, and social health could be operationalized at any level. For instance, physical health could entail measurements of physiology; mental health could focus on diagnoses; and social health could focus on multiple levels of support from family, friends, and co-workers. Alternatively, physical health could be operationalized in self-reports; mental health could be measured using symptoms; and social support could be focused solely on spousal support. Intersections with forgiveness could be at the trait or state level, focus on decisional or emotional forgiveness, entail assessments of one or many dimensions of forgiveness (e.g. self, others, or God), and examine either forgiveness per se or unforgiveness. In effect, the model offers a high degree of flexibility in measurement. However, it requires precision in examining causal linkages and understanding direct and indirect effects of forgiveness on health.

Other useful contributions to modeling the relationship between forgiveness and health are offered by Offenbächer, Dezutter, Vallejo, and Toussaint (Chap. 9), Webb and Jeter (Chap. 10), Hill, Heffernan, and Allemand (Chap. 11), Miller and Worthington (Chap. 12), Smith and McFarland (Chap. 13), and Elliott (Chap. 18). These models are valuable contributions to the book because they offer specific testable predictions and identify or highlight key variables in specific research areas. Especially for students, researchers, and clinicians who are coming to this book with hopes of better understanding the science on forgiveness and health or wanting to develop their own research or interventions, the models presented here should prove useful.

Moving Forward

As we continue to think about what can be gleaned from the existing literature on forgiveness and health and what can be done to enhance this literature, it behooves us to consider the recommendations offered by each of the expert teams on directions of future work on forgiveness and health. The following include the highlights of what we consider to be some of the most important work going forward.

- Clarify definitions. We've already mentioned that Tucker, Bitman, Wade, and Cornish (Chap. 1) provide some excellent questions to guide our thinking on the definition of forgiveness. It bears repeating that future work should carefully consider how forgiveness is defined. Of particular note might be the distinction between decisional and emotional forgiveness. Decisional forgiveness certainly has its place as a cornerstone in the process of facilitating forgiveness through psychoeducation (Worthington, 2006), but in terms of health effects, emotional forgiveness is likely to be the major player—especially if the stress-and-coping model continues to dominate. Cheadle and Toussaint (Chap. 7) specifically mention the emotional replacement hypothesis (Worthington & Wade, 1999; Worthington, 2006) and summarize it as the means by which the negative emotions of unforgiveness are supplanted by the positive emotions of forgiveness. Bitterness, anger, and hatred are replaced by empathy, compassion, and love. Given the emerging evidence showing the value of positive emotions for health (Fredrickson, 2001; Lyubomirsky, King, & Diener, 2005) that are above and beyond the mere removal of negative emotions, this hypothesis should be given greater attention in work connecting forgiveness and health. Emotion is a planet around which all other processes, including stress, orbit in psychosomatic, psychoendocrine, and psychoneuroimmunological models of health and well-being. We need to know more about what emotional forgiveness is, its process, and its health correlates and consequences. Several research teams also agree that the state-trait distinction is important because of the consistent effects of forgivingness over time. Hence, the chronic effects of forgiving traits may be more important to consider than occasional states. Ideally, future work might offer measures that allow for the examination of trait-*emotional* forgiveness.

- Establish causality. A number of research teams call for more longitudinal research. In essence, what they want is better resolution of the temporal ordering of forgiveness and health. One recent longitudinal study of elderly adults offers some insights on this and showed that initial unforgiveness predicted physical health 3 years later, but initial physical health did not predict unforgiveness later in time (Seawell, Toussaint, & Cheadle, 2014). Thus, while our intersections model of forgiveness and health (see Fig. 19.1) offers the possibility of reciprocal causation, these data do not support that claim. Forgiveness is good for health, not vice versa. Though this study offers some insight on causality, it is far from the final word. Resolving issues of causality in health research remain one of the single most important gaps in the literature that need to be filled. Questions of causality abound simply because participants often cannot be randomly assigned in experimental designs to experience high or low forgiveness (or other health protective traits), and we cannot control who develops health problems and who does not. Longitudinal research can go a long way toward addressing issues of causality, but will not provide the final word because alternative causal explanations can never be fully controlled outside of randomized experiments. More than likely, understanding causal relationships will require a convergence of experimental and longitudinal studies.
- Evaluate the developmental trajectory of the forgiveness-health association. A related issue to that of establishing causality is better understanding forgiveness and health over the life course. Krause and Hayward raise this issue in Chap. 14. Just as it is important to understand how health habits like good diet and exercise early in life impact later life health status, so too is it important to understand the benefits of learning forgiveness early in life. If the unhealthy effects of unforgiveness do indeed accrue over the life course, then learning forgiveness as a coping strategy early in life could offer benefits. Gaining an understanding of life course effects could have implications for religious education, public and private primary education, and parenting. Teaching children strategies for forgiveness at an early age requires age-appropriate curriculums and motivated policy makers, parents, and teachers to implement these lessons. The payoffs might even extend beyond physical health and could influence social health through reduced bullying and higher levels of cooperation in the classroom.
- Increase diversity of samples. This may not be what you're thinking. While several author teams commented that samples in this literature are homogeneous, Griffin, Worthington, Lavelock, Wade, and Hoyt (Chap. 6) point out that in their review of 54 studies that 40 of them used samples *other* than college students. This is good. All too often literatures are dominated by the study of college students and young people. Unfortunately, we still have a long way to go. Leach and Parazak (Chap. 15) indicate that there are no studies that examine forgiveness and health across cultures. That is not to say that forgiveness and health have not

been examined in multiple countries and cultures, but that cross-cultural work hasn't been done and our ability to directly compare is limited by that notable gap in the literature. Furthermore, Friedberg, Tuvia, Alanson, and Cha (Chap. 8) note that examinations of forgiveness and health in patient samples is lacking. We know the most about how forgiveness is related to cardiovascular functioning, but even that literature is in need of development. How forgiveness might help in patients with diabetes, cancer, obesity, chronic pain, and other disorders remains a relatively open question. Webb and Jeter provide a comprehensive review and integration of forgiveness and substance treatment approaches but note that virtually every aspect of their conceptual model is in need of further testing and that virtually no research exists on substances other than alcohol. Certainly forgiveness of self and others is important for individuals struggling with smoking, stimulants, hallucinogens, and the like. These patient samples need further study.

- Improve efficiency, accuracy, and relevance of measurement. There is presently an ample supply of forgiveness measures. Unfortunately, to study forgiveness and health often forgiveness measures need to be collected in healthcare settings or in health-related surveys that offer very little space and time. The Trait Forgiveness Scale (TFS; Berry, Worthington, O'Connor, Parrott, & Wade, 2005) might lead the list of qualifying measures for these circumstances, but even so, at 10 items it may often be too long to use. Epidemiological surveys might offer the best opportunity to connect forgiveness to various health conditions and physiological mechanisms, but may only afford one to three items for measurement. This has made the forgiveness subscale of the Brief Multidimensional Measure of Religiousness and Spirituality (Fetzer Institute & National Institute on Aging Working Group, 2003) a popular choice. Unfortunately, this measure has its limits and attempts to measure forgiveness of self and others and feeling forgiven by God all in three items. A tall—and some might say not a wise—task. Other efficient and accurate measures will likely need to be developed. Measures for use in substance use clinical settings and other healthcare settings where screening items might be necessary will require valid and reliable indices that are no more than one to two questions. Witvliet, Tongeren, and Root Luna (Chap. 4) offer some excellent suggestions in this regard.
- Evaluate forgiveness interventions using randomized controlled trials (RCTs) and measure health and physiological variables as outcomes. Over 60 RCTs have been conducted, and a recent meta-analysis (Wade, Hoyt, Kidwell, & Worthington, 2014) has shown both the REACH Forgiveness (Worthington, 2006) and process model of forgiveness (Enright, 2012) to produce forgiveness and mental health benefits approximately equally. Conducting RCTs on forgiveness interventions and physical health offers two distinct advantages. First, it offers an evidence-base on which to evaluate the effectiveness of different types of interventions in promoting forgiveness and health. At present Worthington's (2006), Enright's (2012), and Luskin's (2002) models would be leading candidates for study in forgiveness interventions and their health benefits. Webb and Jeter (Chap. 10) strongly endorse Worthington's REACH model for use in

substance use/abuse contexts. How these models fair in bringing about physical health benefits has only just begun to be examined. The second advantage of conducting RCTs on forgiveness and health is that such studies could offer some insight into the causal influence of forgiveness on health. Because people *can* be randomly assigned to forgiveness or control conditions, the causal effect of forgiveness on health outcome variables can be evaluated if other non-specific treatment factors are controlled. This type of research offers good insight into the question of whether forgiveness might have a causal effect on health.

- Consider the influence of demographic variables. Chaps. 12 through 15 address a range of demographic variables that influence forgiveness and its relationships to health. Because many of these demographics have influences on both forgiveness *and* health there is all the more reason to pay careful attention to these variables that shape so much of a person's life. For instance, Miller and Worthington (Chap. 12) point out that women appear to have modestly higher levels of forgiveness. But do these higher levels of forgiveness help to reduce depression risk or risk of other mental or physical health problems? Older people experience more health problems and illness, but as Krause and Hayward (Chap. 14) point out, they also experience higher levels of forgiveness. To what extent does the development of forgiveness at this time of life, when health challenges become more prevalent, offer advantages for overall health and health behavior? Leach and Parazak (Chap. 15) consider culture and its effects on forgiveness and health. Clearly some cultures are more forgiving than others, and some cultures are completely avoidant of forgiveness. For all cultures, though, there are ways that help deal with offenses and transgressions to restore personal and social harmony. These alternatives to forgiveness deserve investigation. Finally, Smith and McFarland (Chap. 13) provide evidence that Blacks are more forgiving than Whites, but little research has examined how this might offer Blacks protection from illness and disease.
- Examine third-party forgiveness. Third-party forgiveness is forgiveness offered by close friends or family of a victim (Green, Burnette, & Davis, 2008) when a loved one has experienced a hurt. Third-parties often struggle to forgive offenders even more so than the victims themselves. Davis, Green, Reid, Moloney, and Burnette (Chap. 16) discuss the reasons for this, but perhaps most relevant to our purposes here is that difficulty with forgiveness on the part of third-parties may mean that the health consequence of offenses radiate from the victim to individuals close to the victim. Because it appears to be more difficult for third-parties to forgive, the health toll of an offense may actually be greater and wider for third-parties than for victims. Parents, spouses, and friends of victims may hold silent grudges toward offenders long after the victim has forgiven. The health consequences of this are unknown at this point. This may be especially true for social, cultural, and ethno-political conflicts where offenses are widespread and the impact is felt by hundreds if not thousands of like-minded comrades and neighbors. People who have never been directly harmed by someone from an out-group might still feel intense unforgiveness for other members of that group. They perceive that their group, tribe, or family has been harmed, and they

share a sense of collective identity with members of their group, so in a way, a harm to one group member is a harm to the identity of the third party; hence, unforgiveness and even health consequences.

- Examine forgiveness and health in committed relationships where forgiveness of self may be equally important as forgiveness of others. Davis, Green, Reid, Moloney, and Burnette (Chap. 16) and Fincham (Chap. 17) discuss the unique aspects of offenses that occur in ongoing romantic, friend, family, and married relationships. Interestingly, these researchers have found that often the health consequences of the offense are not reserved solely to the victim. Perpetrators struggle with feelings of guilt and remorse, and self-condemnation and subsequent self-forgiveness issues are common. These researchers conclude that we need to examine how a victim's forgiveness of the offender and the offender's self-forgiveness are intertwined and how the joint resolution of the offense through reconciliation can influence the mental, physical, and social health of both parties.
- Examine forgiveness of self in substance use/abuse and "preventable" illness and disease. Many illnesses and diseases are considered preventable. For instance, lung cancer and skin cancer risk can be dramatically reduced by limiting exposure to smoke and the sun, respectively. Obesity is often preventable through proper diet and nutrition. Likewise, hypertension, diabetes, substance abuse and addiction, and HIV/AIDS all are affected by personal responsibility. When people experience these health problems they may blame themselves—more or less—for their plight. As Friedberg, Tuvia, Alanson, and Cha (Chap. 8) point out, self-forgiveness may be an especially useful coping mechanism. Some research suggests that self-forgiveness is related to health, and several chapters of this book have reviewed this work. Knowing this, it is incumbent upon forgiveness scholars and counselors to help healthcare providers to consider options for patients experiencing self-condemnation. This can be difficult to address because condoning unhealthy behavior and offering self-forgiveness lightly could easily prove iatrogenic (Worthington, 2013). Nonetheless, responsible self-forgiveness and well-tested and proven methods for self-forgiveness need to be developed and integrated into these healthcare contexts. Griffin (2014) and Toussaint, Barry, Bornfriend, and Markman (2014) have developed and tested workbook interventions to promote self-forgiveness that have proven to be efficacious in randomized clinical trials.

Closing Thoughts

This present book represents a multinational effort to bring together cutting-edge research on forgiveness and health with the aim of capturing the current state of the literature and guiding future research and practice in this area. As we consider the important themes running throughout this book, it is good to keep in mind that issues of construct definition, conceptual modeling, and measurement will always be present. Progress has been made in each, but (as always in science) more work is needed. Nonetheless, we have sought to provide empirical and theoretical architecture to support sustained work in forgiveness and health. As healthcare costs continue to rise, the population continues to age, and economic and social challenges come from every angle, it is imperative that we consider new, promising, and exciting ways to promote health and assist in coping with illness. Forgiveness, in its various shapes and sizes, benefits not only individuals but also the greater good. In some circumstances forgiveness may not be an appropriate choice, but in many cases if offers healing where little else can. Our future work will require that we can identify those offenses, stressors, and events that offer the best opportunities for forgiveness-related health benefits to be realized. No method of coping with life's hardships is applicable in all circumstances, but identifying the appropriate fit between challenge and response goes a long way toward helping people survive and thrive in difficult circumstances. Forgiveness may offer an appropriate healthy response in many circumstances, and it adds to the coping repertoires of individuals faced with life's challenges.

At the outset of this book, we asked, Is forgiveness good for me? The answer to that question appears to be, "yes, but." There are caveats. It depends on who you are, what has happened, and what sorts of challenges and health problems you might be facing. So perhaps the answer might more accurately be, "yes, but—at least we think so at this point." Much remains to be learned about forgiveness and health. We hope that in collecting current state-of-the-science reviews and focusing attention on conceptual frameworks and needed methodological advances, we will soon be better situated to answer this question more definitively. With continued attention and careful work, our growing knowledge will help support health in the broader public as well as in patients with illness and disease.

References

Berry, J. W., Worthington, E. L., Jr., O'Connor, L., Parrott, L., III, & Wade, N. G. (2005). Forgiveness, vengeful rumination, and affective traits. *Journal of Personality, 73*, 1–43.

Enright, R. D. (2012). *The forgiving life: A pathway to overcoming resentment and creating a legacy of love*. Washington, DC: American Psychological Association.

Exline, J. J. (2008). Beliefs about god and forgiveness in a Baptist church sample. *Journal of Psychology and Christianity, 27*, 131–139.

Fetzer Institute & National Institute on Aging Working Group. (2003). *Multidimensional measurement of religiousness/spirituality for use in health research: A report of the Fetzer Institute National Institute on Aging Working Group*. Kalamazoo, MI: Fetzer Institute.

Fisher, M. L., & Exline, J. J. (2010). Moving toward self-forgiveness: Removing barriers related to shame, guilt, and regret. *Social and Personality Psychology Compass, 4*(8), 548–558.

Folkman, S. (1984). *Stress, appraisal, and coping*. New York, NY: Springer Publishing Company.

Fredrickson, B. (2001). The role of positive emotions in positive psychology: The broaden-and-build theory of positive emotions. *American Psychologist, 56*(3), 218–226.

Green, J. D., Burnette, J. L., & Davis, J. L. (2008). Third-party forgiveness: (Not) forgiving your close other's betrayer. *Personality and Social Psychology Bulletin, 34*(3), 407–418.

Griffin, B. J. (2014). *Efficacy of a workbook to promote self-forgiveness*. Unpublished master's thesis, Virginia Commonwealth University, Richmond, VA.
Hall, J. H., & Fincham, F. D. (2005). Self-forgiveness: The stepchild of forgiveness research. *Journal of Social and Clinical Psychology, 24*(5), 621–637.
Krause, N., & Ingersoll-Dayton, B. (2001). Religion and the process of forgiveness in late life. *Review of Religious Research, 42*, 252–276.
Lazarus, R. S. (1966). *Psychological stress and the coping process*. New York, NY: McGraw-Hill.
Luskin, F. (2002). *Forgive for good: A proven prescription for health and happiness*. San Francisco, CA: Harper.
Lyubomirsky, S., King, L., & Diener, E. (2005). The benefits of frequent positive affect: Does happiness lead to success? *Psychological Bulletin, 131*(6), 803–855. doi:10.1037/0033-2909.131.6.803.
Reblin, M., & Uchino, B. N. (2008). Social and emotional support and its implication for health. *Current Opinion in Psychiatry, 21*(2), 201–205.
Seawell, A. H., Toussaint, L. L., & Cheadle, A. C. (2014). Prospective associations between unforgiveness and physical health and positive mediating mechanisms in a nationally representative sample of older adults. *Psychology & Health, 29*(4), 375–389. doi:10.1080/08870446.2013.856434.
Toussaint, L. L., Barry, M., Bornfriend, L., & Markman, M. (2014). Restore: The journey toward self-forgiveness: A randomized trial of patient education on self-forgiveness in cancer patients and caregivers. *Journal of Healthcare Chaplaincy, 20*(2), 54–74.
Wade, N. G., Hoyt, W. T., Kidwell, J. M., & Worthington, E. J. (2014). Efficacy of psychotherapeutic interventions to promote forgiveness: A meta-analysis. *Journal of Consulting and Clinical Psychology, 82*(1), 154–170. doi:10.1037/a0035268.
World Health Organization. (1948). *Preamble to the constitution of the World Health Organization as adopted by the international health conference, New York, 19–22 June, 1946; signed on 22 July 1946 by the representatives of 61 States and entered into force on 7 April 1948.*
Worthington, E., Jr. (2013). *Moving forward: Six steps to forgive yourself and break free from the past*. Colorado Springs, CO: Waterbrook Multnomah.
Worthington, E. L., Jr. (Ed.). (2005). *Handbook of forgiveness*. New York, NY: Brunner-Routledge.
Worthington, E. L., Jr. (2006). *Forgiveness and reconciliation: Theory and application*. New York, NY: Brunner-Routledge.
Worthington, E. J., & Scherer, M. (2004). Forgiveness is an emotion-focused coping strategy that can reduce health risks and promote health resilience: Theory, review, and hypotheses. *Psychology & Health, 19*(3), 385–405. doi:10.1080/0887044042000196674.
Worthington, E. L., Jr., & Wade, N. G. (1999). The social psychology of unforgiveness and forgiveness and implications for clinical practice. *Journal of Social and Clinical Psychology, 18*, 385–418.
Ysseldyk, R., & Matheson, K. (2008). Forgiveness and coping. In W. Malcolm, N. DeCourville, K. Belicki, W. Malcolm, N. DeCourville, & K. Belicki (Eds.), *Women's reflections on the complexities of forgiveness* (pp. 143–163). New York, NY: Routledge/Taylor & Francis Group.

Index

A
Acts of contrition, 80, 91, 195, 210–212, 216, 217
Adaptive identity development, 5, 159
Addiction, 46, 127, 139, 146, 148–151, 279, 299
Age differences, 6, 179–180, 205–210
Allostatic load, 52, 198, 241, 273, 275, 276, 278–280
Anger, 13, 20–23, 30–33, 36, 38, 39, 44–47, 52, 53, 61, 64, 66–70, 72, 73, 80, 84, 91, 92, 95, 99, 108, 110–114, 116, 126–133, 141–144, 148, 174, 176, 180, 181, 183, 185, 196, 198, 199, 212–214, 225, 228, 240–242, 249, 256, 257, 259, 262, 263, 266, 275, 291, 292, 295
Assessment, 3, 37, 43, 45–48, 53–55, 72, 115, 116, 225, 243, 247, 267, 275, 294
Attachment theory, 6, 239, 245, 248
Autonomic nervous system, 20, 61, 273

B
Barriers, 215–217
Bio-psycho-social-spiritual (BPSS), 49, 272, 274, 275, 280
Blacks, 5, 14, 132, 189, 193–201, 298
Blame, 17, 39, 45, 46, 48, 63, 108, 109, 112, 114, 115, 126, 127, 129, 131, 156, 184, 299
Buddhist, 14–16, 226

C
Cancer, 1, 4, 46, 49, 61, 85, 107, 109, 110, 112–114, 125, 132, 277, 297, 299
Cardiovascular disease, 1, 2, 61, 99, 100, 103, 107, 110–112, 115, 193, 200, 258, 279
Causality, 296
Children, 34, 102, 127, 132, 148, 163, 208, 213, 227, 262, 264, 296
Christianity, 15, 16, 84, 99, 195, 213, 225, 226, 262
Chronic illness, 45, 109, 271, 276, 278
Chronic pain, 2, 4, 52, 107, 110–112, 114, 123–133, 184, 297
Chronic widespread pain (CWP), 4, 123–133
Cohort, 6, 205, 207–209, 217
Conceptual model, 5, 6, 29–39, 109, 123, 124, 175–176, 194, 215, 258–259, 290, 293, 297, 299
Coping, 3, 4, 7, 13, 22, 30–32, 35, 39, 44, 45, 65, 72, 78–81, 85, 87, 93, 109, 123–126, 131–133, 143, 145, 146, 151, 178, 185, 186, 195, 248, 258, 272, 275, 292, 293, 296, 300
Coping mechanisms, 4, 31, 32, 35, 36, 38, 123, 124, 131–133, 199, 271–273, 275, 292, 293, 299
Cortex, 62, 183, 199, 274, 275
Cross-cultural psychology, 6, 192, 221, 223–225, 297
Cultural, 6, 13, 18, 54, 148, 184, 189–195, 201, 222, 223, 225, 226, 229–232, 298

L.L. Toussaint et al. (eds.), *Forgiveness and Health*,
DOI 10.1007/978-94-017-9993-5

D

Dating relationships, 239, 242
Definitions, 2, 7, 13–25, 29–30, 34, 53, 77, 82, 102, 108–117, 124, 130, 132, 155–157, 159, 174–175, 190, 208, 223–225, 227, 240, 257, 263, 272–273, 281, 290–293, 295, 299, 300
Demographics, 38, 71, 85, 110, 111, 227, 298
Developmental trajectory, 190, 296
Disease, 1, 2, 4, 29, 31, 45, 47, 53, 61, 92, 94, 98–100, 102, 103, 107–112, 115, 124, 125, 176, 177, 183, 184, 193, 200, 201, 258, 272, 277–279, 281, 291, 292, 298–300

E

Emergent themes, 144, 146, 258, 267
Empathy, 19–23, 30, 36, 39, 44, 62–64, 93, 114, 116, 128, 143–145, 174, 178–181, 185, 186, 192, 215, 229, 242, 248, 295
Empirical, 3–7, 16, 18–24, 29, 50, 62, 64, 67, 71, 77–82, 92, 93, 99–100, 107, 110–114, 116, 139, 140, 142–144, 146–151, 156, 160, 163–165, 196, 206–209, 211–213, 215, 226, 229, 259–264, 276–278, 290, 293, 300
Empirical findings, 95–100, 194
Endocrine, 3, 7, 16, 44, 70–71, 98, 123, 273, 274, 279
Environment, 61, 125, 127–129, 131, 149, 190–194, 198, 201, 249, 260, 266, 273, 274
Evidence-based treatment, 4, 139–141, 143, 144, 150
Evolutionary theory, 2, 6, 239, 245, 247–248

F

Family relationships, 6, 7, 158, 185, 255–267, 299
Fibromyalgia, 4, 107, 123–133, 278
Forgiveness, 1, 13, 29, 43, 61, 77, 91, 107, 123, 139, 155, 173, 189, 205, 221, 239, 255, 271, 289–290
Forgiveness equity, 177, 265
Forgivingness, 16, 22, 23, 30, 32–34, 38, 47, 54, 66–71, 77, 79–81, 91–103, 110–112, 114, 116, 141, 146–149, 155–164, 174, 176–178, 181, 185, 206, 222–227, 231, 232, 240–242, 244, 245, 248, 257, 260–263, 276, 291, 292, 296
Forgiving personality, 32, 35, 52, 262
Friendships, 5, 6, 180, 239, 243, 245–248, 250
Functional magnetic resonance imaging (fMRI), 3, 62, 63, 72

G

Gender-socialization, 175, 176, 184
Gerotranscendence, 209
Guilt, 36, 46, 48, 69, 83, 84, 92, 100, 108, 109, 112, 114, 128, 129, 131, 146, 147, 159, 174, 181, 210, 216, 217, 225, 229, 231, 232, 291, 299

H

Happiness, 2, 84, 155, 157, 160–162, 165, 166, 247
Health, 1, 13, 29, 43, 61, 77, 91, 107, 123, 139, 161, 174, 189, 205, 229, 239, 255, 271, 289
Health behaviors, 36, 51, 77, 99, 110, 111, 141, 142, 162, 199, 298
Hindu, 14–16
HIV/AIDS, 4, 46, 50, 53, 71, 107, 112, 113, 184, 277, 299
Human stress response, 62
Hypothalamic-pituitary-adrenal (HPA), 61, 62, 125, 273

I

Imagined, 63, 65, 69, 241, 242, 262
Immune system, 3, 13, 15, 20, 33, 36, 44, 61, 71, 93, 98, 125, 177, 189, 192, 241, 273–277
Individualism-collectivism, 6, 222, 223, 229, 230
Intergroup forgiveness, 223, 227–232
Interpersonal forgiveness, 2, 47, 49, 54, 189, 191, 193, 195, 196, 222, 223, 226–227, 229, 232
Interpersonal stress, 16, 67–70, 92, 123, 177, 178, 185, 292
Interventions, 2, 4–7, 31, 34–35, 37, 39, 45, 47, 48, 52, 54, 72, 86, 102, 103, 107–109, 111–117, 147–149, 151, 175, 177–186, 217, 229, 243, 244, 250, 256, 262, 267, 271–281, 295, 297, 299
Intrapersonal stress, 123, 292
Investment model of commitment, 6, 239, 245–247
Islam, 15, 16

J
Jewish, 14–16, 217

K
Key questions, 3, 290

L
Lay conceptualizations of forgiveness, 222–224
Life-course, 6, 102, 205, 207–210, 213, 216, 217, 279, 296
Life histories, 208, 213, 214
Life review, 209, 216
Literature reviews, 30, 79, 86, 147–148, 150, 155, 160–163, 176–181, 258, 274
Longevity, 93, 107, 110

M
Marital relationships, 68, 239, 243, 258
Meaning in life, 70, 128, 214–215
Measurement, 3, 48, 49, 55, 62, 86, 96, 241, 256, 280, 281, 294, 295, 297, 299
Mechanisms, 2–5, 7, 29–36, 38, 39, 61, 72, 87, 103, 107, 123, 124, 131–133, 141, 143, 147, 149, 155–166, 199, 201, 208, 210, 239, 241, 248, 258–260, 271–275, 279, 291–293, 297, 299
Mediation, 66, 77, 162, 163
Mediators, 5, 35, 38, 39, 77, 82, 95, 108, 142, 143, 147, 157, 160, 162, 163, 165, 210, 244, 248, 276–277, 280, 294
Medical, 3, 43–49, 55, 94, 95, 107, 108, 115–117, 129, 183, 274, 275, 279
Meta-analysis, 116, 206, 227, 243, 245, 246, 297
Models, 3–8, 15, 17, 21, 22, 29–39, 44, 50, 52, 53, 77, 78, 84, 92–94, 103, 109, 113, 116–117, 123, 124, 139–151, 155, 157–160, 162–166, 175–176, 194, 200, 215, 225, 230, 231, 239, 245–247, 258–261, 263, 271, 272, 274–276, 279, 280, 289–300
Moderators, 2, 101, 143, 147, 179, 184, 239
Mortality, 20, 45, 51, 53, 80, 92, 94, 99, 100, 102, 103, 185, 189, 193, 198, 201, 206, 214, 256, 277, 291
Multidimensional forgiveness, 132, 151, 290, 291, 297

N
National contexts, 222–223, 230–232
National data, 196
National values, 222–223, 230–232
Negative effects of forgiveness, 93, 94, 128, 178, 181, 198
Neuroendocrine, 70–71, 73, 93, 241
Neurologic, 279

O
Old, 6, 32, 50, 51, 80, 81, 84, 95, 97–99, 101, 127, 161, 164, 179, 180, 196, 197, 205–210, 212, 213, 215–218, 229, 261, 262, 276, 298

P
Parents, 66, 96, 126, 127, 129, 130, 140, 163, 191, 213, 240, 248, 257, 260–264, 296, 298
Patients, 3, 4, 7, 43, 45–48, 52–55, 63, 68, 72, 107–117, 123, 125–133, 184, 256, 265, 297, 299, 300
Personality, 22–24, 30, 32, 34–38, 52, 85, 95, 132, 133, 156, 164, 165, 190, 216, 217, 222, 225, 262, 276
Philosophical, 2, 13, 14, 107
Physiology, 2, 3, 21–24, 29, 31, 33–39, 43, 49, 52, 53, 55, 61–73, 79, 92–94, 96, 98, 102, 103, 107, 110, 113–115, 123, 125, 189, 198, 240–242, 256, 258, 264, 271–277, 279, 280, 294, 297
Positive psychology, 1, 34, 93, 152
Positive religious coping experiences, 35
Positron emission tomography (PET), 62, 63
Problematic substance use, 139–152
Process models, 21, 22, 37, 52, 116, 297

Q
Questionnaires, 6, 97, 100

R
Race, 2, 5, 6, 16, 38, 46, 189–201, 210, 276
Race differences, 189–201
Randomized controlled trials (RCTs), 114–116, 297, 298
Recalled betrayal, 64, 66–68
Reciprocal-effects forgiveness-intersections, 294, 296

Recovery, 23, 29, 45, 46, 49, 52, 53, 65, 66, 68–70, 97, 139–142, 145, 146, 148–151, 177, 240–242, 248, 263, 265, 276
Relational well-being, 2, 265, 272
Relationship harmony, 5, 157–158, 163, 164
Relationship mastery/maintenance, 164
Relationship quality, 7, 163, 241, 242, 244, 245, 250, 259–263, 265
Religion, 13, 14, 16, 31, 35, 37, 43, 53, 97, 99, 107, 141, 150, 182, 196, 197, 199, 200, 210, 214, 217, 225, 226
Reparation, 46, 47, 54
Research agendas, 8, 231, 289–300
Responsibility, 38, 46–48, 54, 115, 127, 299
Rumination, 14, 19, 20, 24, 31, 35, 36, 39, 44, 62, 65, 66, 68, 70, 77, 80–82, 84, 92, 93, 100, 132, 133, 141, 157, 175, 177–179, 181–183, 186, 226, 229, 240, 241, 248, 259, 265, 292

S
Sample diversity, 296
Scaffolding self and social systems, 5, 157–160
Scholarship, 14, 271, 272, 276, 278, 279
Screening questions, 48, 184, 297
Self-acceptance, 5, 159, 164, 291
Self-reported health, 20, 33, 66, 110, 189, 193, 200, 263
Self worth, 5, 159, 162, 164
Sex-differences, 5, 162, 173–184, 200
Shame, 46, 83, 84, 92, 100, 108, 126, 127, 131, 144, 146, 147, 174, 181, 186, 291
Socioemotional selectivity theory, 212
Somatic complaints, 97, 132, 178
Somatic nervous system, 64
Sources of stress, 4, 123, 124, 126–131, 133
Spinal cord injury, 46, 51, 81, 85, 111, 132, 265, 277
Spiritual well-being, 33, 36, 198
State, 2, 3, 13, 16, 17, 19–24, 29, 34, 38, 39, 43, 46, 47, 49, 51–55, 61, 66–73, 77, 79, 80, 82–83, 85, 91, 92, 96, 97, 99, 100, 109, 111, 125, 140, 147, 148, 151, 155–165, 174, 176–179, 183, 190, 197, 199, 226, 230, 231, 240–242, 246, 263, 266, 272, 273, 289, 291, 292, 294, 296, 299, 300
12-step model, 8
Stress, 3, 13, 30, 44, 61, 78, 92, 108, 123, 140, 174, 190, 223, 240, 258, 272, 292
Stress and coping model, 30, 44, 78, 84, 93, 185, 258, 274, 275, 292–293
Stroke, 46, 68, 112, 226
Surplus value test, 261, 262

T
Terminal illness, 107
Theoretical models, 92–94, 155, 276
Theories, 1–7, 13, 21, 25, 29, 30, 81, 84, 92–94, 98, 101, 103, 108, 109, 115, 116, 139, 142, 155, 175, 183, 189, 205, 209–212, 214, 222, 230–232, 239, 245–248, 250, 258–259, 273–276, 280, 290, 292, 293, 300
Third-party forgiveness, 249, 298, 299
Trait, 2, 16, 20, 22–24, 30, 32–34, 38, 43, 47, 49–54, 66–71, 77, 80, 81, 85, 91, 92, 95–97, 99, 100, 103, 109, 111, 114, 115, 130, 140, 141, 146, 148, 151, 155–157, 160, 161, 163–165, 174, 176–179, 185, 190, 206, 216, 218, 222, 223, 225, 226, 229, 240–242, 244, 245, 257, 262, 263, 276, 291, 292, 294, 296, 297
Traumatic brain injury (TBI), 107, 109, 111, 114

W
Well-being, 1, 2, 5, 7, 24, 29, 32, 33, 36, 50, 78–80, 84–86, 94, 107, 108, 113, 116, 133, 139–141, 147, 150–152, 155–166, 189, 192, 198, 199, 205, 208, 211, 215, 231, 242–246, 255, 265, 272, 274, 276, 279, 291, 294
Whites, 5, 14, 23, 69, 97, 189, 191, 192, 194–200, 298
Work relationships, 200, 239, 243

MIX
Papier aus verantwortungsvollen Quellen
Paper from responsible sources
FSC® C105338

If you have any concerns about our products,
you can contact us on
ProductSafety@springernature.com

In case Publisher is established outside the EU,
the EU authorized representative is:
Springer Nature Customer Service Center GmbH
Europaplatz 3, 69115 Heidelberg, Germany

Printed by Libri Plureos GmbH
in Hamburg, Germany